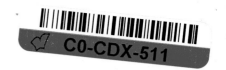
Classification of Nursing Diagnoses

Proceedings of the Ninth Conference

Classification of Nursing Diagnoses

Proceedings of the Ninth Conference

North American Nursing Diagnosis Association

Edited by

Rose Mary Carroll-Johnson, MN, RN

Nurse Editor
Valencia, California

J. B. Lippincott Company

PHILADELPHIA
NEW YORK • LONDON • HAGERSTOWN

Sponsoring Editor: Donna L. Hilton, BSN, RN
Production: Till & Till, Inc.
Composition: The Composing Room of Michigan, Inc.
Printer/Binder: R. R. Donnelly & Sons

6 5 4 3 2 1

Library of Congress Cataloging-in-Publication-Data

Classification of nursing diagnoses : proceedings of the ninth
  conference / North American Nursing Diagnosis Association : edited
  by Rose Mary Carroll-Johnson.
      p. cm.
    Proceedings of the 9th Conference on the Classification of Nursing
Diagnosis, held in Orlando, Fla. in 1990.
    Includes bibliographical references and index.
    ISBN 0-397-54812-5
    1. Nursing diagnosis—Classification—Congresses. I. Carroll-
Johnson, Rose Mary. II. North American Nursing Diagnosis
Association. III. Conference on the Classification of Nursing
Diagnoses (9th : 1990 : Orlando, Fla.)
    [DNLM: 1. Classification—congresses. 2. Nursing Diagnosis—
congresses.   WY 100 C614 1990]
  RT48.6.C57   1991
  610.73—dc20
  DNLM/DLC
  for Library of Congress   91-18391
                                                              CIP

Care has been taken to confirm the accuracy of information presented
and to describe generally accepted practices. However, the author,
editors, and publisher cannot accept any responsibility for errors or
omissions or for consequences from application of the information in
this book and make no warranty, express or implied, with respect to
the contents of this book.

Preface

The Ninth National Conference of the North American Nursing Diagnosis Association seemed to many of us in attendance to be a turning point in our maturity as an organization. We did more than venture away for the first time from our "home base" of St. Louis, Missouri to Orlando, Florida. Our theme, "Create the Vision," seemed more than achievable in the context of the self-examination that was taking place and our willingness to tolerate some ambiguity and to risk forging ahead to achieve our goals. Discussions at the sessions, in the restaurants and hotel rooms, and probably on some of the rides at Disney World, were spirited and productive. Ideas were communicated in many ways and in many forms. As always, the proceedings of the conferences can never fully capture the whole conference, but we have made an effort this time to share with you at least some of the less formal and structured parts of this biennial event.

Much of the conference time and certainly the discussion was devoted to two topics: (1) the considerable work done in the last two years by the Taxonomy Committee on Taxonomy II and the submission to the International Classification of Diseases-Tenth Edition (ICD-10) of "Conditions that Necessitate Nursing Care," and (2) the work of the Diagnosis Review Committee and the NANDA Board of Directors on a working definition of nursing diagnosis. The fine sets of papers presented on these topics comprise the first two sections of these proceedings. Because of the importance of the dialogues that occurred in response to these papers, the transcribed discussions are included at the end of each section.

A selection of high quality scientific papers (Section III) and abstracts of all the posters presented (Section V) is complemented by three excellent overview papers on methodologies for validation research (Section IV). A wide array of nursing diagnosis studies were presented with topics ranging from validation studies to identification of new diagnoses and the processes of education and implementation. The methodology papers represented a wonderful synthesis of the content of a NANDA-sponsored invitational conference held in 1989. Researchers of nursing diagnosis will find a wealth of information here about the methods available to carry out the much needed work of validating the Taxonomy and the diagnoses.

The remainder of these *Proceedings* includes those elements that you have come to expect: minutes of the Business Meeting and the Book of Reports, minutes of the Special Interest Group Meetings, and the new diagnoses accepted for clinical testing. Transcriptions of the discussions generated by the presentations of the two new diagnoses are also included for your interest.

Thanks are in order to Jane Lancour, President of NANDA, Dottie Jones, Chairperson of the Publications Committee, and Donna

Hilton, Lippincott's Nursing Editor, for their help in organizing and structuring this volume. The manuscript was very competently computerized by Catherine Chambers. Judith Miller transcribed the discussion tapes. Debi Folkerts was, as always, very willing to help with any request. Finally, I am most appreciative to all the contributors who submitted their papers, answered my questions, and reviewed the editorial changes. It is the opportunity to work with both neophyte and seasoned authors that makes my job particularly enjoyable.

Contents

SECTION II
Nursing Diagnosis Development and Review

SECTION III
Scientific Papers

SECTION IV
Panel Presentations

Methodologies for Nursing Diagnosis Research

Specialty Organizations: Nursing Diagnosis Use and Issues—
A Panel Presentation

SECTION V
Poster Presentations—Abstracts

Validation Studies

Taxonomy

Diagnostic Reasoning

Diagnosis Development/Identification

SECTION VI
Business Meeting

SECTION VII
New Nursing Diagnoses

   Kathleen C. Sheppard, MSN, RN

   Mary L. Henrikson, MN, RNC, ARNP
   Ginna Wall, MN, RN
   Dona Lethbridge, PhD, RN
   Vicki E. McClurg, MN, RN

SECTION VIII
Group Meetings

Appendixes

Contributors

Marilyn Abraham, BSN, RN

University of South Dakota,
Vermillion, South Dakota

Janet Anderson, BAAN, RN

Sunnybrook Health Science
Centre
Toronto, Ontario, Canada

Cathy Aden, BSN, RN

Visiting Nurse Association of
Omaha
Omaha, Nebraska

Wilda K. Arnold, EdD, RN

Texas Woman's University
Dallas, Texas

Samar N. Assousa, MSN, RN

Veterans Administration
Medical Center
West Roxbury, Massachusetts

**Kathleen Miller Baldwin, PhD,
RN**

Texas Woman's University
Denton, Texas

Genee Brukwitzki, MSN, RN

University of Wisconsin-
Milwaukee
Milwaukee, Wisconsin

**Catherine E. Burns, PhD, RN,
PNP**

Oregon Health Sciences
University
Portland, Oregon

Kitty Byram, RN, CCRN, CPAN

Shawnee Mission Medical
Center
Shawnee Mission, Kansas

Terry Ann Capuano, MSN, RN

The Allentown Hospital–Lehigh
Valley Hospital Center
Allentown, Pennsylvania

Lynda Juall Carpenito, MSN, RN

LJC Consultants, Inc.
Mickleton, New Jersey

**Deborah Caswell, MN, RN,
CCRN**

University of California, Los
Angeles Medical Center
Los Angeles, California

Deb Fischer Clemens, BSN, RN

St. Joseph Hospital
Mitchell, South Dakota

Marga Coler, EdD, RN, CS, CTN

University of Connecticut
Storrs, Connecticut

Marie Cox, MSN, RN

State University of New York at
Stony Brook
Stony Brook, New York

Nancy S. Creason, PhD, RN

University of Illinois at Chicago
(Urbana Regional Site)
Urbana, Illinois

**Carol Lewis Cullinan, MSN, RN,
C, FNP**

Clinical Programs, Ltd.
Providence, Rhode Island

Barbara J. Daly, MSN, RN

Case Western Reserve University
Cleveland, Ohio

Connie W. Delaney, PhD, RN

The University of Iowa
Iowa City, Iowa

Carol A. Dickel, RN

Mercy Hospital
Davenport, Iowa

**Nancy Dudgeon, BSN, RN,
CPAN**

University of Kansas Medical
Center
Kansas City, Kansas

Joan B. Fitzmaurice, PhD, RN

Massachusetts General Hospital
Boston, Massachusetts

Joyce J. Fitzpatrick, PhD, RN, FAAN

Case Western Reserve University
Cleveland, Ohio

Candice Friestad, MS, RN, CCRN, CNA

McKennan Hospital
Sioux Falls, South Dakota

Noreen Frisch, PhD, RN

Humboldt State University
Arcata, California

Phyllis Meyer Gaspar, PhD, RN

South Dakota State University
Brookings, South Dakota

Kay Knox Greenlee, MSN, RN, CCRN

St. Mary's Medical Center
Racine, Wisconsin

Jesse Earl Greene, MSN, RN

South Carolina Department of
Health and Environmental
Control
Columbia, South Carolina

Chanda Harrison, RN, CEN

Veterans Administration
Medical Center
Atlanta, Georgia

Rose Mary Harvey, DNSc, RN

Boston College
Chestnut Hill, Massachusetts

Marilyn Henning, MSN, RN

Sinai-Samaritan Medical Center
University of Wisconsin
Milwaukee, Wisconsin

Mary L. Henrikson, MN, RNC, ARNP

Salem Hospital
Salem, Oregon

Kim S. Hitchings, MSN, RN

The Allentown Hospital–Lehigh
Valley Hospital Center
Allentown, Pennsylvania

Cynthia Holmgren, MSN, RN, OCN

Bellin College of Nursing
Green Bay, Wisconsin

Lois M. Hoskins, PhD, RN

Catholic University of America
Washington, DC

Mary Hurley, MA, RN

Mount Sinai Medical Center
New York, New York

Michelle Jaffe, BS, RN

State University of New York at
Stony Brook
Stony Brook, New York

Janice K. Janken, PhD, RN

University of North Carolina at
Charlotte
Charlotte, North Carolina

Jean Jenny, MSN, MEd, RN

University of Ottawa
Ottawa, Ontario, Canada

Sharon E. Johnson, BSN, RNC

The Bryn Mawr Hospital
Bryn Mawr, Pennsylvania

M. Kay M. Judge, EdD, RN

Harborview Medical Center
Seattle, Washington

David J. Kelly, MS, RN

University of Arizona
Tucson, Arizona

Mary E. Kerr, MN, RN

Case Western Reserve University
Cleveland, Ohio

Mi Ja Kim, PhD, RN

University of Illinois at Chicago
Chicago, Illinois

Susan V. M. Kleinbeck, MS, RN, CNOR

Wichita State University
Wichita, Kansas

Mary Kontz, MSN, RN

Jackson Memorial Hospital
Miami, Florida

Rebecca C. Kuhn, MS, RN, CCRN

Desert Samaritan Medical
Center
Mesa, Arizona

June Larson, MS, RN

University of South Dakota
Vermillion, South Dakota

Anne LeGresley, MS, RN

The Toronto Hospital–Toronto
Western Division
Toronto, Ontario, Canada

Dona Lethbridge, PhD, RN

University of Washington
Seattle, Washington

Christina Lewis, BSN, RN

University of California, Los
Angeles
Neuropsychiatric Institute and
Hospital
Los Angeles, California

Maria Miriam Lima da Nobrega, BS

Federal University at Paraiba
Joao Pessoa, Paraiba, Brazil

Jo Logan, MEd, BScN, RN

Ottawa Civic Hospital
Ottawa, Ontario, Canada

Joan Love, MS, RN

State University of New York at
  Stony Brook
Stony Brook, New York

Regina Maibusch, MS, RN

St. Michael Hospital
Milwaukee, Wisconsin

Eleanor Majewsky, BS, RN

State University at Stony Brook
Stony Brook, New York

Karen Martin, MSN, RN, FAAN

Visiting Nurse Association of
  Omaha
Omaha, Nebraska

Elizabeth A. McFarlane, DNSc, RN

The Catholic University of
  America
Washington, DC

Vicki E. McClurg, MN, RN

Seattle Pacific University
Seattle, Washington

Ann McCourt, MS, RN

Ormond Beach, Florida

Frances A. McHolm, MSN, RN

Kent State University
Kent, Ohio

Rosemary J. McKeighen, PhD, RN, FAAN

University of Iowa
Iowa City, Iowa

Peggy Mehmert, MSN, RN, C

Mercy Hospital
Davenport, Iowa

Sharon Merritt, EdD, RN

University of Illinois
Chicago, Illinois

Norma Metheny, PhD, RN

St. Louis University
St. Louis, Missouri

Winnifred C. Mills, MEd, RN

Alberta Association of
  Registered Nurses
Edmonton, Alberta, Canada

Carol Ann Mitchell, EdD, RN

State University of New York at
  Stony Brook
Stony Brook, New York

Joseph Molinatti, BSN, RN

State University of New York at
  New York
New York, New York

Judith Myers, MSN, RN

St. Louis University
St. Louis, Missouri

Mary Beth Myers, MS, RN

Carle Foundation Hospital
Urbana, Illinois

Angela Maida Nicoletti, MS, RN, C

Brigham and Women's Hospital
Boston, Massachusetts

Rose M. Nieswiadomy, PhD, RN

Texas Woman's University
Dallas, Texas

Juracy Nunes de Farias, MS

Federal University at Paraiba
Joao Pessoa, Paraiba, Brazil

Rita J. Olivieri, PhD, RN

Boston College
Chestnut Hill, Massachusetts

Anna Omery, DNSc, RN

University of California, Los
  Angeles
Los Angeles, California

Vera Lucia de Almeida Peres, MS

Federal University at Paraiba
Joao Pessoa, Paraiba, Brazil

Brooke P. Randell, DNSc, RN

University of California, Los
  Angeles
Los Angeles, California

Donna Loy Ritter, MN, RN

South Dakota State University
Brookings, South Dakota

Barbara C. Rottkamp, EdD, RN

Adelphi University
Garden City, New York

Ellen B. Rudy, PhD

Case Western Reserve University
Cleveland, Ohio

Virginia K. Saba, EdD, RN, FAAN

Georgetown University
Washington, DC

Karen Moore Schaefer, DNSc, RN

Allentown College of St. Francis de Sales
Center Valley, Pennsylvania
The Allentown Hospital–Lehigh Valley Hospital Center
Allentown, Pennsylvania

Nancy Schappler, MSN, RN

Massachusetts General Hospital
Boston, Massachusetts

Mary Ann Schroeder, PhD, RN

University of South Carolina
Columbia, South Carolina

Stephanie Scinta, BSN, RN

Mercy Hospital
Davenport, Iowa

Elizabeth Sergent, BS, RN

State University at Stony Brook
Stony Brook, New York

Kathleen C. Sheppard, MSN, RN

University of Texas MD Anderson Cancer Center
Houston, Texas

Deborah Soholt, BSN, RN

St. Luke's Midland Regional Medical Center
Aberdeen, South Dakota

Sheila M. Sparks, DNSc, RN, CS

Georgetown University
Washington, DC

Cathrine Strauss, BS, RN

State University at Stony Brook
Stony Brook, New York

Sharon Summers, PhD, RN

University of Kansas Medical Center
Kansas City, Kansas

Joseph Thatcher, BS, RN

Massachusetts General Hospital
Boston, Massachusetts

Aileen Thomson, BAAN, RN

The Wellesley Hospital
Toronto, Ontario, Canada

Catherine A. Tracey, MS, RN, CRRN

Northeast Rehabilitation Hospital
Salem, New Hampshire

Suzanne Van Ort, PhD, RN

University of Arizona
Tucson, Arizona

Karen Goyette-Vincent, MS, RN, CS

Veterans Administration Hospital
Brockton, Massachusetts

Ginna Wall, MN, RN

University of Washington Medical Center
Seattle, Washington

Judith Warren, PhD, RN

University of Nebraska Medical Center
Omaha, Nebraska

Janet Weber, MSN, RN

Southeast Missouri State University
Cape Girardeau, Missouri

Nina D. Wilson, RN

Massachusetts General Hospital
Boston, Massachusetts

M. Anne Woodtli, PhD, RN

The University of Arizona
Tucson, Arizona

Maria T. Zickuhr, BS, RN, CPAN

Cleveland Clinic Foundation
Cleveland, Ohio

Shirley Melat Ziegler, PhD, RN

Texas Woman's University
Dallas, Texas

Kay Zingsheim, RN, CPAN

Shawnee Mission Medical Center
Shawnee Mission, Kansas

Taxonomy Development:
Past, Present, and Future

Why a Classification System?

Winnifred C. Mills, MEd, RN

Taxonomy is a term defined as "the science of how to classify and identify" (Fleishman & Quaintance, 1984, p. 22). In addition to taxonomy as a science in its own right, as nurses we are concerned with the influence that taxonomic endeavors may have on the development of our discipline. An exploration of the reasons for generating a taxonomy forms the basis of this discussion. Six objectives for classification in science will be related to nursing as an evolving discipline.

Grouping Entities: The Parts as Pieces of the Whole

Classification is the ordering or arrangement of entities into groups or sets on the basis of their relationships (Simpson, 1961). The result is a classificatory system (Sokal, 1974) and the phenomena of concern, or taxa, are generally grouped on the basis of similarities and dissimilarities. This facilitates description of the structure and relationships of the entities in regard to each other and to similar entities.

As nursing moves forward into the last decade of this century, the conceptual bases for practice in the discipline have been greatly extended. The surge in nursing research occurring in the last two decades has produced a critical mass of information in the functional area of direct care giving.

Members of the North American Nursing Diagnosis Association (NANDA) are particularly interested in the information that describes human requirements for nursing intervention. These requirements have been named nursing diagnoses. They are essential elements in the conceptualization, the language, and the methodology of nursing. A taxonomy should provide a system to identify relationships among these essential elements in both the science and the language of nursing and therefore in the culture of nursing itself.

Hypotheses for Further Investigation: The Discipline Evolves

Fleishman and Quaintance (1984) note that the application of taxonomic principles to a set of observations may result in the emergence of new information. Patterns may be revealed enabling predictions for future action, thus generating hypotheses for further investigation. Rasch (1987) notes that a taxonomy should serve as a heuristic device by which decisions can be made to include or not include specific cases. By their very nature taxonomies change and evolve. Such evolution necessitates theoretical considerations and may include both inductive and deductive approaches leading to further advances in the discipline (Walker & Avant, 1983). At the Eighth NANDA Conference, Hinshaw (1989) reemphasized the importance of building support for each nursing diagnosis, not from one but from a number of studies, in order to establish the reliability and validity of the evidence.

A System to Relieve the Cognitive Burden

Because of the limits of human cognitive abilities, nurses have a need to order nursing diagnoses in an effort "to achieve economy of memory and to facilitate communication" (Fleishman & Quaintance, 1984, p. 24). Language and order are particularly essential in a discipline where practitioners are introduced to knowledge and skills through any one of a number of different conceptual approaches with varying views of person, environment, health, and nursing. The subject matter for classification reflects the enterprise of the whole culture known as professional nursing. Harrington (1988) has stressed the importance of nursing diagnosis as a form of communication in transmitting this culture, our social heritage.

Communication: For Concurrent Care Giving and Also for Research

Brennan and Ramano (1987) suggest that as a first step, nurses must define the domain of nursing and the focus of assessment. By so doing, parameters are established for the subject matter of the taxonomy. The NANDA taxonomy includes only the nursing diagnosis titles or labels. Nursing diagnoses form one part of the language of nursing. In manual systems for documentation of care, many different names can be given to a phenomenon. These names are often inconveniently buried and difficult to identify in the paper record.

With greater and greater demands being made on professional resources, time, and nursing expertise, computerized systems of data management for nursing are becoming more evident. In a computerized system, specified labels are available for selection and data are retrieved under that label. Before a program can be instituted, agreement is necessary on nomenclature or name of a phenomenon. Thus, consistent terminology is necessary not only for improved communication among practitioners but also for ease of retrieval of information, both for care giving and for research purposes. Bringing order to the nomenclature and, thus, to the nursing diagnoses represented is at the heart of classification.

An Expanding Consciousness: Nursing in a New Light

From the beginning in 1973, the efforts to explore nursing diagnoses by the National Group for Classification of Nursing Diagnosis (subsequently named the North American Nursing Diagnosis Association) have proceeded along two paths. One path has been toward identification of new nursing diagnoses and refinement of those extant. The second and parallel path has been toward classification of those nursing diagnoses. Kritek (1978) has referred to identification of diagnoses as a process moving us toward factor-isolating theory and classification as a process moving us toward factor-relating theory generation. She notes that these processes require recognition and review of thinking on the holistic aspects of nursing. Carnevali (1984) states that nursing needs "taxonomists who combine an overall conceptual framework of the domain of nursing with its specific parts to form a logical, cohesive, pragmatic diagnostic classification system." Existing taxonomic principles may not fit comfortably with the overlapping and interacting categories that presently describe nursing's phenomena of concern. This should not, however, prevent continued efforts to classify. New challenges and approaches will emerge. Nursing must not fear the demons of fragmentation and reductionism, but rather overcome them as increasingly complex matrices for classification evolve.

Expanding Borders: Nursing in a Wider World

Other utilitarian objectives are being met by taxonomy development, such as ease of conversion of the taxonomy to a structure acceptable for coding by the World Health Organization for inclusion in the International Classification systems. Recognition and acceptance of this work by the International Council of Nurses will acknowledge the diffusion of nursing diagnosis information and usage that has already occurred. Working with international organizations is essential to prevent fragmentation of efforts and to assist the assimilation of NANDA's work throughout the world of nursing.

Conclusion

The substance of this discussion has focused on the objectives of classification in science as applied to the discipline of nursing. The process of describing the nursing diagnoses and then designing a structure depicting their relationship to each other and to similar nursing diagnoses is a first objective. Through this exercise nurses have become sensitized to the need for criteria for inclusion and exclusion of diagnoses from groups and categories. A result will be the generation of hypotheses for further investigation

as a second objective. An effort to achieve economy of memory and to facilitate communication follows as a third objective. Ease in manipulating observations and relating diagnoses to one another can be achieved. A taxonomy brings order and coherence to the diagnoses, thus related information is more easily retrieved by the computerized systems in practice settings.

The work of taxonomy will proceed far into the future and many changes will result. The challenge will be to support whatever structure emerges with a substantive research base as new patterns evolve.

References

Brennan, P. F., & Ramano, C. A. (1987). Computers and nursing diagnoses: Issues in implementation. *Nursing Clinics of North America, 22,* 935–941.

Carnevali, D. L. (1984). Nursing diagnoses: An evolutionary view. *Topics in Clinical Nursing, 5*(4), 10–20.

Fleishman, E. A., & Quaintance, M. K. (1984). *Taxonomies of human performance: The description of human tasks.* Orlando, FL: Orlando Academic Press.

Harrington, L. W. (1988). The diagnosis dilemma: One preferred remedy. *Nursing and Health Care, 9,* 93–94.

Hinshaw, L. W. (1988). Keynote address: Forging the link between theory and practice. In R. M. Carroll-Johnson (Ed.), *Classification of nursing diagnoses: Proceedings of the eighth conference* (pp. 3–10). Philadelphia: Lippincott.

Kritek, P. B. (1978). The generation and classification of nursing diagnoses: Toward a theory of nursing. *IMAGE, 10,* 33–40.

Rasch, R. F. (1987). The nature of taxonomy. *IMAGE, 19,* 147–159.

Simpson, G. G. (1961). *Principles of animal taxonomy.* New York: Columbia University Press.

Sokal, R. R. (1974). Classification: Purposes, principles, progress, prospects. *Science, 185,* 1115–1123.

Walker, L. O., & Avant, K. C. (1983). *Strategies for theory construction in nursing.* Norwalk, CT: Appleton-Century-Crofts.

Validation of Taxonomy

Mary E. Kerr, MN, RN

There are several types and methods of developing and validating a taxonomic or classification structure. This presentation will highlight those used most frequently by a variety of disciplines including nursing.

Philosophic Considerations Underlying Taxonomic Development

Historical Highlights

As humans, we want to understand the world in which we live. As we attempt to understand this world, there is an immediate separation between a world that we perceive and a world that we do not. We begin to classify that which we can perceive. As we perceive differences among actions, thoughts, or items, classification naturally occurs. The very act of conceptualizing is an act of classifying.

Classification occurred very early in man's cognitive development. The first record of a classification system is the classification of animals by the ancient Chinese. Some of the categories found in this system were

- Those that belong to the emperor
- Embalmed ones
- Those that are trained
- Suckling pigs
- Mermaids
- Fabulous ones
- Stray dogs
- Those included in this classification
- Those that tremble as if they were mad
- Innumerable ones
- Those drawn with a very fine camel's hair brush
- Those that resemble flies from a distance (Aldenderfer & Blashfield, 1984)

The Chinese based this classification of animals on perceptions of an animal world meaningful to the Chinese way of life at that period. Although the ancient Chinese recorded the first classification system, scientists surmise that the ability to perceive similarities and differences was a prerequisite of evolutionary survival (Ricklefs, 1973). Early classifications included male/female, young/old, tribe member/not tribe member, dangerous/not dangerous (Zubin, 1968).

The Greek philosopher Plato classified the world into two systems differing in origin. He described the world as consisting of either phenomena perceived by the senses or concepts and ideas of the mind (Crowson, 1970; Mayr, 1969). Aristotle, building on Plato's basic premise, surmised that the classification of items in and of the world developed from that item's individual characteristics.

Aristotle called an item's individual characteristics its essence. The essence consists of those characteristics that distinguish an item or element from others and provide the item with its identity. The taxonomic strategy based on the logic of Aristotle is the Linnaean taxonomy. This taxonomic strategy assumes every element contains at least one key differentiating characteristic that provides a given element with its identity. It is that key characteristic that becomes the criterion for distinguishing differences and similarities among items.

Immanuel Kant (1724–1804), while not addressing the specific characteristics that identified the essence of an element, differentiated between a world that exists and a world that humans see as a sum of their experience. Kant (1952) groups the world into two categories: a world that is a thing in itself and the world as it presents itself to the person.

William James (1842–1910), with his pragmatic view of reality, rejected the idea that key characteristics provided the essence of an item. James (1955) emphasized the contextual influence on human perception of both sensory items and ideas. Since James's critique, classification systems based on the essence of an element have been called into question. The essence of an element is not constant but alters to fit the perception or purpose of the classifier. The essence of a table to a woodworker may be the quality of wood and manner of construction. However, the essence of a table to an antique dealer may be the age, overall condition, and history of the furniture. Thus, there is no one criterion that determines the ultimate essence of an item.

Adanson, the originator of numeric taxonomy, rejected the a priori assumption that some criteria (criteria that denoted the essence of an item) had more importance than others. He classified based on affinity, or likeness, of a group of criteria. He considered all criteria of an item simultaneously and he weighted the importance of criteria equally.

Thus, he arranged groups based on correlated or highly related criteria (Sokal & Sneath, 1963).

The debate involving the correct designation of criteria for the classification of items persists within all disciplines. Proponents of differing taxonomic strategies (such as subjective disciplinary consensus, evolutionary or hereditary basis, or numeric affinity involving similarity or probability coefficients) maintain that their respective classification method results in the truest representation of reality.

Purposes of a Taxonomy

The purposes of a taxonomy are to (1) understand one's world; (2) communicate with others (Bell, 1967); (3) provide information in a systematic manner; and (4) identify gaps and relationships within knowledge (Fleishman & Quaintance, 1984). A taxonomy helps one understand the world in which one lives. This understanding of the world occurs through naming, identifying, defining, and relating. An initial step in taxonomic development is to give a name to something. The process of attaching a name to a phenomenon disentangles the uniqueness of one item from another.

Defining and redefining items classified within a taxonomic structure is a continual process. As the taxonomist finds a place for new items within an existing taxonomic structure, the delineation of the new item with the old items occurs. This delineation results in a clarification and refinement of both the old and the new item. For example, *constipation* and *perceived constipation* initially appeared related to the family of *altered bowel elimination*. However, when the members of the Taxonomy Committee examined the relevant criteria, very little similarity existed between the criteria of *perceived constipation* and *constipation*. The criteria of *perceived constipation* were closer to those of other altered perception states than the criteria of *constipation*, despite the similarities in the names. Thus, *perceived constipation* may not be a form of *constipation* at all, but more closely related to conditions involving altered perception. This constant comparison between the criteria of the items that require classification and items currently classified results in a clarification both of the definition and of the relationship that exists between and among items.

A second purpose of a taxonomy is to provide a method for people to communicate with each other. A name given to a specific item provides a shorthand method to describe the characteristics of the item without actually describing them. For example, if an item is a chair, immediately the mind sees an item with four legs, a seat, and a back and understands the chair's purpose is to provide a place for someone to sit. Likewise, a taxon (a grouping within a taxonomic structure whose components share similar characteristics but differing characteristics from other groupings) is also a shorthand method that tells you something about that grouping. For example, consider the classification of dogs and cats. This allows a picture of the differences between two sets of animals to come to mind without specifying the differences. Now to separate dogs into Yorkshire terriers and labradors permits a shorthand method that makes finer distinctions between the two taxons. The finer the distinctions, the more knowledgeable must be the person interpreting the classifications.

The same is true in nursing diagnoses. The name given to the items classified provides a consistent representation of the item and provides a shorthand method for identifying an item without specifying all the criteria. As the taxonomic structure becomes more complex, differentiating between specific diagnoses requires an increasing amount of expertise.

A third purpose of a taxonomy is manipulation of data. A classification system provides information in a systematic and economical manner. By providing a name for an item with a specific set of criteria, a consistent language develops. This facilitates retrieval and extraction of information by using this name to merge knowledge from multiple sources. As scientific knowledge accumulates within a discipline, taxonomies provide the organizing medium for new and existing knowledge. The taxonomic language facilitates comparison of findings across fields as well as improving tracking of knowledge within and outside one's discipline (Fleishman & Quaintance, 1984). The submission of a taxonomy of nursing diagnoses for inclusion into the International Classification of Diseases (Revision 10) (ICD-10) represents how a taxonomy provides an international language for nursing.

A fourth purpose of a taxonomy identifies gaps and relationships within knowledge. Before one organizes information, it is difficult to know the completeness of that information. However, after organization, gaps in knowledge become more apparent. For example, NANDA presented two arrangements of nursing diagnoses: the alphabetic list and Taxonomy I. The alphabetic arrangement results in an index of diagnoses for easy clinical access. This index, however, cannot designate relationships between diagnoses. Taxonomy I arranges diagnoses based on the similarity between the nursing diagnoses and a theoretical framework (Roy, 1982). Taxonomy I is a structure that designates the relationship between and among nursing diagnoses. This same taxonomic structure provides a method to deduce missing pieces in the structure.

After the organization of the diagnoses, obvious gaps in knowledge become apparent. For example, there is a gap in diagnosis development under the category of Communicating. The NANDA membership recognized *altered verbal communication* as an accepted nursing diagnosis. After this diagnosis was placed within the taxonomic structure, a gap in information that may require further research became apparent. This gap, illustrated in the earlier taxonomic tree as a "bracketed box," was labeled *altered nonverbal communication* and designated as an area for further research (Kritek, 1984). With the alphabetized list of nursing diagnoses, no gaps were noticeable. Only after the organization of diagnoses based on similar characteristics did the gaps in knowledge become apparent.

Why Validate a Taxonomy?

There is no written assertion that all taxonomies should be valid. However, disciplinary research attempts to define consistently clear categories of knowledge; as these categories emerge, a taxonomy emerges. The issue of the validity of the NANDA nursing diagnosis taxonomic structure has been in question since its inception. The major adversaries of Taxonomy I contend that Taxonomy I is not a true taxonomy of nursing diagnoses (Rasch, 1987); that it was developed unscientifically (Porter, 1986); and that it consists of categoric labels that are not familiar to the disciplinary membership (Jenny, 1989).

Taxonomy I continues to provide interesting material for disciplinary debate. The debate on both sides of the argument stems from differences in opinion rather than from differences in evidence of utilization and structure of alternative taxonomies. The debate requires more substance. Porter (1986) stated that when a diagnosis does not fit into the current taxonomic structure, the entire structure should be reevaluated. A better question may be: How does the usefulness of the taxonomic structure change if that offending diagnosis is placed in a miscellaneous category rather than into the closest fitting, albeit not perfect, category?

Using concept-synthesis techniques, Coler et al. (1989) expanded the definitions of the labels of the nine human response pattern categories of Taxonomy I. They reported an inconsistency between their work on the expanded definitions of the labels for the nine human response patterns and the use of the Taxonomy I categories when organizing the nursing diagnoses. As a result of their work, Coler et al. suggest an alternative taxonomy based on their expanded definitions of the labels for the nine human response patterns. This type of examination of the definitions of the conceptual categories provides a foundation for a validation study comparing alternative taxonomic structures. For example, one study may compare the categoric strength between two taxonomic structures such as the NANDA Taxonomy I and Coler's restructured taxonomy. By using similar statistical techniques, the within-taxon relationships and between-taxon differences between the two taxonomic structures can be compared.

Validation also includes the process of replicating existing relationships, clarifying distinctions between or among very similar items that cannot be classified. Few reported studies validate an entire taxonomic structure unless that structure is very small (e.g., hierarchy of pain) (Turk & Rudy, 1988). Although there is an abundance of smaller validation studies within every discipline, the validation studies do not specify the use of one overriding model used to guide a project. The only general taxonomic development/validation presented here is the Fleishman and Quaintance model (1984).

Fleishman and Quaintance Taxonomy Model

Fleishman and Quaintance identify four steps in taxonomic development:

1. Identify the purpose of the classification system.
2. Identify the criteria used when classifying items.
3. Classify the items reliably.
4. Evaluate the adequacy and utility of the classification system.

The first step is to establish the purpose of the classification system. If the purpose is to develop a classification system that has a specific utilitarian goal, such as prediction of mortality or cost, then the classification stems from a function of its outcome. However, if the purpose is more general and the anticipated use is multidirectional, then the classification of items depends on the characteristics of the items rather than on their functional outcome. The resulting classification system is tested against a myriad of alternative outcomes. In this way, general taxonomies often guide researchers in theory development (Fleishman & Quaintance, 1984).

The second step is to identify the domain of relevant attributes. The evaluation of all relevant criteria is realistic when the total number of relevant criteria is small. When the number of relevant criteria is large, criteria can be randomly selected for use in the classification process. The criteria chosen become the key distinguishing factors for identifying groups.

The third step is to classify the items reliably using the criteria relevant to that item in relation to the other items' relevant criteria. Regardless of the classification strategy chosen, an important concern is the operationalization of the criteria to maximize their usefulness as grouping indicators. Specific operational definitions increase interrater reliability and facilitate consistent categorization of items (Fleishman & Quaintance, 1984). Without clear concise definitions of criteria of the diagnosis, as well as clear definitions of taxonomic categories, the taxonomic placement of diagnoses is merely a conceptual exercise.

The last step is to identify the criteria to evaluate the adequacy and utility of the classification system. The Fleishman and Quaintance model highlights three steps in the validation process: internal validity, external validity, and utilization. An internally valid taxonomic structure results when the criteria are defined so specifically that each item is identified and placed in the same category repeatedly. The issues of reliability embedded in taxonomic validation are similar to reliability issues for all instrument development and usage. The same psychometric principles of instrumentation apply to taxonomic structures. Taxonomic structures, in a sense, are a special type of instrument. An instrument, in order for it to be useful, must be able to measure what it purports to measure consistently.

External validity involves the accomplishment of the taxonomy's stated purpose. The rules of valid taxonomy are designed such that elements placed within the structure consistently have the same placement within the structure upon replication. A taxonomy is designed to provide a consistent standard method of organizing. If the rules for classifying items are unclear or inconsistent, the resultant taxonomy will not be consistent. If the taxonomy is valid, it should be reliable, propose relationships between and among groups, and achieve that which the taxonomic structure was devised to accomplish. Classification systems should be exhaustive, i.e., every item can be placed within the structure. This is frequently unrealistic especially in early taxonomic development. Items may require further research to extract the criteria necessary for proper placement; or the taxonomic structure may require further development before incorporating the new item within the structure.

Since 1983, paleontologists Archer and Godthelp discovered and classified the remains of over 100 pre-Pleistocene-era mammal species in Riversleigh, Australia, more than doubling the number of known prehistoric mammal, reptile, amphibian, and bird species (Park, 1990). Relevant criteria for each species became the basis for categorization of the remains. Conflicting or bizarre criteria were the initiating feature for further investigation of either a mutant or a new class of species. For example, the investigators discovered a marsupial with strange teeth formation. Because this formation did not fit into any other pattern of criteria currently known for marsupials, this marsupial was not classified immediately. After uncovering the skull and more jaw, there were adequate criteria to determine that this was a founding member of a new order of marsupials, *Yalkaparidon* (Park, 1990). Frequently, taxonomic structures contain a catch-all category. This catch-all includes the difficult-to-place items based on conflicting or confusing criteria. Items remain in this category until the discovery of new criteria permits proper placement within the overall structure.

Utilization, the third step of validating a taxonomy, specifies that the structure should make sense or be useful to the informed user. For example, in 1694 the Académie Française, the keepers of the French language, prepared the first edition of the dictionary of purest French. The root of the French words provided the criteria for classification. This resulted in a perfect but useless classification system (Harriss, 1990). Thus, the choice of method for classification is very important and must relate to the overall purpose and usefulness of the classification system.

A major criticism of the existing Taxonomy I is that it does not make sense to the informed user. Levin (1987) contends that the clinical nurse does not understand what the human response pattern Exchanging represents. If that is so, then there may be a problem with the existing taxonomic structure. At the highest level of abstraction, the taxonomic structure should be useful to the minimally informed person, with increased expertise required as one progresses through the structure.

Methods of Taxonomic Validation

There are a variety of ways to validate a taxonomic structure. Four methods presented here include:

1. Overall structural analysis
2. Clarification between specific taxons within the structure
3. Comparing alternative models of discerning criteria for taxonomic development
4. Comparing alternative methods of categorization in taxonomic development.

Overall structural analysis involves identifying the components of the entire structure, and examining it for meaning and consistency. Qualitative methods, such as content and concept-analysis techniques, are useful in evaluating the classification structure's achievement of purpose, clarifying the definitions of classification categories, clarifying definitions of items being classified, identifying consistency among levels of abstraction, and identifying consistency of threads throughout a taxon. The overall validation of an entire taxonomic structure is a lengthy multifaceted project depending on the size and detail of the taxonomic structure. Biologic taxonomists have spent their entire life work on validating one taxon, not considering the entire taxonomic structure.

The second method of validating a taxonomic structure is one frequently identified and used in the literature. This validation method involves the clarification between specific taxons. One clinical study by Turk and Rudy (1988) used different criteria from those traditionally used to distinguish between types of chronic pain. They proposed the use of psychologic criteria to develop a classification of pain. Using a two-phase, cross-validation technique, three types of pain were identified. The relevant criteria for determining types of chronic pain included life interference, psychologic distress, life control, pain severity, and activity level. This example illustrates the identification of categories of chronic pain based on old criteria (pain severity and activity level) as well as new or alternative criteria (life interference, psychologic distress, and life control).

With respect to nursing diagnosis, the work on urinary incontinence is an example of developing and differentiating among types of classification elements. This designation of new or more specific criteria is useful for both the creation of new categories as well as in differentiating and validating existing categories. A taxonomic grouping currently benefiting from improved criteria designation involves the diagnoses *impaired gas exchange, ineffective airway clearance,* and *ineffective breathing pattern.* Is the relationship equal among all three diagnoses, or do any two have a stronger affinity? Are the discriminating criteria consistent when viewed from differing conceptual models? Grounded theory and phenomenology are useful in identifying new criteria among the classifiable items. Quantitative statistical analysis such as discriminant analysis, fuzzy set methods, and probability models are useful in identifying the importance of criteria in classifying items.

A third method to validate a taxonomic strucure is to compare taxonomies that result from the aggregation of criteria originating from alternate models. For example, compare the grouping of diagnoses based on relevant criteria identified from two models (Coler et al., 1989) using an empiric technique such as cluster analysis. The choice of relevant criteria would be designated by the model or theory supporting the underlying classification (Aldenderfer & Blashfield, 1984). If cluster analysis is used, the clustering method chosen as well as the choice of similarity coefficients for both models should be similar to allow for comparison between the models.

A fourth method of validating a classification system involves comparing the taxonomic structures that a result generated with different taxonomic strategies. Rather than comparing the results of alternative models and their respective criteria, one uses one model and one set of criteria, but alternative methods for classifying. There are a multitude of variations of this theme:

- Compare consensus decision making with an empiric method
- Compare an equal-weighted technique with a variable-weighted technique
- Compare two alternative methods of numerical analysis
- Compare two types of cluster analysis (single linkage versus complete linkage)

In comparing alternative methods, no one method is correct but each method provides information about the relationships among the items.

There is a multitude of methods used across disciplines in the development and validation of a taxonomy. How does one decide on the most appropriate validation method? Rather than arbitrarily choosing a validation method, the method often arises from a taxonomic problem or question. It is often the choice of the taxonomic problem, the expertise of the researcher or taxonomist, and the available resources that drive the choice of selection of a validation technique. After the researcher or taxonomist identifies the particular taxonomic problem, his/her energy becomes focused on resolution of the particular taxonomic problem. For example, a common problem occurs when items cannot be easily classified within the existing structure or the new items conflict with the existing classification system. Some classification systems build in a catch-all category where problem items are placed until they are adequately identified. An intense process of scrutinization occurs to examine the rationale for the classification difficulty.

A taxonomy, however, is not stagnant. As one group of researchers works on validating the entire structure, another group is busy defining, or redefining, a smaller section of the structure. This is not to say the work should not be done. This is merely a pragmatic warning to the individuals who take on this task that the work may be obsolete before it is complete.

Conclusions

The work of taxonomic development and validation continues. Every nurse researcher who attempts to clarify or distinguish between diagnoses or groups of diagnoses is facilitating this development and validation process. Numerous methods and strategies are available to the researcher to assist in this validation process. It is an exciting, albeit exhausting and endless task. We will never see it to completion. There is no perfect taxonomy. However, the creation of a taxonomy that is both useful and meaningful to the discipline is a worthy endeavor.

References

Aldenderfer, M. S., & Blashfield, R. K. (1984). *Cluster analysis.* Newbury Park. NY: Sage.

Bell, C. R. (1967). *Plant variation and classification.* Belmont, CA: Wadsworth.

Coler, M. S., Johnson, T., Amaro, A., Johnson, B., Snayd, J., Wiedliger, C., et al. (1989). NANDA Taxonomy I: A preliminary validation/invalidation study. In R. M. Carroll-Johnson (Ed.), *Classification of nursing diagnoses: Proceedings of the eighth conference* (pp. 141–151). Philadelphia: Lippincott.

Crowson, R. A. (1970). *Classification and biology.* New York: Atherton.

Fleishman, E. A., & Quaintance, M. K. (1984). *Taxonomies of human performance.* San Diego, CA: Academic Press.

Harriss, J. (1990). Qu'est-ce que c'est? A social club or a cultural bastion? *Smithsonian, 20*(10), 144–157.

James, W. (1955). *Pragmatism and four essays from the meaning of truth.* Cleveland, OH: World.

Jenny, J. (1989). Classifying nursing diagnoses: A self-care approach. *Nursing & Health Care, 10*(2), 83–85.

Kant, I. (1952). *The critique of pure reason.* Chicago: Encyclopedia Britannica, Inc.

Kritek, P. (1984). Report of the group work on taxonomies. In M. J. Kim, G. K. McFarland, & A. M. McLane (Eds.), *Classification of nursing diagnoses: Proceedings of the fifth national conference* (pp. 46–58). St. Louis, MO: Mosby.

Levin, M. E. (1987). Approaches to the development of a nursing diagnosis taxonomy. In A. M. McLane (Ed.), *Classification of nursing diagnoses: Proceedings of the seventh conference* (pp. 45–52). St. Louis: Mosby.

Mayr, E. (1969). *Principles of systematic biology.* New York: McGraw-Hill.

Park, A. (1990). Giants once ruled Australia, fossil discoveries reveal. *Smithsonian, 20*(10), 133–143.

Porter, E. J. (1986). Critical analysis of NANDA nursing diagnosis Taxonomy I. *IMAGE, 18,* 136–139.

Rasch, R. F. (1987). The nature of taxonomy. *IMAGE, 19,* 147–149.

Ricklefs, R. E. (1973). *Ecology.* Newton, MA: Chiron.

Roy, C. (1982). Theoretical framework for classification of nursing diagnosis. In M. J. Kim & D. A. Moritz (Eds.), *Classification of nursing diagnoses: Proceedings of the third and fourth national conferences.* St. Louis, MO: Mosby.

Sokal, R. R., & Sneath, P. H. (1963). Principles of numerical taxonomy. San Francisco: Freeman.

Turk, D. C., & Rudy, T. E. (1988). Toward an empirically derived taxonomy of chronic pain patients: Integration of psychological assessment data. *Journal of Consulting and Clinical Psychology, 56,* 233–238.

Zubin, J. (1968). *Classification of human behavior.* Paper presented at the meeting of the Canadian Psychological Association Institute on Measurement, Classification and Prediction of Human Behavior. The University of Calgary, Alberta, Canada, June, 1968.

The International Classification of Diseases (ICD): Classification of Nursing Diagnosis

Virginia K. Saba, EdD, RN, FAAN

The Classification of Nursing Diagnoses has been submitted by the American Nurses' Association (ANA) to the World Health Organization (WHO) for inclusion into the Tenth Revision of the International Classification of Diseases (ICD-10). ICD-10 is being prepared and will be available in 1993. This Classification of Nursing Diagnoses is the North American Nursing Diagnosis Association's (NANDA) Revised Taxonomy I that was approved by the Board of Directors of both the ANA and NANDA early in 1989 (Fitzpatrick et al., 1989).

A classification, according to Webster's dictionary, is a systematic arrangement of classes. This definition alludes to the fact that indexing systems, taxonomies, and nomenclatures can also be classifications if they are arranged in a structured framework according to similar groups. Generally, classification systems are developed to facilitate communication within a discipline and used to compare similar findings across groups, countries, and time spans (Gebbie, 1989). Classifications vary depending on the criteria, purpose, and relationships. They are coded using alphabetic or numeric characters.

The International Classification of Diseases

The International Classification of Diseases (ICD) is probably the oldest, most developed, and most commonly used classification in the scientific field. The ICD is the official terminology used for coding causes of death around the world. It is prepared by WHO with input from all their member countries and to date has been revised every 10 years.

According to WHO, the ICD is defined as "a system of categories to which morbid entities are assigned according to some established criteria" (ICD-9, 1977, p. vii). It consists of one axis that provides the basis for comparative statistics in order to generate uniform statistical data. In essence, ICD is the major statistical classification that meets the primary requirements of vital statistics—mortality and morbidity.

The ICD originated as a terminology for indexing medical classification of diseases. It dates back to the 17th century when the British and French attempted to report meaningful causes of death. The first statistical analysis of causes of death was published in the late 1600s by John Graunt in *London Bills of Mortality.*

Graunt's book was followed by François Bossier de Lacroix (1706–1777) who attempted to classify diseases in a systematic manner. However, by the beginning of the 19th century the most widely used system was one developed by William Cullen of Edinburgh (1710–1790) and published in 1785.

The next milestone occurred in 1837 when William Farr (1807–1883), of the General Register Office of England and Wales and the first medical statistician, used Cullen's imperfect classification of disease for his annual report in which he also urged the adoption of a uniform classification. Farr continued to study both nomenclatures and statistical classifications. He focused on their utility as a uniform classification of the causes of death. His focus was finally recognized at the first International Statistical Congress held at Brussels in 1853. At the Second Congress in 1855, William Farr proposed the preparation of a uniform nomenclature that classified diseases by anatomic site (Gebbie, 1989; ICD-9, 1977).

The development of ICD continued when Jacques Bertillon (1851–1922) prepared the classification of causes of death in 1885. It was based on one used by the City of Paris and on the previous work of Farr. Bertillon's Classification was adopted by several countries in Europe. It was adopted for the United States, Canada, and Mexico in 1898 by the American Public Health Association (APHA) at its meeting in Canada. Also, APHA recommended that the classification be revised every 10 years. The ICD as known today emerged as a result.

The first revision was initiated by the French government who convened the First International Conference for the Revision of Bertillon's *International Classification of Causes of Death* in Paris in August 1900. The subsequent second and third revisions (1910, 1920) were also directed by Bertillon. However, following his death in 1922 the responsibility for the revisions shifted to the Health Organization of the League of Nations. It created an International Commission to draft the fourth revision (1929) and fifth revision (1938).

The sixth, seventh, and eighth revisions were prepared by an interim commission and subsequently by WHO in 1946, 1955, and 1965. This marked a new era in international vital and health statistics because it expanded its scope to include both mortality and morbidity statistics. Further, WHO adopted a comprehensive program of international cooperation in the field of vital and health statistics. The purpose of the program was to coordinate statistical activities in member countries and serve as a link between the national statistical institutions and WHO.

Ninth Revision of ICD (ICD-9)

The current Ninth Revision of the International Classification of Diseases (ICD-9) came 75 years after the first revision. It was approved by the WHO International Conference in 1975. The conference was attended by delegates from 46 member countries. ICD-9 was expanded to include not only mortality and morbidity statistics, but also statistics to plan, monitor, and evaluate health services. In addition it was designed for computerization of data—storage, processing, and retrieval—as well as indexing of medical records.

ICD-9 was finally adopted by the 29th WHO Assembly in 1976 and became effective in 1979. It consisted of a detailed list of three-digit categories, four-digit subcategories, and an optional fifth digit for detailed expansions such as anatomic site. Also at that Assembly, six World Health Centers were proposed to assist countries with the uses of ICD. They are located in Paris (French), Sao Paulo (Portuguese), Moscow (Russian), Caracas (Spanish), and London and Washington (English). The Washington Office, located in the National Center for Health Statistics, Public Health Service, U.S. Department of Health and Human Services, serves as the Regional Center for Classification of Diseases for North America. It also serves as a liaison between WHO and the U.S. Government.

The ICD-9 was published by the Department of Health and Human Services for use in the United States. It is called *The International Classification of Diseases 9th Revision: Clinical Modification (ICD-9-CM)* (1980). This version of ICD-9 CM consists of three volumes: Volume 1—*Diseases: Tabular List*; Volume 2—*Diseases: Alphabetic Index*; and Volume 3—*Procedures: Tabular List and Alphabetic Index*. This last volume is another adaptation produced in the United States. It is published separately and contains classification of modes of therapy, i.e., surgical, radiologic, laboratory, and diagnostic procedures. This volume is used to provide statistics of health services provided in hospitals and primary care settings (ICD-9-CM, 1980). This classification is based on anatomy rather than surgical categories. It consists of a two-digit numeric code (no alphabetic characters) with two decimal digits as needed.

Tenth Revision of ICD (ICD-10)

Even as the ninth revision was being prepared, it was apparent that its focus was not clearly agreed upon. The standardization of nomenclature on a multilingual basis was essential for conformity in diagnosis. Yet there was disparity between the broad classifications for international comparisons and the narrow requirements for research. Further,

there were different uses for the classification in a developing country compared to those needed in an highly advanced country with computer processing capability. Finally, there were other statistical uses besides those used for diseases that needed to be addressed, such as economic, social, and health policy.

As early as 1971, a World Health Study Group on Classification of Diseases recommended that WHO conduct a study of classification needs and applications in order to initiate a new alternate structure for the tenth revision. Further, in 1978 when WHO and UNICEF inaugurated a global program to achieve health for all by the year 2000, a renewed impetus was given to develop a population-based approach for organizing health services (Lamberts & Wood, 1987).

The tenth revision was initiated in 1980 by WHO. The first Expert Committee on ICD-10 was held in 1984. The Committee recommended that ICD-10 follow the traditional body-system framework to minimize code-number changes in future revisions. Further, the Committee recommended the use of an alphanumeric scheme instead of a numeric one to provide more space in the framework of the classification. The form finally agreed on was a four-character code with an alphabetic character in the first position, followed by two or three numeric characters. Further it was agreed that the three-character level be mandatory for international comparisons, whereas the fourth character was not (Expert Committee, 1987).

Following acceptance of the four-character-level draft by the first Expert Committee, several successive drafts were circulated to all member countries for review. It is expected that the final version of ICD-10 will consist of 21 chapters, which use 25 of the available 26 alphabetic characters. Further, it is proposed that the title be changed from *The Tenth Revision of the International Classification of Diseases* to *The Tenth Internation-*

al Statistical Classification of Diseases and Health-Related Problems (ICD-10).

ICD-10 is being designed for conventional tabulations of mortality, accurate collection of morbidity, and reporting and analyzing health-related data. Further, it will be used for multipurpose morbidity information systems primarily in the United States with clinical and other levels of detail deemed adequate for specific applications such as reimbursement, resource requirements, quality assurance, vital statistics planning, and monitoring and evaluating health services.

ICD-10 Family of Classifications

The first Expert Committee involved with the design of ICD-10 recommended that a "core," or family of different but related classifications, be developed. This concept emerged once it was determined that ICD could not provide all the information required by its potential users. It was envisioned that the family would encompass established classifications such as the Classification of Impairments, Disabilities, and Handicaps or the Classification of Primary Care. Further it would encompass specialty-based adaptations such as oncology, dentistry, and perhaps nursing.

The first Expert Committee recommended that the family of specialty-based adaptations follow the three- or four-character-level coded framework outlined in ICD-10. They also proposed that WHO be involved in the preparation of the specialty-based adaptations by acting as a clearinghouse for such activities, and by providing the necessary technical guidance to the groups involved. It was agreed that endorsement of the specialty groups would support the information needs of the health-related specialty areas for the implementation of health for all by the year 2000.

Classification of Nursing Diagnosis

The Classification of Nursing Diagnosis was submitted for consideration as a member of the ICD-10 family of classifications of diseases and health-related problems in accordance with the proposed inclusion of specialty adaptations. The Classification of Nursing Diagnosis is an approved nomenclature by the ANA, and provides a new dimension for the traditional mortality and morbidity reporting.

This classification is used by nurses in North America to supplement the documentation and statistical reporting of nursing care of patients. It will assist practicing nurses, administrators, researchers, and educators with the application of labels to the clinical management of patients. It is also being integrated into information systems used to document nursing care of patients as a way to supplement the organization of clinical information on a patient's episodes of diseases over time.

The Classification of Nursing Diagnosis is designed to code "patient conditions that necessitate skilled nursing care." A nursing diagnosis is a clinical judgment about human responses to actual or potential health problems of an individual, and provides the basis for the prescription of definitive therapy toward achievement of actions for which nurses are accountable.

The classification is divided into categories according to the nine human response patterns, numbered from zero to eight: Choosing (0), Communicating (1), Exchanging (2), Feeling (3), Knowing (4), Moving (5), Perceiving (6), Relating (7), and Valuing (8). These nine human response patterns are manifestations of motion or patterns between "man" and his environment, and are characteristic of unity and organization. Together, they make up the total life patterns of human–environment interactions.

To comply with the ICD-10 family framework, an alphanumeric system is used with a three- or four-character code. The proposed framework consists of an alphabetic character "N" (Nursing) in the first position followed by two or three numeric characters. The nine categories are designated as the first digit (second character), while the second and third digits represent a nursing diagnosis in the group.

Example: Human Response Pattern: Moving (Category 5)

N50 Activity, Altered

N50.0 Activity, Intolerance

Summary

The need to classify patients not only by their medical diseases but also by their nursing care requirements is critical for international comparability. The Classification of Nursing Diagnosis, once approved by the World Health Organization as a member of the ICD-10 family, will make possible new comparisons of nursing knowledge around the world.

References

Expert Committee on the International Classification of Diseases. (November, 1987). *Draft Report: 2nd Meeting on the 10th Revision.* Geneva, Switzerland: World Health Organization.

Fitzpatrick, J. J., Kerr, M. E., Saba, V. K., Hoskins, L. M., Hurley, M. E., Mills, W. C., Rottkamp, B. C., Warren, J. J., & Carpenito, L. (1989). Translating nursing diagnosis into ICD code. *American Journal of Nursing, 89,* 493–495.

Gebbie, K. M. (1989). Major classifications systems in health care and their use. In American Nurses' Association (ANA) Cabinet on Nursing Practice (Eds.), *Classification systems for describing nursing practice: Working papers* (pp. 48–49). Kansas City, MO: American Nurses' Association.

Lamberts, H., & Wood, M. (Eds.). (1987). *International Classification of Primary Care (ICPC).* New York: Oxford.

The International Classification of Diseases: 9th Revision: Clinical Modification (ICD-9 CM): Vol. 1, Diseases Tabular List (2nd ed.). (1980). Pub. No. (PHS 80-120). Washington, DC: U.S. Department of Health and Human Services.

The International Classification of Diseases: 1975 Revision (9th) (ICD-9) (Vol. 1). (1977). Geneva, Switzerland: World Health Organization.

The Translation of NANDA Taxonomy I into ICD Code

Joyce J. Fitzpatrick, PhD, RN, FAAN

The goal of introducing nursing diagnoses into the World Health Organization (WHO) International Classification of Diseases (ICD) was not a new one. For some time there has been collaborative planning between NANDA and American Nurses' Association (ANA) representatives. In early 1989, a formal list of nursing diagnoses was submitted by ANA to WHO for potential inclusion in the tenth revision of ICD under a heading of "Conditions that Necessitate Nursing Care." The process and content of the NANDA Taxonomy Committee's translation of nursing diagnoses into ICD code is presented here.

As part of the formalization of the NANDA Taxonomy Committee, objectives were delineated to guide the association in development of the classification scheme for nursing diagnoses. Further, one of the purposes of the Taxonomy Committee continues to be to promote the use of the Taxonomy in collaboration with other groups. As part of the committee goals for 1987 to 1989, the Taxonomy Committee assumed responsibility for leadership in presenting nursing diagnoses to the nursing and health care scientific and professional practice communities.

All previous discussions of NANDA activities in relation to ICD coding had been collaborative with representatives from ANA. Several planning sessions were held in which representatives from each of the organizations (NANDA and ANA) shared joint goals and strategized about means to achieve these goals. In spite of the fact that there was, at times, a difference of opinion on how to achieve the goals, there was consistent agreement that the goal of WHO recognition of nursing diagnoses was central to further disciplinary developments.

In 1986, the NANDA Taxonomy I was endorsed for development and testing and the previously used alphabetic classification scheme was replaced by the hierarchical classification scheme embedded in Taxonomy I. The conceptual structure of the nine human response patterns provided the organizing framework for Taxonomy I. Nursing diagnoses were grouped together at several different levels within the patterns. Taxonomy I was published by NANDA (1987) along with the characteristic "trees" and bracketed diagnoses that represented those yet to be developed. NANDA members, including scientists and practitioners, were encouraged to further refine and develop the diagnoses at all levels of the taxonomic structure.

In late 1987 and 1988, there was formal collaboration between members of the NANDA Taxonomy Committee and ANA representatives of the Council on Computer Applications in Nursing. The joint planning representatives also consulted with outside experts who had had previous experiences with ICD coding.

In Fall 1988, it was decided to develop a translation of nursing diagnoses into the ICD coding format. Some basic decisions were imperative in the early stages of planning. First, it was decided that it would be desirable to propose a separate nursing chapter within ICD-10. Next, to follow the ICD framework, a four-character code was chosen: an alphabetic character (Y) in the first position, followed by three numeric characters.

Two principles were agreed upon by Committee members to guide the work of placement of diagnoses within the coding format. It was determined that labels should first be defined so that each level had a specific purpose and then be clarified to make them more specific and concrete.

The nine human response patterns (Choosing, Communicating, Exchanging, Feeling, Knowing, Moving, Perceiving, Relating, and Valuing) were retained as the overall classification structure. Although there was some consideration of changing this basic conceptual scheme during the Committee discussion, it was concluded that not only had this conceptual structure been useful, but also the more basic conceptual dimensions could best be examined as part of Taxonomy II development. The conceptual issue, then, at this level of abstraction was set aside. For each of the nine patterns a one-digit identifying number was placed immediately to the right of the "Y." Patterns were placed in alphabetic order. Thus, diagnoses placed under Choosing became Y0, Communicating Y1, Exchanging Y2, Feeling Y3, Knowing Y4, Moving Y5, Perceiving Y6, Relating Y7, and Valuing Y8 (see Appendix C). It was concluded that there was not a need to code the patterns separately from any diagnoses.

Thus, the pattern code was embedded in the diagnosis such that one could tell from the diagnosis code under which pattern the diagnosis was grouped. It was concluded that the conceptual structure had direct relevance to the scientific understandings of nursing diagnoses but indirect relevance to its impact on clinical practice. While this issue can be debated, the Committee's conclusions were consistent with the definitions proposed for inclusion in *Taxonomy I Revised 1989* (NANDA, 1989). In this document the level of abstraction of the Taxonomy was further described in relation to abstract and concrete concepts. Abstract concepts were described as theoretical, disassociated from any specific instance, independent of time and space, with general descriptors. Further, it was proposed that abstract concepts may not be clinically useful or directly measurable. Concrete concepts, on the other hand, were described as observable and measurable and limited by time and space. They were understood to constitute a specific category and be clinically useful for planning treatment.

While the decision about retaining the human response pattern conceptualization was important, it was not accompanied by major intellectual debate and disagreement. The more substantive debate occurred regarding the next level of abstraction. For example, a body systems conceptual organizational scheme was considered in order to link together the nursing diagnoses identified under a particular heading. It was concluded that in some instances such headings were necessary. For example, the nursing diagnoses of *dysreflexia, hyperthermia, hypothermia, infection: risk,* and *thermoregulation, impaired* were placed under a Y25 category of Physical Regulation, Altered. It was noted that this label of Physical Regulation, Altered was not a NANDA-approved diagnosis.

In developing the ICD translation, Committee members carefully reviewed NANDA Taxonomy I for inconsistencies in the conceptual basis and lack of clarity and precision in the diagnostic term. As there was already a commitment to development of Taxonomy II as the next stage of programmatic activity, major changes to be proposed were held for future discussions. At the same time some specific changes were necessary. The levels of categorization included within Taxonomy I were collapsed from 4, 5, or 6 levels to only 2 levels of nursing diagnoses. Based on the ICD format, ambiguous terms that had been part of the diagnostic label were refined. More precise terminology was used to replace these ambiguous or value-laden terms. Thus, the qualifier "potential" in a diagnosis was changed to "risk." In all cases "ineffective" as a qualifying label for a diagnostic term was replaced with "impaired" or "altered," which were perceived as more measurable and less value laden. When the terminology was changed from the NANDA-approved terms, every effort was made to label this change in the accompanying literature.

Various examples can be presented to describe the ICD translation of Taxonomy I nursing diagnoses. Within the human response pattern of Choosing, an example of the two levels is Y00 *family coping, impaired* and Y00.0 *compromised*. It is thus assumed that the label "compromised" is in reference to *compromised impaired family coping*. Within the human response pattern of Communicating there is only one formally approved diagnosis, *impaired verbal communication*, coded Y10.0. A label of Communication, Impaired is identified as Y10 with a notation that this is yet to be developed. Within the human response pattern category of Exchanging, there are a number of examples of the two levels. Under the Y29 category of Urinary Elimination, Altered are the various types of urinary incontinence, ranging from Y29.0 to Y29.4, and Y29.5 *urinary retention*. Within the human response pattern of Feeling is included Y31 Comfort, Altered (a category to be developed) and Y31.1 *pain, chronic*. It is important to point out here that the nursing diagnosis of *pain* was further la-

beled as *acute pain* (Y31.0) during this ICD translation process. This refinement of the label was proposed based on a review of the diagnosis definition and defining characteristics. The diagnosis *knowledge deficit* was placed under the human response pattern of Knowing with a further *specify* descriptor. Because of this, this category could be coded from Y40.0 through Y40.9. Under the human response pattern of Moving are the activity diagnoses. The Y50 level is reserved for a label to be developed, i.e., Activity, Altered, with Y50.0 *activity intolerance* and Y50.1 *activity intolerance: risk*, for example. The human response pattern of Perceiving includes codings of Y60 Meaningfulness, Altered (to be developed), through Y62 Sensory Perception, Altered (to be developed). The diagnoses at the more concrete level of abstraction under Perceiving are, for example, Y61.2 *self-esteem disturbance: chronic low*, or Y62.6 *unilateral neglect*. Under the human response pattern of Relating, the *altered role performance* (Y71) and the various subcategories are included. An example here is Y71.1 *altered parenting*. And lastly, under the human response pattern of Valuing, is the Y80.0 *spiritual distress* diagnosis.

In a few instances, previously approved NANDA diagnoses were subsumed under other categories. For example, *body temperature, altered* was subsumed under the category of Physical Regulation, Altered.

In all cases, the same coding principles were used. Efforts were initiated to determine the level of abstraction of the diagnosis and then to categorize it at one of the two levels. Within the Level I category there is the potential for 10 components, ranging from 0 to 9. Thus, one could have Y0 through Y9. It would be immediately clear that with the 0 in the second space of coding, one would be referring to a diagnosis within the Choosing pattern. Then within this Y0 pattern, there could be Level III concepts from Y00.0 through Y00.9, for example, under Y00. It should be readily apparent that this coding format has much potential for inclusion of future nursing diagnoses and yet, due to the constraints of the coding structure itself, there are limits.

This translation of nursing diagnoses into ICD code was viewed by the Committee as a first step in efforts to include nursing language in the broader WHO health care language. Once the initial draft was completed by the Taxonomy Committee, it was submitted to the NANDA Board of Directors for review, revision, and approval. With NANDA Board approval, a new draft was submitted to ANA for endorsement and submission to WHO. The NANDA- and ANA-endorsed document was published in the *American Journal of Nursing* in April 1989 (Fitzpatrick et al., 1989) in an effort to elicit more input from the nursing community and to alert others of this pioneering work. Readers were encouraged to write to the Director of WHO, supporting the inclusion of this coding in ICD-10.

In conclusion, this translation marks an important milestone in the developments in the nursing discipline. It is but another example of NANDA's widespread influence in advancing the profession and, importantly, in influencing health care for all.

References

Fitzpatrick, J. J., Kerr, M.E., Saba, V. K., Hoskins, L. M., Hurley, M. E., Mills, W. C., Rottkamp, B. C., Warren, J. J., & Carpenito, L. J. (1989). Translating nursing diagnosis into ICD code. *American Journal of Nursing, 89,* 493–495.

North American Nursing Diagnosis Association. (1989). *Taxonomy I revised.* St. Louis, MO: Author.

North American Nursing Diagnosis Association. (1987). *Taxonomy I.* St. Louis, MO: Author.

Taxonomy II: Definitions and Development

Joyce J. Fitzpatrick, PHD, RN, FAAN

In 1986 at the Seventh Conference, the NANDA membership endorsed Taxonomy I for further development and testing. Since that time considerable efforts have been invested in the further elaboration of specific diagnoses included within the Taxonomy. At the same time the NANDA Taxonomy Committee has continued to evaluate the taxonomic structure itself. This evaluation has been focused on both internal and external consistency.

At the Eighth Conference, members were asked for guidance regarding taxonomic issues. There was an extensive discussion led by Taxonomy Committee members regarding, for example, the units of analysis to be included in the structure. This feedback was particularly useful to us in formalizing Taxonomy I Revised. In 1989, *Taxonomy I Revised* was published by NANDA with both a brief historical note on taxonomy development within the organization and working definitions that were used to guide taxonomy development. Taxonomy I Revised was always viewed as an interim stage: necessary as a clarification on Taxonomy I and as a means of including new diagnoses approved at the Eighth Conference.

Subsequent to development of Taxonomy I Revised, the Committee turned its attention to two major projects: the translation of Taxonomy I Revised into International Classification of Disease (ICD) code, subsequently endorsed by NANDA and ANA and submitted to the World Health Organization (WHO) and published in the *American Journal of Nursing* (Fitzpatrick et al., 1989); and development of Taxonomy II.

The membership requested that Taxonomy II be a major focus of this Ninth Conference. Toward that goal the Taxonomy Committee has focused considerable time, talent, and energy to delineate the first draft of Taxonomy II. It is by no means a final product, and it is presented here for the purpose of soliciting immediate and continued input. This presentation will provide some background information about the nature and purposes of taxonomies or classification systems, representing scholarly opinions that guided the deliberations of the Taxonomy Committee. In addition, it will describe the principles and processes that were part of the development of Taxonomy II, Draft I, including the new and expanded human response pattern definitions and the first draft of Taxonomy II. Issues are identified for future consideration. It is expected that as a result of this

23

Conference the Taxonomy Committee members' thinking will be enriched and extended.

Taxonomy is the science of identifying and classifying phenomena; it is the study of the bases, principles, procedures, and rules governing such classification (Fleishman, 1975). That which results from the scientific activity is also labeled a taxonomy. Thus, taxonomy is both process and product. What then are the goals of taxonomy development and how can they guide further development of nursing diagnosis? According to Sokal (1974), classification serves that purpose of describing objects in such a way that their true relationships are displayed. From the inherent ordering in a classification system one can infer the laws and principles of ordering. Further, classifications provide a means of summarizing information in order to facilitate communication. Taxonomies enhance scientific communication and assist in identifying the similarities and differences among classified entities.

There are many principles governing classification. As it continued its work to develop Taxonomy II, the Taxonomy Committee paid attention to these principles and made efforts to describe the general guidelines that were used. While engaged in the process of taxonomy development, committee members also remained sensitive to the criteria important for evaluation. Basically, classification systems can be evaluated for

1. Internal validity: whether the system is logical and parsimonious within itself
2. External validity: whether the system is capable of accomplishing its stated purpose
3. Use rate: whether the system is actually used by scientists and clinicians in the field (Fleishman & Quaintance, 1984).

As will be apparent from the discussions, there remain many questions and unresolved issues regarding a taxonomy for nursing diagnosis. One important point of clarification is

necessary here. The taxonomy per se serves primarily a behind-the-scenes role for the clinician. A taxonomy is *not* an assessment tool for clinical use. In fact, the expert clinician may not need to understand taxonomy development and the rules and principles for the classification.

As mentioned earlier, one of the projects following the Eighth Conference was the translation of nursing diagnoses into ICD code. In the process of this challenging task, it became apparent that there were many inconsistencies inherent in Taxonomy I. It was thus imperative not to feel compelled to retain the previous classification system and present only a revision. The Committee functioned within the general guideline to review the approved diagnoses within the human response pattern conceptual structure and reclassify the diagnoses according to rules that were developed. The decision was thus to include components of both inductive and deductive processes in the work. The nine human response patterns were retained based on the evaluation that there was conceptual validity in the process that led to their identification and the subsequent classification of nursing diagnoses within this structure. Although this basic assumption of the conceptual congruence between the human response patterns and the approved nursing diagnoses can be challenged, no obvious alternative paradigm has been identified to date.

In terms of the classification system under development, each human response pattern is perceived as signaling a class of human response patterns. It was therefore considered important that we extend the pattern definitions so that categorization and placement would be more clear and precise and less arbitrary. In particular, the Committee was interested in developing a classification scheme in which there would be less ambiguity. Through a multistage process, extended definitions of the human response patterns were developed. First, definitions of the patterns were culled from the *Oxford English Dictionary*. These were then examined for their fit with general nursing knowledge (theoretical, empirical, and expert clinical knowledge) as expressed by the group of examiners and in the nursing literature. The new proposed definitions are listed in Table 1.

The Committee also considered the newly developed, NANDA Board-approved definition of nursing diagnoses. That working definition was "A nursing diagnosis is a clinical judgment about an individual, family, or community response to actual or potential health problems/life processes which provides the basis for definitive therapy toward achievement of outcomes for which the nurse is accountable." The definition subsequently approved by the NANDA membership at the Ninth Conference is "Nursing diagnosis is a clinical judgment about individual, family, or community responses to actual and potential health problems/life processes. Nursing diagnoses provide the basis for selection of nursing interventions to achieve outcomes for which the nurse is accountable." (See page 65.) In instances in

Table 1: Definitions of Human Response Patterns (October, 1989)

Human Response Pattern	Definition
Choosing	To select between alternatives; the action of selecting or exercising preference in regard to a matter in which one is a free agent; to determine in favor of a course; to decide in acordance with inclinations
Communicating	To converse; to impart, confer or transmit thoughts, feelings or information, internally or externally, verbally or nonverbally

Table 1: (*Continued*)

Human Response Pattern	Definition
Exchanging	To give, relinquish or lose something while receiving something in return; the substitution of one element for another; the reciprocal act of giving and receiving
Feeling	To experience a consciousness, sensation, apprehension or sense; to be consciously or emotionally affected by a fact, event or state
Knowing	To recognize or acknowledge a thing or a person; to be familiar with by experience or through information or report; to be cognizant of something through observation, inquiry or information; to be conversant with a body of facts, principles, or methods of action; to understand
Moving	To change the place or position of a body or any member of the body; to put and/or keep in motion; to provoke an excretion or discharge; the urge to action or to do something; to take action
Perceiving	To apprehend with the mind; to become aware of by the senses; to apprehend what is not open or present to observation; to take in fully or adequately
Relating	To connect, to establish a link between, to stand in some association to another thing, person or place; to be borne or thrust in between things
Valuing	To be concerned about, to care; the worth or worthiness; the relative status of a thing, or the estimate in which it is held, according to its real or supposed worth, usefulness, or importance; one's opinion of liking for person or thing; to equate in importance

which an approved diagnosis was not consistent with the working definition, the diagnostic label was not included in Taxonomy II, Draft I. An example of such an inconsistency is the diagnosis of *decreased cardiac output.* The Committee recommended these diagnoses be revised or deleted from the list of approved nursing diagnoses.

A third major Committee decision was to explore the development of axes to attend to the multidimensional nature of approved and potential nursing diagnoses. An axis was defined as a dimension of the human condition considered in the diagnostic process. As will be elaborated in subsequent papers (see pages 35 and 38), two axes (unit of analysis and age group) are proposed for inclusion in Taxonomy II, Draft I. Four additional axes (wellness, illness, acuity, chronicity) are being examined for their potential relevance to further development of nursing diagnoses. Axis development proceeded from a thorough review and analysis of the nursing literature regarding the variables and an adoption of working definitions. As will be illustrated later, with the adoption of the two axes some of the formally approved diagnostic labels must be changed. For example, *altered family processes* would be included as a coping diagnosis that is evaluated on the individual, family, and community axis.

In placing the diagnoses within a taxonomic structure each diagnosis was reviewed based on its definition. If the definition was sketchy, attention was then paid to the defining characteristics. Then the following evaluations were conducted for each diagnosis:

1. Consistency with NANDA's nursing diagnosis definition. If consistent, proceed to step 2. If not consistent, deletion or revision of the diagnoses was recommended.
2. Review of diagnosis definition for placement within one of the classes (i.e., patterns of human response). Placement

within pattern based on conceptual, empirical, and clinical validation support as reflected in percent agreement among participants engaged in classification.
3. Assessment of level for placement among the two levels based on generality and abstractness of the diagnosis.

Obviously, the review of all approved diagnoses involved major conceptual analyses. The Committee was able to review many significant gaps in the current list of diagnoses. While the amount of work necessary at this time to more fully develop these existing diagnoses is substantial, it is also imperative that it be accomplished now. Such an effort would do much to clarify our professional organization's present and future contributions to the discipline of nursing.

Taxonomy II as proposed in the first draft can be found in Table 2. Some of the diagnostic labels may not be familiar as approved diagnoses. For example, *altered health main-*

Table 2: Taxonomy II, Draft I (Working Draft) 1/15/90

Human Response Pattern	Level
Choosing	2. Coping, Impaired Decisional Conflict Health Management Health Seeking Behaviors 3. Coping, Compromised Coping, Defensive Coping, Dysfunctional Denial, Impaired Noncompliance
Communicating	2. Verbal Communication, Impaired Violence: Risk Self-Directed or Directed at Others 3. Dysreflexia

(continued)

Table 2: (*Continued*)

Human Response Pattern	Level
Exchanging	2. Body Temperature, Altered; Risk
	Breastfeeding, Impaired
	Gas Exchange, Impaired
	Infection: Risk
	Injury: Risk
	Sleep Pattern Disturbance
	Tissue Integrity, Altered
	3. Airway Clearance, Impaired
	Aspiration: Risk
	Breathing Pattern, Impaired
	Developmental Delay
	Hyperthermia
	Hypothermia
	Nutrition, Altered, Less than Body Requirements
	Nutrition, Altered, More than Body Requirements
	Nutrition, Altered, Potential for More than Body Requirements
	Oral Mucous Membrane, Impaired
	Poisoning: Risk
	Skin Integrity, Impaired
	Skin Integrity, Impaired: Risk
	Suffocation: Risk
	Thermoregulation, Impaired
	Trauma: Risk
Feeling	2. Anxiety
	Fear
	Post-Trauma Response
	3. Fatigue
	Grieving: Anticipatory
	Grieving: Dysfunctional
	Pain: Acute
	Pain: Chronic
	Rape-Trauma: Compound
	Rape-Trauma: Silent
	Rape-Trauma: Syndrome
Knowing	2.
	3.
Moving	2. Home Maintenance Management, Impaired
	Urinary Elimination, Altered

Table 2: (*Continued*)

Human Response Pattern	Level
	3. Activity Intolerance
	Activity Intolerance: Risk
	Bathing/Hygiene Deficit
	Bowel Incontinence
	Constipation: Colonic
	Constipation: Rectal
	Diarrhea
	Disuse Syndrome: Risk
	Diversional Activity Deficit
	Dressing Deficit
	Feeding Deficit
	Incontinence: Reflex
	Incontinence: Stress
	Incontinence: Urge
	Incontinence: Total
	Physical Mobility, Impaired
	Swallowing, Impaired
	Toileting Deficit
	Urinary Retention
Perceiving	2. Sensory Perception, Altered
	Sexuality, Altered
	Social Isolation
	Thought Process, Altered
	3. Body Image Disturbance
	Constipation: Perceived
	Hopelessness
	Personal Identity Disturbance
	Powerlessness
	Self-Esteem Disturbance: Chronic Low
	Self-Esteem Disturbance: Situational
	Social Isolation
	Unilateral Neglect
Relating	2. Role Performance, Altered
	Social Interaction, Impaired
	3. Parental Role Conflict
	Parenting, Altered
	Parenting, Altered: Risk
Valuing	2. Sexual Function, Altered
	Spiritual Distress
	3.

tenance has been relabeled *health management*, and *altered sexuality patterns* has become *altered sexuality*. Each of the proposed changes in label can be supported by the classification and clarification guidelines developed by the Committee. Decisions about specific NANDA diagnoses in which significant changes are recommended are as follows. These recommendations will be submitted to the Diagnosis Review Committee.

1. *Potential for violence:* Remove "self-directed or directed at others" from the diagnosis and work to develop new diagnoses within these descriptors.
2. *Pain:* As described in the definition this should be labeled acute pain.
3. *Knowledge deficit:* Recommend revision or deletion.
4. *Unilateral neglect:* Review as a syndrome; develop label and definition to be consistent.
5. *Self-esteem disturbance:* Recommend revision or deletion.
6. *Altered growth and development:* Change to developmental delay.
7. *Altered health maintenance:* Change to health management.
8. *Potential activity intolerance:* Develop actual and potential (risk) diagnoses.
9. *Family coping: potential for growth:* Delete as such, but incorporate under new family axis within health-seeking behaviors.
10. *Ineffective family coping: compromised:* Delete "family" and relabel compromised coping; revise definition.
11. *Disabling coping:* Rename as dysfunctional coping.
12. *Ineffective denial:* Change to impaired denial.
13. *Altered family processes:* Include with compromised coping.
14. *Sexual dysfunction:* Change to altered sexual function based on definition

and develop a new sexual dysfunction diagnosis.
15. *Constipation:* Change to rectal constipation.
16. *Risk for fluid volume deficit:* Recommend revision or deletion.
17. *Fluid volume deficit:* Recommend revision or deletion.
18. *Fluid volume excess:* Recommend revision or deletion.
19. *Altered tissue perfusion:* Recommend revision or deletion.
20. *Decreased cardiac output:* Recommend revision or deletion.
21. *Altered sexual patterns:* Delete "patterns"; change to altered sexuality.

Other important considerations and recommendations have been included in the Taxonomy Committee's report that accompanies this first draft of Taxonomy II. Specifically, the Committee recommends (1) that many of the diagnoses receive attention to develop clarity and consistency; (2) that the modifier "ineffective" be replaced by "impaired" in most circumstances; (3) that all diagnosis definitions be reviewed and many refined or changed; and (4) that several new diagnoses (obviously missing from the list) be developed. In relation to the diagnoses to be developed (TBD) it is suggested that NANDA commission teams of experts to accomplish this necessary work. All the changes have been referred to the NANDA Diagnosis Review Committee and the Board of Directors for further clarification. None of these recommendations should be considered as set in stone. Comments from members are welcome and desirable.

The majority of the approved diagnoses were classified into the new categories (classes or patterns, in this case) with consistency of agreement. While the patterns can be considered "classes" of human responses, taxons within the classification system have not yet been identified. In this first stage of development there is no defined relationship between Level 1 and Level 2, or between the specific diagnoses within these two levels. For example, within the Relating class of diagnoses there are two levels. *Altered role performance* and *impaired social interaction* are placed on one level and *parental role conflict, altered parenting* and *altered parenting: risk* on another level. While there is some apparent face validity to a relationship between *altered role performance* and *altered parenting,* taxonomy development is not at the point where the appropriate taxon label could be identified. It is important to note here that a taxon is a label that is not a diagnosis, but a diagnostic category. Previously in the presentation of nursing diagnoses, the term "diagnostic category" has been used interchangeably with diagnosis. In the present classification system, "diagnostic category" is reserved for a grouping of diagnoses. A diagnostic category may be a taxon but is not a diagnosis. As yet the diagnostic categories have not been named.

Summary

There are many issues to be considered in future refinement and development of Taxonomy II. These include:

1. The relevance of the conceptual framework of human response patterns. While this conceptualization is consistent with the new NANDA definition of nursing diagnosis, questions remain about its relevance as an organizing framework.
2. Axes, including the validity of the two proposed for Draft I and the four under continued development.
3. Development of the taxonomy structure including taxons and possible clusters of diagnoses.

Revisions of existing diagnoses and clarification of terminology for diagnostic labels must be addressed within work groups. And lastly, NANDA must continue the scientific development of the classification system including an evaluation of the clinical validity and the reliability of the system itself.

References

Fitzpatrick, J. J., Kerr, M. E., Saba, V. K., Hoskins, L. M., Hurley, M. E., Mills, W. D., Rottkamp, B. C., Warren, J. J., & Carpenito, L. J. (1989). Translating nursing diagnosis into ICD code. *American Journal of Nursing, 89,* 493–495.

Fleishman, E. A. (1975). Toward a taxonomy of human performance. *American Psychologist, 30,* 1127–1149.

Fleishman, E. A., & Quaintance, M. K. (1984). *Taxonomies of human performance.* New York: Academic Press.

Sokal, R. R. (1974). Classification: Purposes, principles, progress, prospects. *Science, 185,* 1115–1123.

Placement of Diagnoses within Taxonomy II: Development and Process

Barbara C. Rottkamp, EdD, RN
Mary E. Hurley, MA, RN

Placement of approved diagnoses within Taxonomy II can be described as an inferential activity, or making decisions from information that is either known or assumed about each diagnosis.

Placement or categorization of diagnoses is envisioned in the context of diagnosis development, as well as taxonomy development. The model for such a context is depicted as a circle of inferences (see Figure 1). Inferences are made first at the initial conceptualization of a diagnosis, for clarification, for conjunction (or dysjunction) with other diagnoses, and for categorization within the system of classification. It may be possible that reconceptualization or further clarification is necessary before placement in the taxonomy. Because clinical phenomena are continuously under study, the circle of inferences is an open, interactive process of development and refinement by the profession. Each of these processes of development has implications for subsequent and preceding steps. For example, the structure and quality of the diagnostic label, its major characteristics, and its appropriateness to nursing facilitate taxonomy development and enable formulation of criteria for placement.

The major focus of this paper is the conjunction and dysjunction between and among diagnoses and their categorization in Taxonomy II. Conception and clarification are assumed to have taken place in the submission process of the Diagnosis Review Committee. Conjunction might be defined as the apparent similarity and differentiation of two or more diagnoses as represented by the shared characteristics or by other shared properties and relationships (Mussen & Rosenzweig, 1973). The characteristics of a diagnosis have links or lack links for conceptual consistency with other diagnoses (see Figures 2 and 3). Categorization of classification refers to the systematic arrangement of diagnoses in groups or categories according to established criteria or based on relationships with other phenomena in the system.

Taxonomy II Development

Three methods used to examine conjunction and categorization of nursing diagnoses in

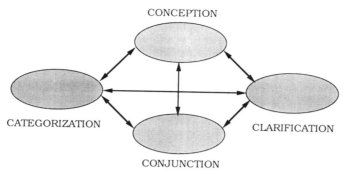

FIGURE 1 Circle of inferences for placement of nursing diagnoses within a taxonomy

Taxonomy II development are pattern analysis, collective consensus, and displays. These methods will be described and illustrated.

Pattern Analysis

Pattern analysis is defined as the examination of the configuration of relationships among the elements of a particular phenomenon (Crawford, 1982). Each diagnosis was reviewed for consistency between its label and its definition, the agreement of major characteristics with the definition, and the degree of variation of a diagnosis between lower levels and higher levels within the hierarchical structure of a human response pattern. In addition, the relationship between diagnoses at any one level across patterns was examined. When NANDA's working definition of a nursing diagnosis became available in 1989, current diagnoses were also reviewed for consistency with that new definition.

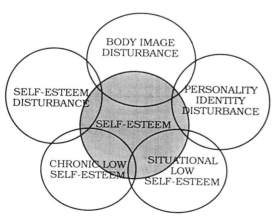

FIGURE 2 A group of Level 3 conjunctive diagnoses in Perceiving pattern

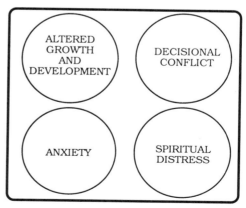

FIGURE 3 A group of Level 2 disjunctive diagnoses in Exchanging, Choosing, Feeling, and Valuing patterns

When new definitions of human response patterns were developed in 1989, each approved diagnosis was again reviewed for consistency with a pattern and its placement at Level 2 or Level 3 within the pattern.

Collective Consensus

A collective consensus process for making decisions about placement of diagnoses was used in 1982 by the taxonomies work group led by Phyllis Kritek, and at subsequent Taxonomy Committee meetings. This method represents the thinking processes of a group based on expert data of the submitter and the clinical and theoretical knowledge of Committee members. A recommendation for placement is proposed by one or more members of the group. Inferences of comparison and contrast for a diagnosis are made by reviewing and analyzing definitions and characteristics and their relationship to the human response pattern. Kritek (1989) claims that collective consensus enables the art of taxonomy and that it is based on the lived experience of nursing practice. She states further that this critical component is the voice of the staff nurse that is often silenced. She recommends that the challenge of collective consensus is a process in which the staff nurse is enabled and accepts the challenge to participate in the multiple phases of diagnosis development.

The consensus process for placement of diagnoses in Taxonomy II in October 1989 took place by vote of 11 members present at the Taxonomy Committee meeting. The new definitions of the human response patterns become the reference point or framework for proceeding with reclassification of each approved diagnosis. Each diagnosis received a vote for agreement or abstention. Agreement meant that the voter concurred that a diagnosis represented the meaning of the assigned pattern.

Displays

Displays are defined by Miles and Huberman (1984) as a spatial format for constructing organized matrices in which each approved diagnosis is placed within a total structure that represents the taxonomy. It is a form of analysis that is immediately accessible so that Committee members can see and discuss a whole structure and its parts in relationship to other parts.

Diagnoses were analyzed in two ways. First, diagnoses were examined for theoretical and clinical conjunction with each human response pattern. In addition, diagnoses were analyzed in vertical and horizontal planes for consistency with levels of abstractness and specificity of diagnoses with each other. This method of placement was used initially by the taxonomies work group led by Phyllis Kritek at the Fifth Conference (1984), and then at each Taxonomy Committee meeting, including the most recent in October 1989. This method can be understood by envisioning a group of people at a table surrounded by large sheets of paper attached to the four walls of a room. Each paper represented a pattern and diagnoses were listed by pattern.

Placement Process

For a better idea of how placement took place, two diagnoses are traced through the process. The diagnosis *sexual dysfunction*, first introduced in 1980, is defined as the state in which an individual experiences a change in sexual function that is viewed as unsatisfying, unrewarding, or inadequate. It was placed in pattern three, Relating, a human response pattern involving establishing bonds.

In 1986 *altered sexuality patterns* was accepted. The definition for this diagnosis is the state in which an individual expresses concern regarding his/her sexuality. This diagnosis was also placed in Relating. In 1989, when the new pattern definitions were developed as part of the Taxonomy II development process, placement of diagnoses was rescrutinized.

When discussing these two diagnoses the Committee first tried to understand what the authors were attempting to describe. It seemed that the placement of the diagnoses in the Relating pattern was based on a preconceived notion of sexual function as a process of relationships. However when you look at the definitions of these diagnoses that the authors had put forward, you see much more than this process being described. In addition, many of the defining characteristics are the same for both diagnoses as are the related factors.

Taxonomy Committee discussion centered around types and levels of sexuality conditions. When discussing the diagnoses in terms of the expanded pattern definitions, Committee members determined that the authors were attempting to get at several different concepts. The word "patterns" was dropped from *altered sexuality* and viewed as a perception of sexuality by the person involved. Regardless of a partner, it was the person's own changing consciousness that created the problem. This is a concept that might be further clarified. The Committee recommended that it be removed from Relating (to connect; to establish a link between; to stand in some association to another thing, person, or place; to be borne or thrust in between things) and placed as a Level 2 concept in Perceiving (to apprehend with the mind; to become aware by the senses; to apprehend what is not open or present to observation; to take in fully or adequately).

Sexual dysfunction describes more than a relationship problem. For whatever reason, the person places a negative value on the sexual experience. This concept seemed to be intertwined with another concept in the defining characteristics. In other words, the definition spoke to one meaning but the defining characteristics spoke to two meanings. The Committee's recommendation therefore was to change the name of the diagnosis (e.g., *altered sexual function*), keep the definition, and place it as a Level 2 concept in Valuing (to be concerned about, to care; the worth or worthiness; the relative status of a thing, or the estimate in which it is held according to its real or supposed worth, usefulness, or importance; one's opinion of liking for a person or thing; to equate in importance). Again, it is a concept that may be open to further clarification. The Committee contends, however, that *sexual dysfunction* does exist as a Level 3 Relating concept and recommends this be developed as such. In this way the two concepts will be separated.

Violence, potential for: self-directed or directed at others was analyzed in the same way. Originally it was placed in the Feeling pattern. This pattern was initially defined as a human response pattern involving the subjective awareness of information. Its new definition became to experience; a consciousness, sensation, apprehension, or sense; to be consciously or emotionally affected by fact, event, or state.

The definition of the diagnosis is a state in which an individual experiences behavior that can be physically harmful either to the self or others. The discussion was difficult. Some members felt Feeling was still the appropriate pattern because the person was experiencing the feeling of violence. Others felt that communicating (to converse; to impart, confer, or transmit thoughts, feelings, or information, internally or externally, verbally or nonverbally) described more fully the concept of violence. These members felt that the violence was the expression of what the person was experiencing and that the expression rather than the feeling itself was the key concept. Still others thought Choosing (to select between alternatives; the action of selecting or exercising preference in regard to a matter in which one is a free agent; to determine in favor of a course; to decide in accordance with inclinations) was the best pattern. These Committee members took the position that the individual was choosing violence as a means of expressing what was felt and that this was the real conceptual meaning of the diagnosis. Communicating won out by consensus, but not by a large margin, and the specificity was designated at Level 2. It is also recommended that "self" and "others" be developed separately and that those separate diagnoses might fit into different patterns.

In conclusion, this was an attempt to show how more information causes one to rethink or reconceptualize the diagnoses. As NANDA develops Taxonomy II, members have begun this reconceptualization of the diagnoses by further refining the human response patterns. Discussion with the authors of the diagnoses, the experience of the clinical experts in the field, and research on the diagnoses are other means of gathering data that would stimulate the Committee to reconceptualize and make inferences once again.

References

Crawford, G. (1982). The concept of pattern in nursing: Conceptual development and measurement. *Advances in Nursing Science, 5*(1), 1–6.

Kritek, P. (1984). Report of the group work on taxonomies. In M. J. Kim, G. K. McFarland, & A. M. McLane (Eds.), *Classification of nursing diagnoses: Proceedings of the fifth national conference.* St. Louis, MO: Mosby.

Kritek, P. (1989). An introduction to the science and art of taxonomy. In *Classification systems for describing nursing practice: Working papers.* Kansas City, MO: American Nurses' Association.

Miles, M., & Huberman, A. M. (1984). *Qualitative data analysis: A source book of new methods.* Beverly Hills, CA: Sage.

Mussen, P., & Rosenzweig, M. (1983). *Psychology: An introduction.* Lexington, MA: Heath.

What Is the Focus of Taxonomy II? Nursing Diagnosis Axes

Lois M. Hoskins, PhD, RN

Introduction

The Taxonomy Committee was officially appointed at the beginning of the Sixth NANDA Conference in 1984. This Committee was charged with the development and regular review of a taxonomic system for the diagnoses approved by the NANDA membership. At the Seventh Conference in 1986, the Committee presented Taxonomy I and won its endorsement for development and testing. The Committee's work has included placement of newly approved nursing diagnoses within the taxonomy, and study of the issues and problems related to the taxonomy. Some of these issues were presented to the membership in an open forum at the Eighth Conference in 1988. Included among these issues were the unit of analysis, the specialty nursing focus, and wellness nursing diagnoses. One clear direction was given to the Committee—nursing is nursing, there should be only one taxonomy for diagnoses. The problem was how to incorporate different units of analysis, that is the individual, the family, and the community; the wellness diagnoses, and along with the wellness diagnoses the issue of growth and development; and differ-

ent specialty interests, such as the physiologic diagnoses.

To begin its task, the Committee observed that some diagnoses addressing each of these issues had been approved and had already been placed in the Taxonomy. There was not consistency, however, in the level of placement; for example not all family or all community diagnoses were at the same level across the different patterns. And there certainly were not family and community versions of all diagnoses. Taking this all into consideration the Taxonomy Committee did some brainstorming, and arrived at the concept of axis.

Theoretical Background for Concept of Axis

From a theoretical perspective Webster's New World Dictionary defines axis as a "real or imaginary straight line on which an object rotates or is regarded as rotating; a real or imaginary straight line around which the parts of a thing, system, etc. are symmetrically arranged or composed." It may also be "a main line of motion, development, etc.," or "a straight line for measurement of reference, as in a graph, the abscissa and ordinate."

Axis, Operational Definition

For the purposes of the nursing diagnosis taxonomy, the Committee operationally defined axis as a dimension of the human condition considered in the diagnostic process. That is, each diagnosis would be evaluated on the identified axes.

Graphically, Taxonomy I is a two-dimensional system consisting of patterns and diagnoses by levels of abstraction. The Committee's problem was to add to this two-dimensional system in such a way that we solved the problems and at the same time eliminated the need for separate and parallel taxonomies, such as a wellness taxonomy and an illness taxonomy. Another way of stating the problem is: Given a certain diagnosis, can it be looked at from many dimensions? Will the result be theoretically valid? Can it be operationalized?

Other related questions were raised. Can it be displayed graphically? The answer is no. Any three dimensions can be displayed in a figure, but more than three at any one time is not possible. The figure the Committee envisages is multidimensional with lines intersecting somewhere in a spherical space. The results can, however, be coded.

Further questions included: How will the defining characteristics and etiologies be affected? How will the interventions be affected? In other words, if the unit of analysis is the community rather than the individual will not the defining characteristics for a given diagnosis be different, etc.? These are issues of application, and will be addressed in a subsequent presentation (see page 38).

Theoretical Definitions of the Nursing Diagnosis Axes

The nursing diagnosis axes that have been identified at this point are the unit of analysis as individual, family, and community; age group; wellness; and illness. These axes are at different stages of development. The development process involves a number of steps. First the Committee brainstormed the issues. After identification of a potential axis, a Committee member developed a paper containing dictionary definitions of the axis and conceptual definitions from authorities. Approval of the NANDA Board of Directors to proceed with the axis development was sought, and the papers containing theoretical definitions of the axes were shared for their comment. The Taxonomy Committee then met as an expanded Committee of new and outgoing members and developed the definitions that are being presented here today. Coding schemas were developed for some of the axes; others are in earlier stages and need more development before coding is begun.

Unit of Analysis

Each diagnosis would be evaluated as to the unit of analysis, individual, family, or community, as follows:

Individual is defined as a single human being distinct from others; a person.

Family means two or more individuals, having continuous or sustained relationships, perceiving of reciprocal obligations, sensing of commonness, and sharing of certain obligations toward others, and often related by blood or law.

Community is defined as a unit of people and the relationships that emerge among them who share common goals, perspectives, interests, or collective needs and some common identity or characteristics; a place and its social and nonsocial resources and structures; communities are many different sizes and types.

The definitions of family and community entailed considerable discussion, and it is significant to this point that there are both family and community health specialists on the Taxonomy Committee. Currently approved nursing diagnoses were reviewed and it was concluded that family and community units could reasonably be expected to present with these nursing diagnoses. The use of a community axis may encourage the development of more nursing diagnoses from that specialty.

Age Group

Another axis is age group. Originally the Committee discussed an axis related to developmental state and an axis related to age. Age was defined in terms of age groups as a segment of the population of approximately the same age. Developmental state was defined in terms of growth and differentiation and the tasks or achievements expected at different stages. The Committee considered that the defining characteristics may be different for a diagnosis at different developmental stages, and also considered that this dimension was more general than an assessment factor that would list the chronologic age. The Committee concluded that the concept of age group, as defined by membership in one of 11 age cohorts, captured the desired dimension. Those cohorts are described as

00 Fetal
01 Neonate
02 Infant
03 Toddler
04 Preschooler
05 School-aged child
06 Adolescent
07 Young adult
08 Middle-aged adult
09 Young older adult
10 Aged adult

Wellness and Illness

The axes of wellness and illness are not fully developed. Definitions exist for each of the concepts, but it is not clear if they are one axis or two.

> *Wellness* is defined as experiencing life processes that reflect expectations concerning a quality of life.
> *Illness* is defined as experiencing or at risk for health problems that affect functioning.

The Committee considered the concepts of health, wellness, and illness. It is not yet clear if there is one axis with a bipolar continuum or two axes. Work is ongoing.

Finally, the Committee discussed acuity and chronicity, and actual and potential or "at risk" as dimensions. There are issues to be resolved before further work can be done.

Summary and Conclusions

The Taxonomy Committee has developed the concept of axis, or axes, to provide a multidimensional nursing diagnosis taxonomy. Axes will address dimensions upon which human conditions may be evaluated. Figuratively and conceptually (because the figure cannot be drawn), the resulting nursing diagnosis or diagnoses will have many dimensions or lines intersecting at the point of diagnosis. This point of intersection will provide a more complete picture of the human condition. Theoretical definitions have been provided for the unit of analysis axis (individual, family, and community), for an age group axis, and for wellness and illness. The axes are in different stages of development. Application and further implications will be addressed in a subsequent paper (see page 38).

Implications of Introducing Axes into a Classification System

Judith J. Warren, PhD, RN

The introduction of axes within the nursing taxonomy can have a far-reaching impact. As with any innovation, one must carefully consider the impact or implications of proposed changes. This paper will highlight some possible implications for the diagnoses and for the users of Taxonomy II. The proposed four axes are unit of analysis, age group, wellness, and illness. By no means are these all the axes that can be identified. They are just those that the Taxonomy Committee identified as major concerns of the membership at the last conference.

Taxonomic Implications

Unit of Analysis Axis

The first axis to be discussed is unit of analysis. Currently, three categories exist on this axis: individual, family, and community. A proposed coding schema might consist of a single digit: 0 = other, 1 = individual, 2 = family, and 3 = community. A "0" category or code for "other" is included to allow for

the identification of new categories. Conceivably this could be expanded at a later date to include state, country, planet, and so forth. The major concern of this axis is to determine whether all diagnoses can be made at the level of individual, family, or community. Is it necessary that each category within the axis exist for each diagnosis for the axis to be valid? For example, does a community have *rape-trauma syndrome, unilateral neglect, altered growth and development,* or *impaired swallowing*? Other diagnoses that have not been viewed from a community perspective are very relevant—*anxiety, powerlessness, potential for violence, altered nutrition,* and *decisional conflict*—just to mention a few. There are similar examples for family: Does a family have *decreased cardiac output, urinary retention,* or *impaired gas exchange*? However, a family may have *altered role performance, noncompliance,* or *altered nutrition,* diagnoses that have not been used this way before. These diagnoses have not been evaluated within our nomenclature from a family perspective; yet they are ideal diagnoses for this evaluation. A diagnosis may have some defining characteristics at each level, but may not have these characteristics on all levels. Is that going to

The author would like to acknowledge Kay Avant, PhD, RN, FAAN, for her thoughtful review of this paper.

be a valid concern within the Taxonomy? Do we want to grapple with some of this ambiguity?

One cluster of diagnoses that has received work identifying individual and family concerns is *ineffective individual coping* and *ineffective family coping*. If the axes were in place, would the words "individual" and "family" be dropped from the diagnoses, leaving only "ineffective coping"? If this rule were applied to all diagnoses, what would happen to the diagnosis *altered family processes*? Does this label give us clues as to what is being diagnosed or generate a meaningful label for the cluster of defining characteristics? Or is this diagnosis the family level of an existing diagnosis that is focused on the individual? This demonstrates some of the conceptual problems this approach generates.

The second concern leads to the question of whether or not the defining characteristics will be the same for a diagnosis in all three categories of the axis. The prevailing thought has been that if the defining characteristics were different, it was a different diagnosis. Yet if the definition of the diagnosis is basically the same across all three categories, then only one diagnosis exists with the influence of the unit of analysis creating subtle differences in the defining characteristics. These issues are timely and should lead to some discussion or research about how information is organized in nursing science concerning individuals, families, and communities. The axis may become a pointer to areas requiring further study and research.

Age Group Axis

The second axis for discussion is age group. A possible coding schema would consist of two digits: 00 = fetus, 01 = neonate, 02 = infant, 03 = toddler, 04 = preschool child, 05 = school-aged child, 06 = adolescent, 07 = young adult, 08 = middle-aged adult, 09 = young older adult, and 10 = aged adult. At prior conferences, questions have been asked about pediatric diagnoses, geriatric diagnoses, or other developmental-group diagnoses. Upon review, most of the diagnoses seem to apply to all age groups. Yet nurses stated that diagnoses were missing for their specialty areas. Because diagnoses describe the independent domain of nursing and capture the essence of human responses, have these diagnoses not been identified or have current diagnoses not been completely developed?

Some recent research with the elderly indicated that both problems (diagnoses not identified and diagnoses not completely developed) exist (Buckwalter & Maas, 1989; Warren & Haight, 1990; Weekes & Rankin, 1988). The research demonstrated that the defining characteristics for a diagnosis in an elderly population were a little different from those for children or young adults. The cues found in the literature on this phenomenon differed from the cues identified in the research, which involved discussion, expert nurses, and observations of patients. Upon review of the literature it was found that most of the findings were generalized to the entire population from information that was gained from studying college freshmen. There have been other articles published in the newsletter of the Council of Gerontological Nursing pleading for development of the psychosocial nursing diagnoses because current diagnoses do not apply to the fragile elders and some of the other aged population. These clients exhibit the phenomena in question very differently.

The Taxonomy Committee reviewed the defining characteristics of several other diagnoses and noted that many of them were age related, predominantly for the adult. For example, if an infant cannot "verbalize an inability to cope," how can it demonstrate ineffective coping? The definition of the diagnosis for *impaired adjustment* reads as if it can work across all age groups, yet a major defining characteristic for *impaired adjustment* is unsuccessful ability to be involved in goal setting. Is this a behavior that would be seen in a toddler who has impaired adjustment? Can a toddler be diagnosed with *impaired adjustment* in the absence of the "ability to set goals"? The concern, then, is: Which of the defining characteristics of a diagnosis must be present to make a diagnosis? This discussion implies a need to describe how each diagnosis is manifested in each age group. There is probably a core of commonalities, but there also may be critical differences depending on age.

Wellness and Illness Axes

The third and fourth axes are wellness and illness, respectively. These two, though defined, are the least developed. Wellness is defined as experiencing life processes that reflect expectations concerning a quality of life. Illness is defined as experiencing or being at risk for health problems that affect functioning. Do these axes have discrete or continuous values? How would an axis with continuous values of wellness and illness be coded? A possible coding schema for discrete values might be based on a Likert Scale format. An example of the coding might be 0 = axis not used or not applicable, 1 = small amount of wellness or illness, 2 = moderate amount of wellness or illness, 3 = great extent of wellness or illness. Operational definitions for each category would need to be developed to ensure reliable and valid coding.

The major concern here is: Are these one or two axes? A case can be made for two separate axes at least with respect to chronically ill adults. These clients will always have symptoms of disease and impaired function, but they may have a moderate to high quality of life or demonstrate wellness in some areas of their lives. Again, the major concern is: Does each diagnosis have a wellness axis? Martens (1986) and Popkess (1981) have encouraged diagnosis of client strengths, to focus on the health or wellness of the client in addition to the health problems. At the last NANDA conference, Pender (1989) suggested two taxonomies, one for wellness diagnoses and one for illness or problem-focused diagnoses. Does the addition of the wellness axis solve this conceptual dilemma? Other authors suggest that only one multidimensional axis representing the pattern of health-ease and dis-ease exists (Antonovsky, 1987; Moch, 1989). Newman (1986) believes that health and illness are not separate but part of the life-style pattern and are considered together. If these three authors' recommendations are followed, then only one axis would exist in the Taxonomy. The determination of whether to have one or two axes that describe the wellness and illness perspectives is a taxonomic decision that requires further study and an active dialogue within the NANDA membership.

User-Group Implications

Use of the axes has implications for each of the user groups: taxonomists, researchers, and practitioners.

Taxonomists

There are two major implications for taxonomists when axes are used in a taxonomy. First, the taxonomic structure becomes a blend of hierarchical and nonhierarchical components. Taxonomy II proposes that the diagnoses be classified in a structure that contains three levels of complexity (see the ICD-10 translation coding scheme) (Fitzpatrick et al., 1989). Once the relationships between Level 2 and Level 3 are identified, a hierarchical structure will exist. After the hierarchical structure is identified, then axes are considered and these are nonhierarchical.

A nonnursing example may help to clarify how axes are supposed to work. A faculty member shares a secretary with other faculty. The secretary has devised a taxonomy to organize her computer files so that she can locate any document (see Figure 1). First, because she shares the computer terminal with other secretaries, she accesses her "pattern"

Wordperfect Example

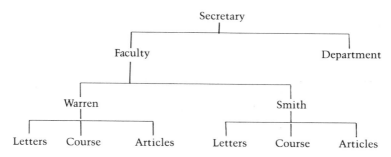

FIGURE 1   A nonnursing example of axes

—Debbie. Next, she selects from the second level—faculty or department. Then the specific faculty member is selected—Warren. So far this is a hierarchical structure. These relationships are at different levels of abstraction. But under the faculty name, everybody has the same categories/axes. An example might be that the faculty member wants to write a letter and get a guest speaker to come and give a presentation in a course. How is that classified? At this point letters, courses, and articles are taxons. These are the names for the boxes where things are going to reside. Decisions are made about what file to put something in. Letters are put in the letter box, but letters, courses, and articles are all at the same level. They can be considered in any order—letters do not have to be accessed be-

fore getting to courses. However, it is possible to see the relationship between letters and courses and which is being used where. Information can be accessed and merged as desired, thus capturing a wide diversity of data. These categories can be viewed as axes. A relational axis system assists in keeping the focus on the phenomenon of concern (Warren) while capturing the diversity or dimensionality of that work (letters, courses, or articles).

Figure 2 offers an example of how this system works in Taxonomy II. To classify a diagnosis it must be matched with the right pattern. The diagnosis *ineffective denial* is classified in the Choosing pattern because the definitions agree and the rules of classification are followed. A Level 2 concept of *inef-*

Taxonomy II Example

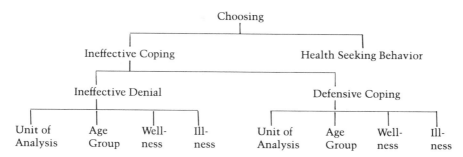

FIGURE 2   Nursing diagnosis example of axes

fective coping is also in place. At this point a hierarchical structure has not been created because the names/taxons of those levels (i.e., relationships) are not known. Once the relationships are identified, then a hierarchy will exist. *Ineffective denial* is at a more concrete level than *ineffective coping*; therefore, it is classified at the third level. The next level contains the axes. Now the diagnosis must be evaluated on unit of analysis, age group, wellness, illness, and whatever other axes are identified. The axes are not hierarchical because they must be considered simultaneously while describing and classifying the diagnosis. While this is difficult to diagram, try to imagine the axes emerging from the surface of a globe. The essence of the diagnosis would be located at the point where the axes intersect, yet the entire structure must be evaluated when classifying the diagnosis. A concern of this particular structure is that the axes are not independent nor are they mutually exclusive. One example of the lack of independence occurs between the axes age group and unit of analysis. The category of individual must be linked with an age group. If an individual is coded on unit of analysis, various age groups must be considered. How should family development and community development be considered? What would be a parallel axis to age group for family and community development? This demonstrates how new axes could be generated for future research exploration.

A major purpose of taxonomies is to identify gaps in knowledge. This is the second major concern about the use of axes in Taxonomy II. If each diagnosis is evaluated on each axis, gaps in knowledge about the diagnosis appear. The essential characteristics of the diagnosis also become more apparent, and facilitate the task of classifying the diagnosis. The rules for classification are then applied to the diagnosis without the confusion of information overload, which is handled by the axes.

Researchers

The researcher, as a taxonomy user, may benefit the most from the addition of the axes to the taxonomy. The axes identify information that must be specified for each diagnosis. They define the dimensions to be explored for each diagnosis. Do the defining characteristics change with the unit of analysis, age group, wellness, or illness? Which axes are appropriate for the diagnosis, either an accepted diagnosis or a proposed diagnosis? Are the etiologies the same for a given diagnosis independent of the axes or are the etiologies subtly different for a diagnosis as modified by the axis of interest? Which interventions and patient outcomes are appropriate for each diagnosis? Do they change when the axes are considered? The diagnoses and the axes may provide a structure to organize nursing knowledge and, thereby, provide a guide for future research into the areas that are poorly defined—rather like a score-keeping mechanism for keeping track of what is known and what still needs to be explored. Another purpose of a taxonomy is to be heuristic. And indeed the deliberations about and study of the Taxonomy identified a number of areas to be explored, gaps in knowledge, etc.

Practitioners

The practitioner user has two roles: administrator and bedside clinician. The administrator is responsible for describing the types of nursing services provided to the client. Do the axes assist in this task or do they complicate the task? Is the coding for the diagnoses and its axes the most practical and parsimonious? Because the administrator must compile various reports (e.g., nursing minimum data set, quality assurance) to document various measures of resource utilization and effectiveness, what are the implications of the axes of nursing diagnosis on this process? Can this coding method be handled in small hospitals where handcoding is the norm, at a reasonable cost? How do axes impact on current computerized hospital information systems and care planning packages? To be useful, the axes should be more effective and efficient at coding and facilitating retrieval of the specific nursing resources consumed by the client. The role of a diagnosis and its axes is to summarize the raw clinical data into information that can be efficiently understood and used by the administration and staff in organizing and facilitating the delivery of quality patient care.

The impact of axes on the practice of the individual clinician remains unclear. Must the clinician be aware of or use the axes in determining a diagnosis? Should these axes be included or considered by the practicing nurse? Axes are *not* assessment categories. These axes are developed to assist taxonomists in accurately classifying the diagnoses. That is why the Committee is still unclear about the implications for the staff nurse. Are the axes only used to capture the essential information from the assessment and diagnosis of the client and is this done by a coder or a clinician? It is important to clearly separate diagnostic reasoning and taxonomic reasoning. These are two separate cognitive processes that are very similar. The taxonomist engages in classification or a process of identifying the location of where a diagnosis should be placed. The clinician uses clinical judgment to determine which diagnoses apply to her or his patients. Although both individuals are dealing with nursing diagnoses, they are involved in very different processes.

Summary

Four axes were proposed and their implications within the taxonomic structure discussed. First, can all diagnoses be made at each level of the axis? Second, will the defining characteristics be the same for the diagnosis at each level of the axis? Third, which of the defining characteristics of a diagnosis must be present to make a diagnosis? Fourth, do the axes have discrete or continuous values? Fifth, are wellness and illness one axis or two axes? Does each diagnosis have wellness and illness values on these axes?

Implications of axes were also discussed for the users of Taxonomy II. The taxonomists have four concerns. First, the taxonomic structure becomes a blend of hierarchical and nonhierarchical components instead of a total hierarchical structure. Second, the essence of the diagnosis would be located at the point where the axes intersect, yet the entire structure must be evaluated when classifying the diagnosis. Third, the axes are not independent nor mutually exclusive. Fourth, a relational axis system assists in keeping the focus on the diagnosis while capturing the diversity or dimensionality of the diagnosis.

The researcher is affected three ways. First, the axes identify information that must be specified for each diagnosis. They define the dimensions to be explored for each diagnosis. Second, the diagnoses and the axes may provide a structure to organize nursing knowledge and thereby provide a guide for future research. Third, the taxonomy becomes heuristic.

The administrator may use the codes for axes to summarize the raw clinical data into information that can be efficiently understood and used by the administration and staff in organizing and facilitating the delivery of quality patient care.

Finally, axes are not assessment categories, though the data in the axes appear similar. It is important to clearly separate diagnostic reasoning and taxonomic reasoning. The axes, though they appear to solve many taxonomic problems, must be tested for their usefulness as part of Taxonomy II (Fleishman & Quaintance, 1984). All users of Taxonomy II must assume accountability for testing the new structure—patterns with axes.

References

Antonovsky, A. (1987). *Unraveling the mystery of health: How people manage stress and stay well.* San Francisco: Jossey-Bass.

Buckwalter, K. C., & Maas, M. (1989). Development and testing of psychosocial nursing: Diagnoses and interventions for the dependent elderly. *Oasis: Council of Gerontological Nursing Newsletter, 6*(3), 1, 3.

Fitzpatrick, J. J., Kerr, M. E., Saba, V. K., Hoskins, L. M., Hurley, M. E., Mills, W. C., Rottkamp, B. C., Warren, J. J., & Carpenito, L. J. (1989). Translating nursing diagnosis into ICD code. *American Journal of Nursing, 89,* 493–495.

Fleishman, E., & Quaintance, M. R. (1984). *Taxonomies of human performance: The description of human tasks.* Orlando, FL: Academic Press.

Martens, K. (1986). Let's diagnose strengths, not just problems. *American Journal of Nursing, 86,* 192–193.

Moch, S. D. (1989). Health within illness: Conceptual evolution and practice possibilities. *Advances in Nursing Science, 11*(4), 23–31.

Newman, M. A. (1986). *Health as expanding consciousness.* St Louis, MO: Mosby.

Pender, N. J. (1989). Languaging a health perspective for NANDA Taxonomy on research and theory. In R. M. Carroll-Johnson (Ed.), *Classification of nursing diagnoses: Proceedings of the eighth conference* (pp. 31–36). Philadelphia: Lippincott.

Popkess, S. A. (1981). Diagnosing your patient's strengths. *Nursing 81,11*(7), 34–37.

Warren, J. J., & Haight, B. K. (1990). *Loneliness in the elderly: A proposed nursing diagnosis.* Unpublished manuscript.

Weekes, D. P., & Rankin, S. H. (1988). Life-span developmental methods: Application to nursing research. *Nursing Research, 37,* 380–383.

Discussion

ICD-10

NOT IDENTIFIED: Based on the definition of the ICD as a system of categories to which morbid entities are assigned, I'm wondering where the proposed wellness-oriented diagnoses are going to fit in.

VIRGINIA SABA: Well, as I stated, that was the original and major focus of ICD-9. ICD-10 has changed in scope and it's not only going to be used for morbidity and mortality, but it's going to be used to codify health services and the management health services. So, I see that the family of classifications, which is broader in scope, will therefore encompass the providing of health services. [For] those who have been working with ICD-9, the last chapter, Chapter 21, which deals with signs and symptoms, and there's another chapter, 22, which deals with reasons for encounter with health professionals—is anybody familiar with that chapter? There's one word in that chapter saying nursing care and it's got a code—encounter with nurses, I believe is the term. We struck that out of Chapter 22 because we want a whole chapter, which is what our original intent was, or a whole supplement on nursing care. These chapters have been growing by leaps and bounds, and the definition has changed so much that it is no longer a classification of [just] morbid entities. The Health Care Financing Administration wants to use it to reimburse. Blue Cross wants to use it to reimburse. Research

is funded by categories. And the list goes on and on, so that original narrow focus has been expanded to include services, health services, the reason for health services that are provided to patients in, across settings.

NOT IDENTIFIED: I still don't see how that relates to wellness, though, health services.

VIRGINIA SABA: We only do health services to well people. We don't do health services to people we don't know are in our arena. The only time you do prevention is when you are providing a service for prevention of disease, and that service may be wellness service but it's also a health service of teaching wellness. To me, a *knowledge deficit* or a *noncompliance* requires that you teach. And so the diagnosis is *noncompliance* or *knowledge deficit* but you teach on the other side wellness to, or, knowledge deficit of lack of understanding of normal diet. You still have to teach or provide a procedure or a health service. So I don't see wellness as being a problem at all because we only provide service to those who are well. We provide a service, we aren't providing an intangible nothing. We do have something we do when we provide a service to a well client.

NOT IDENTIFIED: I guess we have a difference of a point of view.

MI JA KIM: Is there still room for any type of support that can be given by, let's say, WHO regional officers, primarily nursing officers, and by ICN? You did not address that aspect and I would be curious to know whether ICN has supported this notion. And the reason why I'm asking the first question is because we have about 15 WHO collaborating centers, nursing collaborating centers in the globe. The person who is in charge from Denmark is in the audience, and, you know, there is a mechanism that we could provide, perhaps stronger support along with ANA and NANDA, and I just wonder whether you would like to make a comment on those.

VIRGINIA SABA: For your information, the ICN has the nursing diagnosis on its agenda in April. In April it's having its regional meeting and the classification of nursing diagnosis will be presented and it will start. As you know we did start the international focus last summer at ICN in Korea, and now it has been taken up and put on the agenda for the ICN meetings that are being held. We see, or it is felt, that the classification of ICD-10 is firm, so, therefore, we did not get the Y chapter. But the family of health-related conditions is evolving and we have time to get it circulated around the world and to get the regional WHO offices to vote on the family members when the vote comes up. At this point, I understand the vote is not apparent until the big edition is finalized, but it will be soon. I don't have a date on that as yet. I am told that we will know about the dates for the family after the meeting that's coming up at the end of this month in London.

MI JA KIM: I would like to suggest that official communication go to all the WHO regional nursing officers for their support, and also to the collaborating centers on the WHO so that all of them also can give their support toward this end.

VIRGINIA SABA: I believe Margaret McLaughlin is here from the American Nurses' Association and she is responsible for transmitting all the formal correspondence to WHO and to ICN headquarters.

MARGARET MCLAUGHLIN: Dr. Greta Styles is the chairperson of the Professional Services Committee at ICN and she is working with ANA right now, and with Connie Halloran to

get this information shared and to get cooperation with all of the WHO offices.

MI JA KIM: That gives us the connection because the Collaborating Centers Network is meeting in April. And the 15 Collaborating Centers representatives will be there and Greta Styles is coming as an ICN representative. So all I want to say then at this point is that we do have a mechanism.

VIRGINIA SABA: I believe she has planned to present it at that meeting.

KRISTINE GEBBIE: One of the things I think needs to be underscored, Virginia, in your presentation, and I think that while you said it, people who haven't followed this process could miss it, is the stately procession of development of the whole ICD system. And for an observer it's hard to appreciate the degree of work you have contributed to making this progress as rapidly as has been made. It is very rare for an entirely new section to be developed in the short time that this has, and we all need to thank you for that. One of the issues then becomes something to which you referred only briefly toward the end, and that is that cross-translation that will happen between ICD-9 and ICD-10 so that people can see how an item has moved. Now that we have officially put forward from this country a possible classification for nursing, Conditions in Need of Nursing Care, into that system, how will we make certain that as we do revisions from our own work we deal with that cross-tabulation, because that system will be in circulation in the world, and as we put new things forward it will have to be cross-tabbed into it; and we're not used to that formal dance and progress that has to happen to make sure pieces aren't lost along the way.

VIRGINIA SABA: That's one of the benefits of having an international classification of diseases/health-related conditions. We will be in the queue and we will then be able, and there may be funding available for the redesign and the revision of subsequent editions. At this point in time, that has not been addressed. But I can see that as ICD gets revised, and as computer systems get remapped, we will be in the queue and have this part of the formal structure alleviating some of the problems that we may have to address as we go along with our revisions and with the problems that Taxonomy II will be addressing in deliberations as they plan their next step.

PHYLLIS KRITEK: Virginia, the other thing I thought you alluded to that ties into what Mi Ja observed, and I really think we may want to focus on that, is the "Health for All for the Year 2000" initiative of WHO, because I think the language system we're introducing is extremely compatible with an international effort, not only of WHO but very specifically of nursing. I think the way things are moving would indicate that these concepts we're bringing forward will be very attractive to larger and larger groups of people. And I think that gives a reason for hopefulness in the midst of what I know is a very difficult struggle, and I join Kris in commending you on the work you've done.

VIRGINIA SABA: Thank you. I think the critical issue is going to be that the WHO regional centers also approve and endorse this classification, and bring it to the voting body or get the vote in our favor. The USA is just one vote in the world assembly, and there are many, many other countries that have a chance to veto what we propose. So, therefore, the need to expand to the international horizons is critical and that is why we're very glad that it will be taken up at the April meeting and that ICN and WHO regional nurses are starting to take up the mandate.

KATHLEEN MCMILLAN: I'm also an anthropologist as well as a nurse, and I'm concerned that some of these descriptions of responses to illness may be heavily culture bound. And I'm not entirely sure whether they will apply cross-culturally. I think it's very important that we do get input from other members of nursing throughout the world, because when we're talking about responses to illness,

we're talking about heavily culturally influenced behaviors; and I think it'd be extremely important for us to get input from other nurses to ensure that we are talking about phenomenon that apply cross-culturally.

VIRGINIA SABA: When we gave this similar presentation at ICN in Korea, many of the foreign nurses described and gave similar opinions and views; but in principal they were in favor of a common terminology. I think that's the beginning and then we can iron out the details later. I think our goal is to have, in principal, a language that we all want to agree on; and then how we codify and what we codify will follow. If we [don't] keep that focus in mind we'll never get there, and I think we have to begin and make concessions and start with something. And I believe that's the opinion of NANDA and of the Taxonomy Committee. A lot of concessions had to be made and, of course, Joyce Fitzpatrick will describe how we agreed and what we agreed on.

REGINA MAIBUSCH: I am confused about the Y chapter. I thought I heard Virginia Saba say that we could not have the Chapter Y for some reason or other. Did I misunderstand that?

JOYCE FITZPATRICK: No, you did not. But this work was done and was submitted to WHO for possible inclusion as a Y chapter knowing that the timing was such that it may not be included; it was concluded that this was a first step, that we needed to move forward with this on the chance that some aspects would be included in ICD coding.

SHARON SUMMERS: I had heard that Blue Cross, in particular, and maybe some of the other insurance carriers were really opposed to the word "risk" and would not reimburse for that term. Does anybody know anything about that or has anybody heard anything about that?

JOYCE FITZPATRICK: Has anybody in the audience heard about reimbursement from third-party payers in relation to the risk concept?

DONNA LOSEY: I had attended a program done by a medical records person, because I do a lot of ICD coding for my husband's office. You're not supposed to code to get reimbursement. So when medical records coders give seminars on how to code for an office or for a hospital, they teach you how to code properly, not how to code for reimbursement. And when you go to these seminars, they don't tell you how you're going to get your reimbursement. But, off the record, [the presenter] told us for a lot of these risk things and a lot of health prevention, you're not going to get reimbursed. I had another question. When you code now in the system using the ICD-9 coding, you're to code up to the most specific number. Using the present system of coding, I would not be able to use Y23 (what used to be *potential for injury* or *risk for injury*). I would have to use one of the more specific ones, the Y23 would not be accepted. How would that stand in the future?

VIRGINIA SABA: Following the same logic as ICD-9, you can code either very specifically or very broadly. And so with the three digits you are coding more specifically than with the two digit, which is a broader coding methodology. And it depends on whether you are going to look at your cases in a broad way or in a narrow way. And you can get as specific as you like or keep the categories as broad as you like. So I think at this point, the scheme has to be tested and tried, and it is a first cut as we said. It is working. We have tried it. And I will verify that in a project that I am working on, and I have been able to code 40,000 nursing diagnoses with ease and without too much difficulty.

NANCY CREASON: I need some help understanding how "risk" is a better non-value term than "potential."

JOYCE FITZPATRICK: I didn't talk specifically about that as a value label. The implication was that "risk" was a more specific label than "potential for" because there is always potential for, there are not always high-risk situations that we can identify in relation to

the diagnoses. Whereas "potential for" is a broader label.

NANCY FLYNN: My question is also about risk, but I wondered why you didn't choose to use the fourth number so that *skin integrity, impaired* would be Y27.1 and *skin integrity, impaired, risk* would be Y27.12. So that all of those that had a risk associated with them would have that fourth number.

JOYCE FITZPATRICK: We debated this issue and it certainly is not closed, and we need ideas about how to deliberate this more. One of the questions we addressed, for example, is do all diagnoses come in both forms, and that is "actual" and "risk for" particular problems. That is something we are continuing to discuss in relation to Taxonomy II, and you will hear more about this in the discussions later this morning as we deliberate the "actual" and "potential" components of all nursing diagnoses. We chose to take this interim step and we said to ourselves we have to impose some structure on areas that still have some ambiguity, including this area of "risk." We made some decisions about how to classify these nursing diagnoses in relation to the framework of ICD coding, and chose to go with two levels of coding. Therefore, what you see is that *skin integrity, impaired* and *skin integrity, impaired, risk* are at the same level. And those are just based on some interim decisions that we made knowing that we had to more fully address the whole area of "risk" and "actual" problems at some later time. We'll debate this and discuss it again today.

CECILE LAMBERT: I would like to address the question of the human response patterns. I must say I was a little bit disappointed when I saw that we were going to have this pattern for many years. I think at previous meetings we've always said this was going to be discussed, we'd be talking about this; and we're really going into cement with this thing now, this human response. I would just like to bring a cultural difference point of view. We have been working a great deal on the translation of these things. We couldn't find the words. These nine categories, as someone has pointed out, are really value-oriented. So we had to simply override the nine response patterns. We went to what you call Level 2, because we still wanted to respect NANDA. For example, we don't have a problem on *anxiety* any more because it belonged to the emotional integrity level. And that was the way we got around it.

JOYCE FITZPATRICK: Well, please don't be disappointed and stop there. Please help us to figure this out. What you will notice from the ICD coding is that the patterns themselves do not get coded. I mean, we have been clear that the patterns are up for consideration in our future development. We just did not have enough data to change the conceptual structure. They are coded indirectly but you can change the label of the coding because it's indirect. There is some flexibility in the way that the system is coded. You never identify what the patterns are in the coding.

CECILE LAMBERT: That's the problem, you do. If I'm in 3, I'm in Feeling. When you go into another language, you're caught with this and you have to be, there's no way of your getting around it.

JOYCE FITZPATRICK: Well, I understand your point, but what I'm say is, let's take the category of Feeling. If we put a different label, [if] we just called that Category 3, didn't label it Feeling and tried to figure out what those diagnoses underneath that category had in common, we could figure out whether they needed to be placed together or whether they should be shifted somewhere else. Our decision was in some way, these diagnoses under that category fit together more than they fit somewhere else. So we have some flexibility for future development.

LENORE BOLES: We were wondering how impaired or altered is less value-laden than ineffective. And specifically, my concern is under Choosing. *Individual coping, impaired* is not really the same thing as *individual coping, ineffective,* at least not to my mind. And

that's a diagnosis that I use very frequently. Impaired means that the person is not able to cope. Ineffective to me means that the coping mechanisms they are using are not sufficient to handle the situation. The other thing that I think is perhaps even more important is under *denial, impaired.* Now, as a psych person, that does not make sense to me at all. In denial, which is a defense mechanism, if it's used excessively to rule out any reality, that's a problem. If on the other hand, one is unable to continue to deny, that implies a confrontation with reality or decompensation. So, to me, to say *denial, impaired* is impossible. I'm not trying to be difficult, but I think that you have to take all concerns in. I know that there is also the project phenomena concern, I'm very well aware of the Psych-ANA project. But I don't think that we have to set up roadblocks here that make any combination impossible for us.

JOYCE FITZPATRICK: Well, we did have the list from the psychiatric nursing group in working with this coding, and we did include some components of that. We very much want your input, so I would encourage you to let us know, and if you could write down some of your specific concerns, we would be glad to take those back to the Taxonomy Committee and to all the groups that are deliberating the future refinement and generation of nursing diagnosis.

LENORE BOLES: My suggestion regarding *denial* is to just leave denial without the qualification. I think that will then allow the clinicians to identify why denial is a problem.

JOYCE FITZPATRICK: I do appreciate the concern. We had a great deal of discussion about that specific label.

BRENDA DUTIL: I was wondering what you did with the diagnosis *family coping, potential for growth.* Are health-oriented diagnoses eliminated from this coding system?

JOYCE FITZPATRICK: We did not in any way want to imply exclusion of health-related diagnoses. But we had to make some cut at what we had, and we thought that [diagnosis] was already included.

Taxonomy II

PHYLLIS KRITEK: I want to first of all commend the Taxonomy Committee. And I think what they did today was advise us on the extraordinary complexity of the task. And, as someone who has worrisomely thought about that a lot, it's nice to see the entire body grapple with those tough questions. In addition to that, I want to just observe that it seems to me [that] part of what we're struggling with is the dimensions of taxonomy. Virginia's observations on the urgency of having something usable today versus a discussion on the conceptual clarity probably highlight that. What Mary Kerr said about the purpose is part of what we're struggling with and we need to get clearer on that, I think, that this is both a conceptual task, a scholarly task, a social construction, a language system, a fiscal or billing system, a research tool for both concept development and databases, a political tool internal to the NANDA operation and external to the larger world, and I think that's part of our problem. And interestingly under all of that is the tough question of what works for the practicing nurse. That may be the issue that we still don't have on the table, however. I think we need to make a decision that we do need to let this Taxonomy grow and develop and move to its next phase. It seems to me, though, that we do need to distinguish between political expedience and political wisdom, and I think that's part of what the membership is struggling with and we need to say that out loud. The practitioners that are struggling need to be heard. And when I go around, I hear the practitioners saying two things, either the nine patterns are totally impossible and should be shot at dawn, or they're absolutely wonderful and who would change them. But the proposed Taxonomy II retains that which is usually the point of intense debate and eliminates some of the subsequent levels, and that, I think, needs discussion. The perception of that as a hierarchical system, I

think, is also a misconception, because I don't think it's hierarchical so much as it's an attempt to capture sets or categories. These are the suggestions I have. I'd like to see the journal used as a place for dialogue on this. And some other people have mentioned that. I think some of the materials that Joyce is saying she has would be a useful article for us to all have an opportunity to sit and ponder. I think "think tanks" could be created so some of the people that have strong feelings on this could come together in groups of 15, 20, 25, and 30. The initial Taxonomy I was really generated with a group of about 35 people. It was not a committee structure so much as a group of people that wanted to do a "think tank" on it. We may benefit from a public and a working document, that is, one document we use for the kinds of things Virginia's speaking to—this is our public document, we take it everywhere, we carry it in our pockets—and one we're working on to enhance. And I think we do need a detailed framing of every shift we make. We can't make shifts until we detail them and struggle with them as a collective for some time.

CONNIE PINKLEY: I feel I'm standing here with one foot in two worlds because I think the work of the Taxonomy Committee is really challenging and exciting. I think that the axes create an opportunity to address many of the issues from the last conference, looking at the scope of health and wellness. On the other hand, working with database development in information systems I can appreciate Virginia's comments about the practical issues. And there are two things that I'd like to point out on the revised Taxonomy I. Under the category of *Injury, Risk,* what we have done is rule out Actual Injury. If we look at things like disease syndrome, because the categorization applies at different levels, we've implied that everything under that is a risk. And that certainly is not the case in terms of what we manage. I would suggest that perhaps when we look at the more abstract level in there, the broader category, that we should try to take away the value statements. Instead of saying, for example, risk or impaired, that if we had said altered, we would be able to encompass on a very practical level in our systems a broader range, until we get to the point that Taxonomy II really does address those. So, if we took, for example, family coping, instead of saying impaired, if we had altered family coping [or] altered individual coping. As Joyce suggested, when we get to fuller development of Taxonomy II, those may all fit under *health-seeking behaviors*, but we don't have that at this point. In the area of injury, I think that is too much related to a deficit. If we looked at altered physical integrity, it would be a much broader category and operational at this point in time.

CLAUDIA KLINE: I have a question for Dr. Fitzpatrick about the diagnosis of *altered cardiac output* and those others that were listed that were going to be removed. I'd like to know if direction is going to be provided in those areas as to what the critical care people are to do without those diagnoses.

JOYCE FITZPATRICK: Let me say again what I said this morning and that is that those diagnoses do not fit Taxonomy II. And we recommended that they be deleted based on this Taxonomy II structure that is currently proposed. Taxonomy II as a structure, however, is only in draft one. It is not our responsibility as a Taxonomy Committee to delete diagnoses from the approved list, and there is a mechanism that will be discussed that is part of the Diagnosis Review Committee's charge. That group will look at our recommendation and there is a whole set of activities that must occur in order to revise or delete a diagnosis from the NANDA-approved list. So don't take them off your list, they are on the approved list. As we struggle with the conceptual and the practical issues of development of both the Taxonomy and the diagnoses, we hope that this will all be clear and we will come up with better definitions of diagnoses, better defining characteristics, better labels, and

ultimately a better way of describing what we do in our clinical judgments in nursing practice, and put that all together in a taxonomy. So it's an important point, and, yes, in answer to your question, there will be some way of further discussing that and nothing will happen until a formal process is initiated and completed. So we're looking for research, we're looking for clinical validation, not just of those diagnoses but explorations of all those components. Encourage all your [critical care] friends to let us know what data they have to support or not to support various diagnoses, various interpretations of them, whether it's clinical data, whether it's research data, whatever is available. We need that kind of input now.

CINDY DOUGHERTY: I'm dismayed and rather disturbed by some of the things that have been said. My comments would be directed towards the major changes that were supposedly made in the area of the Exchanging human response pattern. It seems to me like there was a commitment in the past on the part of NANDA as well as the committees that diagnoses are not going to be lopped off without some evidence of research. And I am really disturbed by what's been done, especially in the three categories of cardiac output, fluid volume, and tissue perfusion. I understand how that's happened now, because of the application of the new definition of nursing diagnosis, and while I'm not in favor of that, I can understand how that's happened. What I would like to say is, I am intimately involved with some of the nursing diagnoses, especially in the physiologic area, and I think we're going to be doing a big disservice to the people, at least the 65,000 people I know who practice in critical care, where these areas of physiologic nursing diagnosis have not been well-developed anyway, and now they're even lopped off further. And I would also like to say I know of at least seven studies, five that are published, which give support to the use of the diagnosis *decreased cardiac output* and three which specifically identify nursing interventions that are used for that diagnosis. I would also like to suggest that we stop pretending that all of our interventions are independent and give more credence and recognition to the fact that we do have collaboration with other health care professionals.

JOYCE FITZPATRICK: We are not proposing the deletion of any diagnoses; it is not our authority to do that. We are recommending to the Board that within this new structure of Taxonomy II, there be consideration of deletion of some diagnoses and refinement of some diagnoses, because it is not consistent. There are inconsistencies if you take all of those assumptions and you work with those assumptions. So that you should not conclude that you should delete those diagnoses. This is stage one in our development. We're recommending that various groups look at this so that we can come up with the scientific support to justify these changes. So if you are to use any list of nursing diagnoses, the current list is Taxonomy I—Revised, includes all of the current list with the current approved diagnoses and the current definitions. We think we need to do a lot of work to further develop nursing diagnoses. The Board has commissioned certain work groups, including the Diagnosis Review Committee and the Taxonomy Committee as well as the Board, to look at some of these recommended changes. We would like to see more structure around the further development, not just of the Taxonomy, but of the refinement of diagnoses and the new development of diagnosis. Thirdly, your perception that some of these diagnoses are not consistent with the new definition is accurate. Some of them are not and, therefore, were recommended for consideration for either change, refinement, or deletion from the current structure.

DAWN BARBIERI: I was just wondering how did the Committee decide which nursing diagnosis would fit under Level 2 or Level 3? If I understand you right, you said that there was no discernible relationship. So, I can't seem to see any ties.

JOYCE FITZPATRICK: The comment I made was that there was no relationship between Level 3 diagnoses and Level 2 diagnoses. The decision as to which level a diagnosis was placed at had to do with generally the level of abstraction of the diagnostic label, the definition, and the defining characteristics. Now it is quite possible that as we further develop some of these diagnoses and more clearly specify defining characteristics and the definitions, which is the work that we've recommended as the next stage, that the level in which that diagnosis would be placed might change as it's further developed. So the basic factor determining the level placement has to do with the level of abstractness of what is currently available for us to evaluate. This includes what is in the published grey book which is called *Taxonomy I Revised 1989*.

LIZ HILTUNEN: I wanted to address a question about some of the differences between the new proposed Taxonomy II Draft One and the proposed ICD-10 version that was addressed earlier in the morning. If the ICD-10 is accepted and Taxonomy II is approved, what mechanism will there be to resolve the differences in placement of diagnoses within human response patterns and within levels between those two documents? And specifically, I'm always tracking the diagnosis of *decisional conflicts* since I have a vested interest in that particular one, and I notice in one document in the ICD-10, it's in Level 3 and in the new Taxonomy II it's in Level 2. Will there be a resolution of that and how will that happen?

JOYCE FITZPATRICK: What we have presently submitted to ICD, we believe must stand as the submission because we are at such an early state in the development of Taxonomy II. It would not be appropriate to recommend these changes yet for the ICD coding list. In order to move forward, we recommended that the ICD coding list go as it was even though we knew we would be looking at some of these issues within Taxonomy II. It's a question of having to move forward even though you don't have all the answers to all the questions. It is our expectation that we will submit materials refining what has already been submitted to WHO for ICD coding, as we are prepared to do that. At this time we think it's premature to include any of the recommendations that are included in Taxonomy II, Draft One. We have so much more work to do—developmental work, conceptual work, and work on clarifying the existing classification system as well as the list, that it would be premature to submit that. Which list should you use? I would say the ICD coding list is more reflective of what has been approved because it has been approved by the NANDA Board and by ANA and has been submitted to WHO.

LIZ HILTUNEN: In the future, if there are differences in those two documents, when and if they are approved, how would there be a reconciliation between the two?

JOYCE FITZPATRICK: Well, we will submit the list as it's approved by the NANDA Board, by ANA, and we will submit it for a formal process and we will make that be known, we will publish that. But it is a very formal process that we went through in developing the ICD coding list in working with ANA, and that will occur again in order to make the changes in the list.

DONNA VER STEEG: I need first to say that the sophistication of this group at this conference is so far beyond where this group was in the first conference that we all need a pat on the back for that. I think we also need to look at the fact that when we made some of those early decisions, we did not have the level of sophistication that we have now. And I was thinking today a couple of things. One is my nurse practitioners and I, finally having struggled womanfully with Taxonomy I, went back and looked at Gordon and revised it to fit into the computer, because that's one of the major problems with Gordon. The second problem with the Gordon Taxonomy is it was using language which in our work we've discovered is sloppy. Potential is a bad word. I didn't realize how vague potential was until I had ten people tell me what potential meant, and I came up with ten different definitions. So that

we, instead of using potential, we looked at the purpose of the taxonomy in terms of diagnoses guiding interventions and we used "risk," and we used "possible," which meant that we were trying to generate more data; and we used presumed which meant that we had a pretty good idea this is what it was and we were going to treat it as that until we found out differently. That helped us a lot in our thinking. And I think, you know, some of those dictionary problems . . . and you have to remember that there's a conceptual gap and a time gap between what gets used in a hospital and what finally ends up in Webster's, and Webster's is old hat by the time it gets into print. I think we have in this room the capability of answering most of the questions that were being dealt with. I think you have to think about the fact that most of the textbooks that go out to the clinician include both the Gordon Taxonomy, which, as I say, in its current form is not computerizable, and the NANDA Taxonomy I, and that ought to tell us something: that clinicians conceptually understand the Gordon responses. Most of them out in the "real" world are not too clear on the Taxonomy unless they come from one of our more theoretically based programs. They don't have the tools to use it, and we have to think about that.

MI JA KIM: First I'd like to thank the Committee who are brave enough to raise all those questions and take some actions. I think it's a very, very difficult task. I for one have been really wanting to refine what we have had in our taxonomy, and so I am delighted that the Committee has taken one step further. Part of the pain we are experiencing perhaps is really sort of the growing pain that may be necessary and probably essential, but there are some fundamental questions that I have that I would like to address. I perceive that these are recommendations coming from the Committee, therefore, that we have room for these thinking. Am I correct? (Correct.) Also the Diagnosis Review Committee came up with the official definition for our discussion and consideration and I think that's going to be very helpful. But one thing that we really have to be mindful of is that even though we will have a definition clearly black and white, that it's the interpretation of the definition or the application of that definition that still is going to be somewhat of a problem, because, as we know, the definition does not have weights and scales and thermometers, etc., so that it's difficult to objectively say and have 100% reliability. Therefore, there will be a subjective application and interpretation—that's going to cause some pain to us. Perhaps this is one of the pains that I am going to share with you. It is extremely important [to remember that] the very essence of nursing being the applied science with pluralistic view that's necessary. In other words, we have to preserve nursing as a biopsychosocial science. It is extremely important that what you do not necessarily know because you are not in a particular setting doesn't necessarily mean that they are not nursing diagnoses. Unless you really are one of the geniuses who are experts in everything, I just don't see that's humanly possible. Therefore, we have to have a reliance on clinical experts who say that these diagnoses are useful in their practice. And I think this organization better listen to them very carefully. Otherwise we will invite problems, that we will not have one organization but many, and that's something that I want to prevent. Nursing should be inclusive at this point, not exclusive. We are not ready to be exclusive, particularly when clinicians are saying [these diagnoses] are useful. This is not the time to be exclusive. We cannot afford that.

This piece of information has some bearing to our further thinking. Just two weeks ago, NCNR—the National Center for Nursing Research—had called a biological task force. The purpose of that task force was to discuss the domain of nursing or the importance of the biological sciences in nursing. There will be a recommendation or set of recommendations coming from this particular task force.

The essence of the task force's recommendation is that nursing simply, currently as it stands, does not have enough biological sciences. Therefore, we have to increase that component in terms of research. Now, you may choose to think that that's NCNR, that we can ignore. You may not want to do that [if] you who are in academia, because that's where the decisions for budget allocation comes, and that is a real issue for nursing. We have to really restore the credibility of the biological aspect of nursing to the people outside of us, particularly NCNR needs to demonstrate that to NIH for our credibility and existence. This is not the time to make some decisions that's going to be viewed otherwise. The other [point] is that, as Taxonomy I was submitted for ICD-9 or ICD-10 consideration, we simply have to think about the professional integrity. What type of communication are we going to give, never mind to nursing, but to others?

JOYCE FITZPATRICK: We deliberated whether or not this work was ready to present at this time. And as you can appreciate, there are some concerns that we have about where we are in the development of the work that leads to the discussion of issues right now. We chose to present our work, even though it is not finished, even though there are some hard decisions that have to be made in the future that aren't yet made because we needed this feedback from this group, and we need the feedback from the larger nursing community including the specialty groups. We do not have as much feedback as we would like in order to move forward, so again I encourage all of you to let us know what's happening and we'll develop a vehicle. Secondly, it is our full intention to be inclusive rather than to be exclusive. Toward that goal, we need to look at all the work that's been done and know that we're in the process of developing Taxonomy II but what is public is Taxonomy I Revised, 1989. And that's what we're recommending be used in the public arena including clinical practice. We're stepping back from that and we're saying "Where are we going next?" and we're raising questions about that. We're not saying we're down the road to Taxonomy II. So please appreciate that we're telling you we think we should go forward with Taxonomy I Revised, including the translation in ICD-10. So I think I'm supporting what you're saying, Mi Ja.

KRISTINE GEBBIE: I think the last point that Joyce made needs to be said about every 20 minutes just to remind us all of where we are in these processes. A process observation and then a request to the Committee: we've said since the beginning, this organization indulges in two processes, one of naming phenomena and the other of classifying or sorting them. The naming process is a little more regularized and we know a little more about how to revise that. We are now experiencing the first iteration of the revising of Taxonomy informing the naming process, just as the naming process has informed the organizing. And they should be feedback loops, but they're still two separate processes. I think what happened this morning is that in having the feedback to the diagnosis-labeling process called out, people were somewhat distracted by that and by that list of labels that your Committee has found problematic in the revision of Taxonomy, and, therefore, did not hear some of the rationale for other things that were done in moving to Taxonomy II. Hence, my request that the Committee might provide all of us at some point with a little more clearly, preferably written, rationale for the movement to these Level 1, Level 2, and Level 3, because it looks like we've moved back to mere alphabetical lists which were a real problem to the organization at one time, and there's no indication of how to relate things from Level 3 to things in Level 2 that look very similar. Absent a real grasp of the rationale, it's hard for me and I suspect others to make informed comments on whether this is progress, regress, or just something new and different to react to. So, if the Committee could look at how to give us,

to look at and struggle with you, some of that rationale for this change, I think it would help inform us on the Taxonomy side as well as on the diagnosis side.

ANNA OMERY: I'd like to follow up just briefly with the comment from Mi Ja Kim and I'll do it in the form of a charge I got from my colleague as I came here. What she said to me was that from her point of view, nursing diagnoses without physiological diagnoses were a lot like communism. They worked well in theory but they just weren't going to work in practice. So I ask you to take that into your consideration as we address the issues surrounding them.

JUDY WARREN: One of the things you need to really clearly look at as we're trying to explain our deliberation, when we reevaluated those diagnoses, we looked at the new definition of nursing diagnoses that you will be looking at tomorrow in the business meeting. Please look at that definition. If you are worried about the physiologic diagnoses or any other kinds of diagnoses, see whether or not it fits in the definition that the organization is supporting. I mean, that is your opportunity to influence what goes on because all further work—acceptance of new diagnoses, revision of the taxonomy—hinges on what a nursing diagnosis is. We need to come to consensus on that. We need some criteria that we can hold up or a ruler or a measurement or something to see whether or not this really is a diagnosis. Some of the issues that we're speaking of have to do with the whole domain of nursing and how we interact within the health care team. I think it's valuable for us to dialogue on that and be very clear what nursing diagnoses are, and then we can go forward. As far as deletion of physiologic diagnoses, if you will check your Bylaws, all diagnoses are added, modified, and deleted by a vote of this membership. They are not capriciously gotten rid of by a committee or the Board. So you still have that power to determine what diagnoses we're classifying. What we've done by evaluating those diagnoses is identify the problems within the structure, and we've tried to present those to you. So take a look at the definition and really try to conceptualize it so that you can come to that meeting and really have a meaningful dialogue and make an informed type of comment or contribution.

BONNIE WESORICK: I want to tell you that our critical care areas in 10 different hospitals in eight different states stopped using *decreased cardiac output.* Without the rest of the story that might not make any sense, but if anybody would like to discuss it I'd be more than glad to. We did delineate out and became clear about the difference between the definition of a nursing diagnosis and collaborative or what we call interdependent standards of care. And [the nurses] on their own got rid of it, do not use it. I think it goes back to what Judy said about the differentiation and what are we trying to do here and it's so critical. So I'd be more than willing to, for those who had concerns, to show you how we did that and what.

KAY GREENLEE: As an active critical care nurse and somebody who's been in critical care for approximately 12 years, I guess I want to reiterate what Bonnie said in that we have to go back to the presentation of Linda Carpenito and, I believe, Joyce Fitzpatrick addressed it as well in that all that we as nurses do is not a nursing diagnosis. Therefore, I on a daily basis treat patients who have an alteration in their cardiac output, and yet that is not the nursing diagnosis that I chose to put on my care plan. I think we need to clarify that while we may be treating it as a nurse, it is not independently that part of our practice that we address in the terms of a nursing diagnosis.

JOYCE DUNGAN: My concern is related to both the definition and how the definition then will shape the inclusion in the taxonomy, in Taxonomy II. And then listening to the critical care nurses, the definition does recognize that there is a collaborative part of our practice, not only with medicine but with other disciplines, and that a great deal of the very important nursing judgments that we use are within the scope of collaborative practice. And those judgments, while they may be related to biological domain which has been associated with the medical model for a long time, while those collaborative judgments are related to that shared domain, they are independent judgments and the response to them is executed independently [because] nurses in critical care monitor the patient in the absence of other personnel. I would hate to see that not recognized as a part of the independent domain of practice of nursing because we would lose a big part of the importance of our practice. If we recognize that we have these collaborative concerns that are kind of not a part of the taxonomy, they exist someplace outside our classification, we're going to lose a part of the essence of nursing. I don't know that's going to come about and whether collaborative things can fit into the taxonomy. But I hope that somehow they can.

JOYCE FITZPATRICK: Let me respond to that specific comment by giving an analogous situation. We could also include the diagnoses under DSM-3 within the NANDA Taxonomy, taking that same logic. I as a psychiatric nurse can diagnosis schizophrenia in its various manifestations, and I can treat that independently or interdependently, depending on how you interpret that. It is an important critical juncture that we're at in developing nursing diagnosis to decide whether or not to include some of those specialty-based diagnoses that are used across disciplines within the NANDA Taxonomy. I see that as a very similar issue as some of the issues that have been raised today, although they have not specifically been addressed in relation to DSM-3. So, we don't have closure on that. All we used to guide our development at this point was the definition of nursing diagnosis that was approved and is presented for discussion here. Having made that decision, we might come to the same conclusion about some of the diagnoses that could be better included in that collaborative area that happened to be psychiatric diagnoses.

JOYCE SHOEMAKER: What I have been hearing

today has brought to mind, and Mary Hurley's presentation again reinforces it, that we have a taxonomy of human responses that doesn't seem to be working. And I think [Mary's] examples made it clearer and clearer where we take a diagnostic label and try to figure out what kind of a human response we're talking about, and there's so much overlapping and lack of clarity, and the definitions of the human responses are not helping. Now what I'm hearing is maybe we need to change the diagnoses. I'm wondering whether in all of the deliberations that the Taxonomy Committee has been engaged in, and obviously it's been engaged in a great deal of work over the past two years, whether there was any consideration to changing the taxonomy?

MARY HURLEY: There's been a lot of discussion and talks about changing the taxonomy that never goes far away from the discussions. But I think that the point I was trying to make today is that we don't have enough data to say that the human response patterns don't work. But we *do* have enough data to say that we've started this work a long time ago. We haven't done an awful lot of work on some things; we've done a lot of work on other things; we've grown, we've matured; our thought processes are different; and we have to keep going back from time to time to refine. I think that was the message I was trying to get across today. Everything changes over time, and what we did 15 years ago has got to change, be impacted on by our practice today. That was the major thrust of the discussions. Changing the taxonomy at some point in time, if we have the data that tells us that, is an open, not a closed, issue. But that was not the message I wanted you to get today. I wanted you to get the message that as we grow and mature we have to rethink the work we've done as well as the work that we're going to do.

CONNIE PINCKLEY: I would appreciate an explanation just of the redefinition process. The definitions are helpful, but there's also some areas that I have difficulty differentiating part of the concept. For example, between Feeling and Perceiving: How were the revised definitions arrived at and is there further work that really needs to be done over the next years in looking at concept clarity?

MARY HURLEY: We took a look at the nine human response patterns. The original definitions came from the theorist group, and they had not really been relooked at through all of the taxonomy meetings that I was privileged to attend. We went back to the definitions, went back to the dictionary as Joyce said this morning. We looked up every one of those words in the Oxford Dictionary, in Webster's Dictionary, and in one other dictionary. Then we brought all that information to the meeting. In addition, we each had a pattern to look at and we looked at the pattern and the diagnoses under the pattern and we looked to the definitions that we had plus the old definition. We also looked in nursing textbooks, theorist books, any book that had nursing information that we could then use in with the regular definitions of the word. We took a look at some of the diagnoses—where we would change them—and how we would collapse different patterns. We looked at each pattern and came up with a new definition based on the old [definition], based on what was coming out of the dictionaries, based on what was coming out of the nursing literature, obviously based on our own perceptions of how we saw the patterns evolving, and based on what was in the definitions and defining characteristics of each of the diagnoses. So a lot of work was done before we even came to the meeting. I can remember the original two I had (Perceiving and Feeling). I collapsed the diagnoses, I changed the levels around and whatever. It was just a growing process, a maturing process of thought that brought us to this finally, in a consensus of eleven people and the work that they had done, the many hours of work they had done at home. I don't know if that answers your question, but that really is where the definitions came from.

I think we've always felt [that given] the

human being and his complexity, there's an overlapping of some of those patterns, and there may always be unless we get rid of the patterns and then, and find something that's totally exclusive. But mutually exclusive patterns are going to be hard to find, at least in the current terminology that we use. But it does need further conceptualization and certainly a lot more work. It was just the second step. The first step was done how many years ago?, and then this step today.

NANCY CREASON: I appreciate the toughness of trying to do this and some of you know that I have had a long-standing concern about the lack of definition of anything in the nursing diagnosis process. It's about time that we're paying good attention to that. However, I also hope that we're going to be careful about not changing before we've checked out what we already have. I think that's one of our dilemmas in figuring out how to move forward on a couple of fronts at the same time. We don't have research that says whatever we did before was wrong in the first place or wasn't quite right. And so I think we really must pay attention to getting people going. You've sort of just outlined a nice research program for a lot of people, I think, in terms of moving forward now and looking at some of those definitions and looking at the literature and looking at it in actual clinical practice. And that is the point I want to get around to. We can spend a lot of time with the literature and a lot of time talking to each other, but until we get to the clinical practice arena it's for naught, and I hope we will go on to do that before we do too much changing.

DONNA VER STEEG: I don't think anybody in this room isn't honoring the Committee for the amount of work they've done because anybody who's been involved with this knows that it's a tremendous amount of work. The problem is we seem to be treading water in a forward direction. The analogy that comes to mind is "if it looks like a duck and it walks like a duck and it talks like a duck . . . " What we've got here is a flamingo.

It's elegant and it's aesthetically pleasing, but it doesn't well represent the whole family of water fowl, and I think that's what you're hearing today. Some of the rest of us aren't flamingos, we're geese and mud hens and mallards, and a few of us are swans, not very many. And unfortunately our ecological needs are not being met in this particular bird sanctuary. Some of us make nests out of sticks and some of use mud and some of us use feathers and we all ought to be able to live together as water fowl. But some people, and I think we've heard them here today, feel that they're in a hostile environment at the moment. And that's preventing us from building on the very wonderful kind of work that's being done and going to the next step. Sometimes words get in the way of getting ahead. We need to find a common thing that we can work with comfortably and get out of this nesting around problem. And I'm not sure how we go about doing that.

BRENDA LYON: I would just like to suggest that I think that one of the things that we're experiencing, and this is a suggestion for a fix that we might want to talk about tomorrow in the Business Meeting, is that while we're responding to external publics and feel a sense of urgency to do that, the ICD-10 being an example, what we haven't had sufficient opportunity to do yet is to respond to our own urgencies in dealing with the conceptual issues that we keep setting aside. I think tomorrow that we all need to think about setting up for ourselves next year, not two years from now, but next year, working debate groups where we can deal with the issues that we really need to deal with.

BONNIE WESORIK: I work with hundreds of practitioners who day in and day out are trying to figure out what nursing diagnosis to use. Last week on one of the units, there was a discussion with three nurses at the bedside saying "Well, I don't know, I think this is *spiritual distress*," and the other one said "No, this is definitely *grieving*." And the other one says "Well, I think this is *ineffective coping*."

And I was sitting here all day long and thinking, wherever you go, the questions are always there. I want you to know that today I am so impressed with the work that each of you have done. I would like to ask the committees how we might help. I have contact with 4,000 clinicians each day. I was thinking when I heard each one of you ask very hard questions and very thought-provoking questions, that maybe the committees ought to take those questions that are the end of a 2- and 6- and 10-hour discussions and narrow it down to critical questions. Send them to us, the very countable members of this organization, and say "Can you get us some feedback on them?" Not only what we think, but what might the practitioners think about these questions. You've come with such important issues and how might you feed them back to us so we might give you feedback to sort through it. Because the work in your groups must be profound and I know you all have ten thousand other jobs. So might you think about that and how we could help.

MARY KERR: It seems like the journal is a perfect vehicle for disseminating some of the problem diagnoses, the possible questions for research, the problems that we're having within the taxonomic structure. That was one of the purposes of the journal, and I'm hoping that we can use that to its fullest extent.

BONNIE WESORIK: There should be a component of the journal that has a formal feedback mechanism. I think we would all help.

Axes

STEPHANIE RICHARDSON: I'm wondering how [the Committee] considered gender, although I know gender doesn't exist along an axis, a continuum. It looks like these axes 1 and 2 are placed as categorical levels, and would you consider gender as an issue?

JUDY WARREN: We had a dialogue about that because I know that right now there is a lot of interest in research about how women respond, what those female responses are to a variety of health problems. At this point, when we were discussing this, we were looking at a dichotomous variable. Is that just assessment data because it's recorded for everybody? We probably may have to reconsider that as research comes out, especially if the research tells us that the defining characteristics for women would be different.

STEPHANIE RICHARDSON: So, you're considering that as an axis perhaps for development.

JUDY WARREN: At this point in time, we are not, because we are trying to really work with what we've worked on. We had a discussion and at that point we decided that was assessment data and we left it there. Now that does not mean that it has to stay there. Certainly if there are people that are really interested in that axis and want to work it up, please contact the Committee and that work can go forward. We want to hear what do you want, what's missing, what would you like to do. Then we're going to ask you to help us do it.

JEAN JENNY: I'd just like to tell you of my great interest in these papers. They certainly reflect questions that my colleague and I are grappling with in our own research. First of all, I think we might agree that all diagnoses arise from basically two focal points—the individual and the context or situation. Now, it seems to me that these axes could be preliminarily, roughly, sorted into both client axes and situational axes, so that might be something that we would like to pursue, because the diagnosis occurs in situ—it's not an encapsulated reality. The second thing that I would suggest is that it's really the first time that our discussion has reapproached a point of concern that arose at least eight years ago in my memory, and that was the debate as to whether nursing diagnoses are continuous or categorical states. This is bringing us closer to something that interests us very much, the idea that many nursing diagnostic states are not categorical states, they are continuous states. I would like to suggest that a possible axis to think of in the future would be in line with the continuous nature of our diagnostic states and that we look at level of severity as a possible client-related axis rather than as a situational-related axis.

JUDITH WARREN: We were trying to get at that in looking at acuity and chronicity. Basically we tabled that because of all the issues of the variety of patient classification tools that are out there. We wanted to deal with the axes that we could deal with fairly quickly and successfully, and to try to figure out what the issues were. We chose unit of analysis and age group, and then uncovered a lot of issues coming out of that, and then began work on the wellness, because we heard loud and clear last time that wellness was a big area. Now some of the issues with severity is the difficulty that when we collaborated with ANA and the World Health Organization, we had to negotiate words and ideas, and we couldn't just impose NANDA's view of the world. We had to give a little and take a little, and it was politic for us to make some concessions so that we could get our information out there. Now, with the issue of the continuousness and discreetness, I think that's another one of those types of issues that we need to grapple with. But we also have the real world, and computers are fast coming in, and so the other part of my brain says, well, if it's a continuous variable, how are you going to code that? How are you going to capture that information so that you can retrieve it for whatever purpose? That brings another implication that was brought up by Virginia Saba. Many times, people develop taxonomies for one use, [and] other people start looking at it and using it differently than what it was designed for. So that we keep having to come back and reevaluate the taxonomy to see if it meets the criteria of usefulness.

DONNA VER STEEG: I just wanted to congratulate you and encourage you in pursuing this [axis] approach, because we found that kind of a modification in diagnostic categories to be extremely fruitful. It opens up whole new ways of looking at it, and I think it's very powerful.

Summary

JOYCE FITZPATRICK: I wanted to try to sum up our concerns and our issues for further discussion and also to say to you that we are interested in all of your ideas about how to carry on this dialogue. We think there are major issues about inclusive versus exclusive; how we define the work that we do as nurses is an important component of developing this taxonomy and an important component of developing nursing diagnoses. Secondly, the scholarly work juxtaposed with the clinical work that has to be done and juxtaposed with the political agenda that we all have to concern ourselves with. Now, I once learned that you solve political problems with political solutions. You don't solve political problems with scientific solutions. And I think we also need to keep that in mind and remember what we're doing for what purposes. We tried to be very cognizant that our task as the Taxonomy Committee was not to solve the political problem when we developed the first draft of Taxonomy II, but rather to develop a scientific problem or to respond to a scientific problem if you understand taxonomy development as the science of classification. When we developed the ICD coding of Taxonomy I Revised, we were very cognizant of the fact that we were doing something different than addressing a scientific problem. What we were doing there was responding to the public, to those people outside of ourselves as well as within the organization and within the discipline of nursing, to be more clinically relevant as well as more responsive to the health care arena and address such issues as classification within a standard format as well as reimbursement. So we think we have been jumping back and forth in these various arenas and sometimes perhaps jumping in the wrong one at the wrong time or jumping in the wrong one at the right time. So it's a very, very important agenda that we have in front of all of us, not just as the North American Nursing Diagnosis Association, but as members of the discipline developing our discipline for health care more broadly. We have a number of suggestions that have come forward today, including an important one of using our new publication, NANDA's new publication, for some of the debate. We've already taken some notes about aspects of our presentation that we hope to communicate in that journal. All of you know that the presentations today will also be included in the proceedings, so they will be available to you soon. We hope that you will help us by giving us all your comments, not just the ones that have been made here on tape, but also any comments you wish to [write] down and send to us. I thank you for your input, I thank the Committee for their work and everybody for their tolerance of all the ambiguities that are there for all of us.

II

Nursing Diagnosis Development and Review

The NANDA Definition of Nursing Diagnosis

Lynda Juall Carpenito, MSN, RN

"We know what we do, but we cannot put it into words. It became necessary to state more clearly the reasons that some persons were receiving care from two professionals" (Gebbie & Lavin, 1975, p. 1). These words were spoken by Gebbie at the First National Conference for the Classification of Nursing Diagnosis in 1973. At this conference, nursing diagnosis was defined as a judgment or conclusion that occurs as a result of a nursing assessment (Gebbie & Lavin, 1975). The same definition was used at the Second National Conference. In the proceedings of the Third and Fourth Conferences, seven definitions of nursing diagnosis were utilized. Needless to say, the number of published definitions of nursing diagnoses has dramatically increased with each national conference.

During the diagnosis-review cycle of 1986 to 1988, the Diagnosis Review Committee discussed NANDA's dilemma: There was no approved definition of nursing diagnosis. At the Eighth Conference in 1988, this issue was raised and a motion presented and passed requiring a working definition of nursing diagnosis be submitted to the 1990 General Assembly.

The following definition represents the outcome of a joint effort between the NAN-

DA Board of Directors and the Taxonomy Committee:

A nursing diagnosis is a clinical judgment about an individual, family, or community response to actual or potential health problems/life processes which provides the basis for definitive therapy toward achievement of outcomes for which the nurse is accountable.

The remainder of this paper explores the elements of this definition drawing from both lay and nursing literature.

Clinical Judgment

Judgment is defined by *Webster's* (1976) as the action of mentally establishing a relation between two or more terms, a formal expression embodying such a logical conclusion. Gordon (1982) describes three types of judgments involved in the diagnostic process. Perceptual judgment determines if a sign is present or not. Inferential judgment affirms that a relation exists between the collected data. Finally, a third type of judgment concludes that the cues in the cluster fit the name of the cluster—the nursing diagnosis label.

65

Webster (1984) reported at the Fifth National NANDA Conference that "complete success in naming coordinate species and mutually exclusive and jointly exhaustive classes is possible only in the formal and not in the empirical sciences" (p. 15). Nursing is an empirical science; thus clinical judgments called nursing diagnoses will be the result of weighing and evaluating conflicting information. They will be probabilistic (Gordon, 1982). It is not possible for nursing diagnoses to represent mutually exclusive classes; overlap will exist. The accuracy of diagnostic judgments should be augmented as the scientific process of clustering defining characteristics increases.

Central to the issue of a definition of nursing diagnosis is what types of judgments are nursing diagnoses: all nursing judgments or only some. It is interesting to note the following lawyer's perspective of nursing diagnosis published in the Proceedings of the First Conference.

Except in an emergency situation where a physician is not available, it is unlawful for a nurse to medically diagnose a patient's condition for the purpose of instituting positive treatment or therapeutic measures. This is clearly the province and function of the physician. However, the professional nurse is always authorized to make a nursing diagnosis, in order to evaluate those factors (physical, mental, sociological, and economic) which may have an influence on the patient's recovery. She may then take appropriate steps based on such diagnoses to prevent complications or anything which might worsen the patient's condition (Bernszweig, 1969).

Aspinall and Tanner (1981) wrote that nurses make two types of inferences or judgments about the state of the patient: (1) those health problems that ". . . nurses, by virtue of their education and experience, are licensed and able to treat" (p. 4), nursing diagnoses, and (2) those health problems that must be diagnosed and treated by other members of the health team, but that require continued nursing observation, assessment, and implementation of the therapeutic regimen. These differences will be discussed later.

Nursing Diagnosis Defined

Individual, Family, and Community Response

Response is defined by *Webster's* (1976) as a corresponding act or feeling to a motive force or situation. In 1980, the American Nurses' Association (ANA) published the ANA Social Policy Statement: "Nursing is the diagnosis and treatment of human responses to actual or potential health problems." The inclusion of individual, family, and community represents the populations that nurses treat. The proposed axis on the Taxonomy of individual, family, and community should further help to facilitate development of diagnoses for the family and community.

It is important that nursing diagnoses represent responses to situations or processes, not situations in themselves. Our history in nursing education and practice is laden with nursing interventions linked to situations. Nurses learn that the client with a myocardial infarction should receive care directed at reducing anxiety, monitoring for complications, implementing the medical orders, and teaching the client and family. All these interventions were linked to a myocardial infarction. The situation is myocardial infarction, some of the responses being treated were nursing diagnoses. We will fail again to explain the science of nursing if we define nursing diagnosis as a situation. The following are examples of this:

- Sensory-Perceptual Alteration: Visual (for blindness)
- Impaired Skin Integrity (for laceration)
- Altered Patterns of Urinary Elimination (for urostomy)
- Sensory-Perceptual Alterations (for spinal cord injury)

- Altered Cerebral Tissue Perfusion (for CVA)
- Impaired Gas Exchange (for tuberculosis)

. . . Actual or Potential Health Problems/Life Processes . . .

Nursing's phenomena of concern can run the gamut of responses from pathophysiologic states and treatment-related situations to personal situations, environmental factors, and maturation issues. Examples of actual or potential health problems include loss of vision, diabetes mellitus, trauma, or surgery; while examples of life processes or events include pregnancy, relocation, financial problems, dying, or child rearing.

. . . Definitive Therapy . . .

Definitive is defined by *Webster's* (1976) as serving to supply a final answer, solution, or evaluation; to end an unsettled or unresolved condition; most authoritative, reliable, and complete. The term "definitive" will be discussed later with outcome achievement.

Therapy is defined as reaction to the treatment of disease or disorders by remedial agents or methods. According to Gordon (1976), "to treat or the provision of treatment" refers to the initiation of accepted modes of therapy. Gordon continues that these exclude "prescription of drugs, surgery, radiation, and other treatments that are defined legally as the practice of medicine" (p. 1299). The term "therapy" can be described as a set of interventions prescribed by nurses for a specific purpose. Bulechek and McCloskey (1989) define nursing interventions as "any direct care treatment that a nurse performs on behalf of a client. These treatments include nurse-initiated treatments resulting from nursing diagnoses, physician-initiated treatments resulting from medical diagnoses, and performance of the daily essential functions for the client who cannot do these" (p. 25). This definition expands on their pre-vious definition of nursing interventions being related only to nursing diagnoses and their goals (Bulechek, 1985).

Bulechek and McCloskey's research (1989) has identified seven types of nurse activities as

1. Assessment activities to make a nursing diagnosis
2. Assessment activities to gather information for a physician to make a medical diagnosis
3. Nurse-initiated treatments, in response to nursing diagnoses
4. Physician-initiated treatments, in response to medical diagnoses
5. Daily essential function activities that may not relate to either medical or nursing diagnoses but are done by the nurse for clients who cannot do these for themselves
6. Activities to evaluate the effects of nursing and medical treatments. These are also assessment activities but they are done for purposes of evaluation, not diagnosis.
7. Administrative and indirect care activities that support the delivery of care.

Figure 1 represents the relationship of six of the seven types of nursing activities to nursing diagnoses and medical diagnoses. Figure 2 is an adaptation of the previous seven nursing activities into two types of nursing interventions for nursing diagnoses and nonnursing diagnoses.

Nonnursing diagnoses are those situations where nurses may intervene but are not accountable to prescribe the definitive therapy: Definitive therapy is the most authoritative—the complete and final solution. These situations require both nursing- and medical-prescribed interventions. Two authors have proposed solutions for this nonnursing diagnosis category: Gordon (1982) proposed using a medical diagnosis label; Carpenito (1983) defines nonnursing diag-

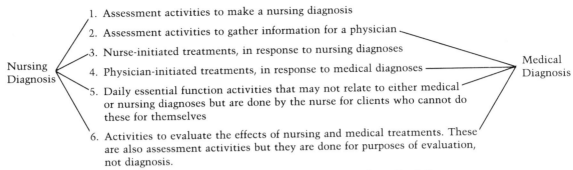

1. Assessment activities to make a nursing diagnosis
2. Assessment activities to gather information for a physician
3. Nurse-initiated treatments, in response to nursing diagnoses
4. Physician-initiated treatments, in response to medical diagnoses
5. Daily essential function activities that may not relate to either medical or nursing diagnoses but are done by the nurse for clients who cannot do these for themselves
6. Activities to evaluate the effects of nursing and medical treatments. These are also assessment activities but they are done for purposes of evaluation, not diagnosis.

FIGURE 1   Relationship of nursing interventions to nursing and medical diagnoses

noses that nurses treat as collaborative problems (formerly called clinical problems).

There are only two types of nursing interventions: nurse-prescribed and physician-prescribed. Nurse-prescribed interventions are prescriptions formulated by nurses for themselves or other nursing staff to implement. Physician-prescribed interventions are prescriptions formulated by physicians for nurses to implement. Both types require independent nursing judgment (Carpenito, 1987). Both are scientific and critical for client well-being. It is important to note that nurses can and should consult with other disciplines, such as social workers, nutritionists, or physical therapists. However, this relationship is consultative and if interventions result for nursing diagnoses from this consultation, the nurse will place these orders on the nursing care plan for other nursing staff to implement.

. . . Achievement of Outcomes. . .

At the Sixth NANDA Conference, McCourt stated "How better to assess the effectiveness of nursing care than to evaluate outcomes of health problems which nurses diagnose and treat?" (1986, p. 133). The literature is full of definitions of outcome criteria or client goals, including

- Statements describing a measurable behavior of client/family/group, which denote a favorable status (changed or maintained) after nursing care has been delivered (Alfaro, 1986)
- Changes in health status resulting from nursing interventions (McCourt, 1986)
- Standards used to determine the responses to or results of nursing interventions (Pinnell & Meneses, 1986)

Expected outcomes serve as criteria on which to judge the success of nursing interventions (Gordon, 1982; Carpenito, 1983; Field & Winslow, 1985; McCloskey, 1985). They serve as indices to evaluate the quality and efficiency of nursing interventions. The nurse must assess the client's or group's present response and compare it to the projected desired response or outcome criteria. If no progress toward outcome achievement is seen, the nurse must reevaluate the situation: Is the diagnosis correct? Has the goal been mutually set? Is more time needed for the plan to work? Does the goal need to be revised? Does the plan need to be

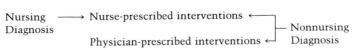

FIGURE 2   Relationships of nursing interventions to type of diagnoses

revised? Are physician-prescribed interventions needed?

Outcomes for nursing diagnoses will not serve to evaluate the effectiveness of nursing interventions if physician interventions are also needed.

. . . for Which the Nurse Is Accountable . . .

Accountable is defined as subject to giving an account, to explain, to be liable; to furnish substantial reasons or a convincing explanation (*Webster's*, 1976).

Nurses are intricately involved in the diagnosis and treatment of many problems and situations. For example, a nurse can diagnose dysrhythmias, a cerebral vascular accident, and Lyme's disease, but the nurse cannot assume accountability for the treatment; physician-initiated interventions are needed. Certain diagnoses may involve several disciplines—anxiety, for example. The physician may prescribe a medication, the occupational therapist may provide diversional activity, and the nurse may prescribe several anxiety-reducing interventions such as relaxation exercises or problem-solving strategies. Gordon wrote that "saying a nursing diagnosis is a health problem a nurse can treat does not mean that nonnursing consultants cannot be used" (1982, p. 4). The critical element is whether the nurse-prescribed intervention can achieve the outcome established with the client.

Legally, nurses have been held accountable to diagnose problems that are beyond the domain of nursing (Fortin & Rabinow, 1979). Gordon writes that "interpreting signs and symptoms and judging how to treat them (nursing diagnoses) or making referrals (tentative medical diagnoses) are nursing responsibilities" (1982, p. 267).

Gordon (1982) described three types of definitions of nursing diagnoses: conceptual, structural, and contextual. Conceptual definition communicates the meaning of nursing diagnoses (diagnostic responsibility and

focus). Structural definition describes the components of a nursing diagnosis statement. Contextual definition describes the relationship of the nursing diagnoses to other ideas or concepts as "the nursing process." The proposed NANDA definition represents a conceptual definition. Shoemaker (1984) presented the essential features of a nursing diagnosis resulting from a Delphi study and grouped them into three categories: generic features, differentiation features, and condition features. Table 1 represents Shoemaker's essential features and the type of definition they would be associated with. Table 2 repre-

Table 1: Essential Features of a Nursing Diagnosis Grouped under a Conceptual, Structural, or Contextual Definition

Definition	Generic Features Considered Essential
Conceptual	A nursing diagnosis is a statement of a patient-client problem.
Conceptual	A nursing diagnosis refers to a health state.
Conceptual	A nursing diagnosis refers to a potential health problem.
Contextual	A nursing diagnosis is a conclusion resulting from identification of a pattern or cluster of signs and symptoms.
Contextual	A nursing diagnosis is based on subjective or objective data that can be confirmed.

Definition	Differentiation Features Considered Essential
Conceptual	A nursing diagnosis is a statement of a nursing judgment.
Conceptual	A nursing diagnosis refers to a condition that nurses are licensed to treat.
Conceptual	A nursing diagnosis refers to physical, psychologic, sociocultural, and spiritual conditions.
Structural	A nursing diagnosis is a short, concise statement.

(continued)

Table 1: (*Continued*)

Structural	A nursing diagnosis is a two-part statement that includes the etiology, when known.

Definition	Condition Features Considered Essential
Conceptual	A nursing diagnosis refers to conditions that can be treated independently by a nurse.
?	Nurse practitioners who function in expanded roles should clearly differentiate between the nursing and the medical diagnoses they make.
?	A nursing diagnosis should be validated with the client whenever possible.
?	Diagnosing is an independent nursing function.

SOURCE: Essential features from Shoemaker, J. (1984). "Essential Features of a Nursing Diagnosis," in M. J. Kim, G. McFarland, & A. M. McLane (Eds.), *Classification of Nursing Diagnosis: Proceedings of the Fifth National Conference.* St. Louis: Mosby.

Table 2: Essential Features for a Conceptual Definition of Nursing Diagnosis

A nursing diagnosis is a **clinical judgment** . . .
   [A nursing diagnosis is a statement of a nursing judgment.]
   . . . about individual, family, or **community responses** . . .
[A nursing diagnosis is a statement of a patient-client problem.]
   [A nursing diagnosis refers to a health state.]
   [A nursing diagnosis refers to a potential health problem.]
   [A nursing diagnosis refers to physical, psychologic, sociocultural, and spiritual conditions.]
to actual or potential health problems/life processes that provide the **basis for definitive therapy** toward achievement of outcome for which the nurse is accountable.
   [A nursing diagnosis refers to a condition that nurses are licensed to treat.]
   [A nursing diagnosis refers to conditions that can be treated independently by a nurse.]

sents only those essential features that apply to a conceptual definition of nursing diagnoses and their representation in the NANDA definition.

NANDA has been recognized as the official organization to classify nursing diagnoses, but has been engaged in approving and classifying nursing diagnoses without an official conceptual definition for 17 years. A NANDA definition of nursing diagnosis is not just desirable, it is imperative.

References

Alfaro, R. (1986). *Application of nursing process: A step by step guide.* Philadelphia: Lippincott.

American Nurses' Association. (1980). *Nursing: A social policy statement.* Kansas City, MO: Author.

Aspinall, M. J., & Tanner, C. (1981). *Decision making for patient care.* Norwalk, CT: Appleton-Century-Croft.

Bernzweig, E. P. (1969). *Nursing liability for malpractice.* New York: McGraw-Hill.

Bulechek, G., & McCloskey, J. (1985). *Nursing interventions: Treatments for nursing diagnosis.* Philadelphia: Saunders.

Bulechek, G., & McCloskey, J. (1989). Nursing interventions: Treatments for potential nursing diagnoses. In R. M. Carroll-Johnson (Ed.), *Classification of nursing diagnoses: Proceedings of the eighth conference* (pp. 23–30). Philadelphia: Lippincott.

Carpenito, L. J. (1983). *Nursing diagnosis: Application to clinical practice.* Philadelphia: Lippincott.

Field, L., & Winslow, E. H. (1985). Moving to a nursing model. *American Journal of Nursing, 85,* 1100–1101.

Fortin, J. D., & Rabinow, J. (1979). Legal implications of nursing diagnosis. *Nursing Clinics of North America, 14,* 553–561.

Gebbie, K., & Lavin, M. A. (1975). *Classification of nursing diagnoses: Proceedings of the first national conference.* St. Louis, MO: Mosby.

Gordon, M. (1976). Nursing diagnosis and the diagnostic process. *American Journal of Nursing, 76,* 1276–1300.

Gordon, M. (1982). *Nursing diagnosis: Process and application.* New York: McGraw-Hill.

McCourt, A. (1986). Nursing diagnoses: Key to quality assurance. In M. Hurley (Ed.), *Classification of nursing diagnosis: Proceedings of the sixth national conference* (pp. 133–138). St. Louis, MO: Mosby.

Northrop, C., & Kelly, M. (1987). *Legal issues in nursing.* St. Louis, MO: Mosby.

Pinnell, M., & Meneses, M. (1986). *The nursing process.* Norwalk, CT: Appleton-Century-Croft.

Shoemaker, J. (1984). Essential features of a nursing diagnosis. In M. J. Kim, G. McFarland, & A. McLane (Eds.), *Classification of nursing diagnoses: Proceedings of the fifth national conference* (pp. 104–112). St. Louis, MO: Mosby.

Webster, G. (1984). Nomenclature and classification system development. In M. J. Kim, G. McFarland, & A. McLane (Eds.), *Classification of nursing diagnoses: Proceedings of the fifth national conference* (pp. 14–24). St. Louis, MO: Mosby.

Webster's Third New International Dictionary (Unabridged). (1976). Springfield, MA: Merriam.

Signs and Symptoms, Etiologies, Diagnostic Labels: What Do We Mean and Where Do We Want to Go?

Brooke P. Randell, DNSc, RN

Signs and symptoms, etiologies, diagnostic labels, where does one begin and the other end? How can we tell when we have one or the other? On the occasion of our visit to Orlando and our proximity to the "Magic Kingdom," I find the characters of Fantasyland offer some apt analogies to our experience.

Remember *Alice in Wonderland?* At the tea party Alice talks with the March Hare and the Mad Hatter; Alice is asked a riddle and replies:

"I believe I can guess that!"
"Do you mean that you think you can find out the answer to it?" said the March Hare.
"Exactly so," said Alice.
"Then you should say what you mean," the March Hare went on.
"I do," Alice hastily replied; "at least—at least I mean what I say—that's the same thing, you know."
"Not the same thing a bit!" said the Hatter. "Why, you might just as well say that 'I see what I eat' is the same thing as 'I eat what I see'!" (Carroll, 1946, p. 78).

It has been the experience of the Diagnosis Review Committee (DRC) that submitters, like Alice, do mean what they say, but do not always say what they mean.

In reviewing submissions, the DRC must constantly deal with issues of differentiation and are confronted with questions regarding the nature of the diagnostic statement. We must be clear on when a sign or symptom ceases to be such and becomes a diagnostic statement. It has also been emphatically stated that a diagnostic statement can never be an etiology! But a diagnostic statement can be an etiology for another diagnostic statement. Hence the relevance of *Alice in Wonderland.*

While the DRC constantly grapples with the question of whether the diagnosis truly says what is meant, the submitter must often feel as if dealing with the DRC comes close to dealing with the Mad Hatter. As an outsider I often wondered about the process and felt that the solutions I had would solve the problems of this troubled process. The experience of working with the DRC has extinguished my belief in simple solutions.

The person and his or her human responses represent a set of extremely complex and ever-changing phenomena. The process of capturing this elusive complexity is a difficult task. Because the process of creating diagnostic labels is largely driven by a diverse and ever-evolving nursing practice, DRC solutions or guidelines emerge out of experience and therefore are difficult to anticipate prior to their occurrence.

What is being proposed is the latest and most definitive perspective on what counts as a diagnostic label, as well as what constitutes an adequate defense of that label. It is the intent of the DRC to create a circumstance where it is possible for Alice to say what she means by defining what it is that the DRC currently needs to know. The DRC intends to clarify issues around signs and symptoms and etiologies so that the submitter can then address these dilemmas prior to submission, thereby facilitating the review process.

A sign, by definition, is a signifier of something. In the generic sense the word 'sign' is considered as an object, action, event, pattern, etc., that conveys a meaning (*The Random House Dictionary of the English Language*, 1987). In the technical sense, a sign is an entity that signifies some other thing and may be interpreted (*McGraw-Hill Dictionary of Scientific and Technical Terms*, 1984). In medicine, a sign is any objective evidence of disease (*Dorland's Illustrated Medical Dictionary*, 1988).

The generic definition of a symptom does not differ remarkably from that of a sign. According to the Random House dictionary, any phenomenon or circumstance accompanying something and serving as evidence of it is a symptom. While a sign is thought to represent objective evidence of a phenomenon, a symptom, as defined technically and medically, reflects subjective experience. A symptom is a phenomenon of physical or mental disorder or disturbance that leads to complaints on the part of the patient (*McGraw-Hill Dictionary of Scientific and Technical Terms*). More specifically, a symptom is any subjective evidence of disease or of a patient's

condition, i.e., such evidence as perceived by the patient (*Dorland's Illustrated Medical Dictionary*). Finally, etiology is universally understood as the cause or origin of disease.

How are these terms then used in the nursing diagnosis literature? A diagnostic statement is a two- or three-part statement consisting of a diagnostic label, related factors, and signs and symptoms. These diagnostic statements may also be called nursing diagnoses.

An actual nursing diagnosis is written in three parts: a diagnostic label related to etiologic or contributing factors as evidenced by validating signs and symptoms (e.g., *impaired skin integrity* related to pressure and shear as evidenced by a 2-cm lesion on the left trochanter). A high-risk nursing diagnosis is written in two parts with the term 'high risk' preceding the diagnostic label and the related risk factors (e.g., *high-risk impaired skin integrity* related to immobility and incontinence).

While signs, symptoms, and etiology are usually associated with disease, the generic definitions of these words, with the exception of etiology, allow for the broader interpretation used in the nursing literature. Generally when a single nursing diagnosis is examined, signs and symptoms are cited as evidence of the health problem and related factors are considered contributory or causal. On other occasions, when the existing list of nursing diagnoses as a whole is examined, it would appear that some diagnoses are themselves signs, symptoms, or etiologies.

Given the new definition of nursing diagnosis and these definitions of signs, symptoms, and etiologies, how will the DRC review diagnostic submissions and draw these essential boundaries?

First, the DRC will determine if the label is consistent with the NANDA definition— that is, does the label represent a clinical judgment about individual, family, or community responses to actual or potential health problems/life processes, and do these nursing diagnoses provide the basis for the selection of nursing interventions to achieve outcomes for which the nurse is accountable?

Diagnoses have been submitted that are not consistent with this definition. For example, miscarriage or spontaneous abortion does not represent a response for which the nurse can be held accountable for outcomes. From the perspective of the DRC, such a label clearly deviates from the definition, but given the number of submissions that reflect this deviation, there are many submitters who might disagree. A submitter who knows his or her diagnosis is likely to be considered in this light should be prepared to offer evidence in support of the diagnosis as a nursing phenomenon for which a nurse is accountable.

The second determination will be whether the diagnosis represents a cluster of critical descriptors that clearly label a health problem. In this instance the issue is scope. Is the diagnosis sufficiently broad to describe a problem, or is it so narrow that it represents only a sign or symptom? Gordon (1982) states that a single sign or symptom does not represent a diagnostic label. In general, such a label is too narrow in scope and does not state the problem in a manner that guides nursing intervention. Signs and symptoms should represent a cluster of critical descriptors that permit the nurse to identify the client's particular health problem (Gordon, 1982).

When the current list of diagnoses is reviewed, certain labels are quite narrow while others appear overly broad. For example, the diagnostic label of *fatigue* is also a defining characteristic associated with the diagnostic label of *activity intolerance*. Clearly both labels represent discrete phenomena that often require nursing activities. At what level is nursing activity directed? Do nurses intervene with fatigue per se, or is fatigue not a defining characteristic or etiologic factor associated with many diagnostic labels?

Looking at a broader scope, consider the diagnostic label of *altered growth and development*. As a child psychiatric nurse who has dealt with developmentally disabled populations for many years, I cannot dispute the validity of the label, but I must question its utility. Does the nurse truly intervene with the alteration in growth and development, or are our activities more accurately targeted at some of the defining characteristics associated with this diagnosis (e.g., inability to perform self-care)?

What is involved here is the level of specificity. If the diagnostic label to be submitted exists in another diagnosis as a sign or a symptom, how will the increased specificity of an additional diagnosis be useful to nurses? How does the submitter defend separating out a portion of another diagnosis? The nursing diagnosis *fatigue* is a diagnostic label itself and is also a defining characteristic associated with another nursing diagnosis, *activity intolerance*. When is *fatigue* the correct diagnosis, and when is *activity intolerance* appropriate? Would it be necessary to use both diagnoses to characterize a problem when the broader diagnosis would have been sufficient? It would seem if one diagnosis represents a major defining characteristic of another diagnosis, the higher-level problem will always exist and the nurse will need to diagnose and intervene with both problems.

Gordon (1982) states that nursing should seek a middle ground between overgeneralization and overspecificity. Diagnoses should not be so broad as to provide no useful direction for intervention, nor so narrow that applicability is limited (Gordon, 1982). What we are seeking reminds me of Goldilocks and her visit to the three bears. We want diagnoses that are not too broad, not too narrow, but just right. In the current process of diagnostic proliferation, we have paid little attention to each diagnosis within the context of other diagnoses. The multiple levels of specificity must be consciously addressed or we will have an enormous and unwieldy list that has no utility or meaning for anyone.

Finally, there is the question of etiology, an issue alluded to in this discussion on diagnostic specificity. Is an etiology ever a diagnosis? It depends. When an etiology is a human response then it could be a diagnostic label (e.g., *impaired physical mobility* related to *activity intolerance*). This particular inconsistency in the diagnostic process, as well as the differentiation of signs and symptoms from diagnostic labels, is a product of our commitment to wholism. The process of diagnostic labeling takes apart that which we understand to be an inseparable whole. The process of taking apart is engaged in for the purpose of explaining relationships and communicating our understanding of those relationships. Simultaneously we recognize that the separations are somewhat arbitrary and inconsistent with our belief in wholism. Where to draw the lines and how to differentiate between signs and symptoms and etiologies will therefore remain a problem to which we must constantly attend. The current three-level system proposed by the Taxonomy Committee would provide direction for definitive work in determining what counts as a "just right" diagnostic label.

Gordon (1982) describes etiologic factors as subcategories of a diagnostic category, factors that suggest the primary reasons for the problem and the focus of the nursing therapy. Frequently, diagnostic labels are submitted because they are the focus of nursing therapy, not because they are the problem or the human response (e.g., inadequate surgical preparation). The human response might be *noncompliance* while the etiologic factor was inadequate surgical preparation.

A final issue related to etiologies is encountered when the etiology is embedded in the diagnostic label. For example, if written correctly a diagnosis might read *stress incontinence* related to weakened pelvic muscles as evidenced by reported or observed dribbling. This is a redundant statement. There-fore the current structure of the diagnostic statement leads us to question the appropriateness of the label.

We must proceed with care for we have reached a critical juncture. It is the position of the DRC that all diagnostic label submissions must be (1) consistent with the NANDA definition of nursing diagnosis, and (2) defended in relationship to existing diagnoses or represent a modification or extension of an existing diagnosis. Lack of consistency with the definition should weed out submissions that do not represent phenomena of concern to nurses. Identification of the diagnostic label's relationship to other labels will require attention to level and scope and the clear differentiation among label, signs and symptoms, and etiologies. If this burgeoning body of work is to survive, clinical utility and relevance to clinical practice remain critical aspects of the decision-making process, but nursing must also attend to conceptual issues and scientific rigor. The DRC invites your comments and dialogue regarding this proposed course of action. In conclusion, I suggest we heed the words of the Cheshire Cat:

"Would you tell me, please, which way I ought to go from here?" Alice asks.

"That depends a good deal on where you want to get to," said the Cat. (Carroll, 1946, p. 71)

References

Carroll, L. (1946). *Alice's adventures in wonderland.* New York: Random House.

Dorland's illustrated medical dictionary (27th ed.). (1988). Philadelphia: Saunders.

Gordon, M. (1982). *Nursing diagnosis: Process and application.* New York: McGraw-Hill.

McGraw-Hill dictionary of scientific and technical terms (3rd ed.). (1984). New York: McGraw-Hill.

Random House dictionary of the English language (2nd ed.). (1987). New York: Random House.

Defining Characteristics: General or Population Specific

Karen Goyette-Vincent, MSN, RN, CS

There have been varying debates within the profession about nursing diagnosis since its "birth" in the 1970s. These include debates of "whether" nursing diagnosis, "why" nursing diagnosis, "can nurses diagnose?" and "where are physiologic and other specialty-specific nursing diagnoses to be placed within a holistic taxonomy?" Some issues continue to be the focus of question and analysis in many arenas: academia, the clinical setting, and within the organization of NANDA. As the nursing diagnostic taxonomy has become more sophisticated, the questions have become more complex.

The purpose of this paper is to describe yet another debate: Should the defining characteristics within a diagnosis remain general or should they identify population-specific differences? This issue arose during the Diagnostic Review Committee (DRC)'s discussions about several diagnoses in this review cycle. For example, during one review the Committee used the American Nurses' Association (ANA) document "Standards of Addictions Nursing Practice with Selected Diagnoses and Criteria" (1988). These standards utilize NANDA-approved nursing diagnoses. However, the defining characteristics of several diagnoses are identified as being different for patients in this particular specialty and setting.

The issue arose a second time when several reviewers questioned the applicability or appropriateness of the defining characteristics for a particular diagnosis for different age groups. Often, the diagnostic categories did not include signs and symptoms or behaviors that reflected the same problem for patients across the life span. This issue was raised separately by the Taxonomy Committee and discussed in an earlier paper (see page 38). This presentation provided further evidence that there is a pattern emerging for several issues. From the DRC perspective, what should be our response to these questions when they are presented by reviewers over time and with different proposed diagnoses? The DRC cannot answer this important question in isolation. The input of the membership is needed for development of clearer guidelines for diagnosis submission and, ultimately, increased refinement of the taxonomy. The goal of this presentation will be to frame the choices—the argument for specifying population differences within a diagnosis, and the position supporting keeping the defining characteristics general. In this discussion, 'population' will refer to either specialty, health care setting, or age.

Acknowledging the behavioral differences for specific populations within diagnoses has been proposed. At present the defining characteristics of several diagnoses are viewed as too broad and abstract. For example, the most common complaint with the diagnosis *ineffective individual coping* is that the defining characteristics are so broad (e.g., inappropriate use of defense mechanisms), that it is difficult to describe actual patient behaviors and to use the diagnosis to plan specific interventions for the patient. If the defining characteristics classified patient behaviors specifically according to setting or specialty (e.g., the addicted patient in a rehabilitation setting), this diagnosis could potentially be much more helpful in identifying patients at risk and in planning care.

There also may be diagnoses that are present in both the elderly and adolescent, but the behaviors exhibited are different for the two age groups. For example, the phenomenon of failure to thrive is found in both nursing and medical literature. Yet the behaviors, or potential defining characteristics, for this diagnosis may be quite different for the elderly versus infants. The diagnosis should reflect those differences. Similarly, the diagnosis of *dysfunctional grieving* is manifested differently by small children, who may exhibit specific age regression behaviors, severe withdrawal, or exaggerated activity. These behaviors are much more specific than the general behaviors currently identified.

If each nursing diagnosis contained the behaviors or signs and symptoms exhibited by patients in various populations, then each diagnostic category would more likely be inclusive of all patient phenomena to describe the human response. The result could then be less likelihood of diagnostic error across specialty or health care setting, and with different age groups. Research on the validation

of diagnoses across populations would also be enhanced. Although the amount of nursing diagnosis research has increased dramatically in the last five years, there has not been sufficient research to validate the diagnoses with different populations in the clinical field. Perhaps enlarging the specificity of the diagnosis would guide research in this area.

The Diagnostic and Statistical Manual III (Revised) (DSM-III–R) of the American Psychiatric Association (APA, 1987) provides an example of how one profession accounts for age-related differences in diagnostics. DSM-III–R classifies age-related differences in two ways. Disorders that manifest themselves in children during infancy, childhood, or adolescence are listed separately within the taxonomy. The manual also includes age-specific features within the text of the diagnostic category. For example, the patient behaviors indicative of major depressive episode are listed with age-specific features to describe how major depressive episode is manifested in children or adolescents (APA, 1987). How would population-specific defining characteristics appear in a nursing taxonomy? One suggestion is that the nursing diagnosis indicate *nursing diagnosis (specify population)*. For example, upon submission of the proposed diagnosis, specifying age would delimit the boundaries of the diagnosis and facilitate the work of the Committee. It is not yet clear how population-specific differences would appear within the diagnostic category. It is clear, though, that several deficits within the nursing taxonomy may be resolved by including defining characteristics that are population specific within each nursing diagnosis.

There is the option of keeping the defining characteristics within the diagnosis general and not specific to population. Are diagnoses with age-range, specialty, or setting differences actually different nursing diagnoses? The argument in support of this position is founded in the belief that nursing diagnosis reflects the holistic nature of nursing. The purpose of taxonomy development has been to provide a common language so that a description of patient phenomena by nurses working with different populations enables a reciprocal understanding of the problem (Carnevali, 1974; Gordon, 1987). Nursing diagnosis provides a model that can be generalizable across specialty, age range, and setting (Hinshaw, 1989). It may then be important to keep the defining characteristics general and, instead, add to the taxonomy those phenomena that have not been described as diagnoses. When the clusters of behaviors or signs and symptoms that describe a human response are behavioral and generic, they apply to patients with that specific problem response. If differences exist in the patient/client presentation, then a different nursing diagnosis may exist. For example, a hypothetical diagnosis of *family caregiver strain* pertains to caring for the elderly patient at home. If the patient being cared for were a child, this diagnosis would then more appropriately be named *alteration in parenting*. In this way the diagnostic label clearly involves a patient within a particular age range.

Again, there is a paucity of research validation studies available to compare the validation of defining characteristics of diagnoses across populations. The majority of research presented at previous NANDA conferences has studied nursing diagnoses with either the same patient population or with nurse expert consultants. Whitley (1989) summarized the reports of two separate clinical validation studies conducted on the diagnosis *anxiety*, utilizing patients in medical-surgical settings and patients in their third trimester of pregnancy. The frequency of occurrence of the defining characteristics with different populations was analyzed. The studies showed no agreement in the critical defining characteristics that are present for this diagnosis. If specialty-specific research is conducted, then the yield of this research may again be more specific parameters of defining characteristics within the diagnosis. Those behavioral clusters found outside the parameters would then be separately labeled diagnoses.

After having assessed both perspectives of the question of population differences in diagnoses, the question may be posed, "Are the behaviors of certain age groups or patients in specialty settings so different? If so, do they represent completely different human responses to health problems?" The DRC invites the guidance of NANDA's membership as it continues the process of diagnosis review and acceptance.

References

American Psychiatric Association. (1987). *Diagnostic and statistical manual of mental disorders* (3rd ed. rev.). Washington, DC: Author.

American Nurses' Association. (1988). *Standards of addictions nursing practice with selected diagnoses and criteria.* Kansas City, MO: Author.

Carnevali, D. L. (1984). Nursing diagnosis: An evolutional view. *Topics in Clinical Nursing,* 5(4), 10–20.

Gordon, M. (1987). *Nursing diagnosis: Process and application* (2nd ed.). New York: McGraw-Hill.

Hinshaw, A. (1989). Nursing diagnosis: Forging the link between theory and practice. In R. M. Carroll-Johnson (Ed.), *Classification of nursing diagnoses: Proceedings of the eighth conference* (pp. 3–10). Philadelphia: Lippincott.

Whitley, G. (1989). An analysis of the nursing diagnosis anxiety. In R. M. Carroll-Johnson (Ed.), *Classification of nursing diagnoses: Proceedings of the eighth conference* (pp. 371–375). Philadelphia: Lippincott.

Syndromes in Nursing: A Continuing Concern

Ann E. McCourt, MS, RN

Syndromes in nursing are a continuing concern of the Diagnosis Review Committee (DRC). Does a syndrome differ from other nursing diagnoses? How are nursing syndromes being used? Why are they being developed? These are the concerns of the Committee.

What is a syndrome? There is a field of study known as syndromology. Landau (1986) described syndromology as the interdisciplinary study of the causes, mechanisms, and manifestations of syndromes or of aggregates of signs and symptoms suspected of being associated by more than chance occurrence. The DRC's concern is not with individual health-related syndromes, of which there are more than 2,700, but rather with how a syndrome is defined.

The word *syndrome* is derived from Greek and means "running together." Definitions of syndrome found in dictionaries, encyclopedias, and texts (*Blackiston's Gould Medical Dictionary*, 1979; *Dorland's Illustrated Medical Dictionary*, 1981; Jablonski, 1969; Landau, 1986; Magalini & Scrascia, 1981; *Melloni's Illustrated Medical Dictionary*, 1985; Miller & Keane, 1983; Roper & Boorkman, 1984; Skinner, 1961; *Taber's Cyclopedic Medical Dictionary*, 1985; *Webster's*

New World Dictionary, 1980) were reviewed to determine any consensus on the definition and characteristics of a syndrome. There was consensus that a syndrome (as used in medicine and related fields) is a cluster or group of signs and symptoms that almost always occur together. Together, these clusters represent a distinct clinical picture. Jablonski (1969) stated that a syndrome usually incorporates three or more symptoms occurring together. There were several etiologic considerations, ranging from syndromes always having a single cause (Miller & Keane, 1983) to syndromes being used when there is no known cause (Landau, 1986). Nonmedical definitions of syndrome include a group of related or coincident things, events, or actions; a predictable characteristic pattern of behavior (*Random House Dictionary of the English Language*, 1987); or any set of characteristics regarded as identifying a certain type of condition (*Webster's New World Dictionary*, 1980).

A limited Med-Line search, although primarily detailing specific syndromes, revealed that new medical syndromes are being described at the rate of one or more per week (Toriello, 1988).

In addition to the literature review, the National Library of Medicine in Washington, DC, was contacted to determine whether the World Health Organization (WHO) had officially defined syndrome. The reference librarian indicated that insofar as she could determine, neither WHO nor its International Classification of Diseases group has published a definition for syndrome. She did provide additional references, noting that as early as 1900 Dorland defined a syndrome as "symptoms running together." This is not unlike the current definition.

As previously mentioned, the DRC needs to know how nursing syndromes differ from other nursing diagnoses, how nursing syndromes are being used, and why additional syndromes are being developed. As present, two nursing syndromes have been approved by NANDA—*rape trauma syndrome* in 1980, and *potential disuse syndrome* in 1988. Others, including *relocation syndrome* and *translocation syndrome*, have been proposed but require further development.

During the NANDA approval process, the DRC solicits the opinion of several reviewers. Their comments and suggestions are compiled and presented to the Committee for discussion and further consideration. While reviewing a recently submitted syndrome, it became clear to the Committee that confusion exists over the difference between the defining characteristics of a syndrome and those of other diagnoses. NANDA's Taxonomy I Revised (1989) states that defining characteristics are clinical criteria that represent the presence of the diagnostic category. This is not particularly helpful in differentiating between syndromes and less complex diagnoses. The reviewers' concern was whether the defining characteristics of a syndrome represent a cluster of signs and symptoms or a cluster of other nursing diagnoses or health problems. Recently submitted syndromes appear to represent a cluster of nursing diagnoses.

The clustering of problems (specific diagnoses) into a single label can be clinically useful. Esposito, Tracey, and McCourt (1989) developed and submitted *disuse syndrome, actual and potential.* This diagnosis grew out of a rehabilitation nursing practice, where nurses were observed separately documenting problems that almost always occurred together and that shared a common related factor (etiology). For example, *potential for impaired skin integrity, potential for contractures, potential for constipation,* etc., were separately documented but were all related to prolonged immobilization and disuse. These and other problems that usually occurred together were combined into *potential disuse syndrome.* This is a label that clinicians find understandable, meaningful, and efficient. Not only did the new syndrome decrease the number of problems being documented, the same interventions (e.g., turn and position every two hours) were not continually repeated. These are strong arguments for the development of nursing syndromes.

The next question considered similarities shared by the current syndromes. In looking at the diagnostic labels, the syndromes would seem to be etiologically defined. That is, the diagnostic label contains the primary etiologic factor for the cluster of diagnoses represented in the category. *Rape trauma syndrome, disuse syndrome,* and *translocation* and *relocation syndrome* clue us not only into the problem but also into the related factor or probable cause.

As noted, the defining characteristics of the syndromes tend to represent a cluster of nursing diagnoses or other health problems: that is, certain diagnoses almost always occur together forming a cluster or set that is given a syndrome label. *Rape trauma syndrome* was submitted many years ago when fewer labels existed. Today, the defining characteristics of *rape trauma syndrome* could be represented by several nursing diagnoses as well as other health problems.

Of two previously submitted syndromes, *potential disuse syndrome* and *disuse syn-*

drome, only the former was approved by the DRC. Thus the characteristics of *actual disuse syndrome* are not available and therefore are not part of the classification. In Taxonomy I, an attempt is made to resolve this problem by placing an asterisk after the diagnoses and then listing the complications that might ensue. Perhaps the real problem is that there cannot be a "potential" syndrome. Rather, there are stages or phases of syndromes, with potential represented in the initial phase. In this case, *disuse syndrome* would be the diagnosis and the defining characteristics would be a set of high-risk states. If major complications arise, such as level 3 to 4 pressure ulcer, the DRC suggests that they should be listed separately or referred to other health care professionals.

Rape trauma syndrome, as approved, has both an acute phase and a long-term phase. *Disuse syndrome*, as originally submitted, had short- and long-term stages and there is supporting evidence that *translocation syndrome* also has initial and long-term stages (Rantz & Eagan, 1987). The presence of stages or phases might represent another differentiating characteristic of syndromes.

In comparing the syndromes mentioned in this paper, it was also apparent that their defining characteristics represent physical, social, and emotional components. One thing is certain: Nursing diagnosis syndromes represent complex clinical conditions requiring expert nursing assessments and expert nursing interventions.

In summary the following can be said:

- Nurses are submitting diagnostic labels that include the term syndrome.
- A syndrome is defined as a group or cluster of signs and symptoms that almost always occur together.
- The two currently approved nursing syndromes are *rape trauma syndrome* and *potential disuse syndrome*.
- Common characteristics of reviewed syndromes would appear to be

1. Syndromes represent a cluster of nursing diagnoses.
2. Their labels give clue to the cause.
3. Syndromes have initial and long-term phases.
4. Syndromes have emotional, social, and physical components.
5. Syndromes represent complex clinical conditions requiring expert nursing assessment and expert nursing interventions.

In the future, the DRC and NANDA must consider a number of issues: Should we continue to support the use of nursing diagnosis syndromes? If we continue to use syndromes, how should they be defined? Can there be a "potential" nursing syndrome? Are there existing nursing diagnoses that should be nursing syndromes? Where would syndromes fit in the Taxonomy if the related diagnoses represent more than one human response pattern? The answer to these and other questions will be forthcoming in the years ahead.

References

Blackiston's Gould medical dictionary (4th ed.). (1979). New York: McGraw-Hill.

Dorland's illustrated medical dictionary (26th ed.). (1981). Philadelphia: Saunders.

Esposito, M. C., Tracey, C., & McCourt, A. (1989). Nursing diagnosis: Potential for disuse syndrome. In R. M. Carroll-Johnson (Ed.), *Classification of nursing diagnoses: Proceedings of the eighth conference* (pp. 464–468). Philadelphia: Lippincott.

Jablonski, S. (1969). *Illustrated dictionary of eponymic syndromes and diseases and their synonyms.* Philadelphia: Saunders.

Landau, S. (Ed.). (1986). *International dictionary of medicine and biology* (Vol. 3). New York: Wiley.

Magalini, S., & Scrascia, E. (1981). *Dictionary of medical syndromes* (2nd ed.). Philadelphia: Lippincott.

Melloni's illustrated medical dictionary (2nd ed.). (1985). Baltimore: Williams & Wilkins.

Miller, B., & Keane, C. (1983). *Encyclopedia and dictionary of medicine, nursing and allied health* (1983). Philadelphia: Saunders.

North American Nursing Diagnosis Association. (1989). *Taxonomy I revised.* St. Louis, MO: Author.

Random House dictionary of the English language (2nd ed.). (1987). New York: Random House.

Rantz, M., & Eagan, K. (1987). Reducing death from translocation syndrome. *American Journal of Nursing, 87,* 1351–1352.

Roper, F., & Boorkman, J. (1984). *Introduction to reference sources in the health sciences.* Chicago: Medical Library Association.

Skinner, H. (1961). *The original of medical terms.* Baltimore: Williams & Wilkins.

Taber's cyclopedic medical dictionary (15th ed.). (1985). Philadelphia: Davis.

Toriello, H. (1988). New syndromes from old: Evaluation of heterogeneity and variability in syndrome definition and delineation. *American Journal of Medical Genetics—Supplement, 4,* 55–70.

Webster's new world dictionary (2nd college ed.). (1980). Springfield, MA: Merriam.

Discussion

Definition of a Nursing Diagnosis

Editor's Note: Additional information and discussion regarding the working definition of nursing diagnosis can be found in Section VI in the Minutes of the Business Meeting and the submitted report of the Diagnosis Review Committee.

VICTORIA COLE SCHOENLAU: I'm speaking on behalf of the Wellness Interest Group. We were very pleased to see the definition include "life processes" because of our concern about wellness in promoting health. We did have some concerns about the way that some of [the definition] was worded. Since the focus of nursing is really to look at preventing a lot of health problems, we would like to see the definition worded "response to life processes and risk or actual health problems," so that the focus was on prevention first and restoration second. We also looked at the word "therapy" and looking at definitions, it really was much more of a medical model in terms of treating illness or disability. We thought that the word "actions" really was more encompassing of a broader spectrum of what nurses do including treatment and therapy. Action is a much less discriminatory word and implies much more what nurses do as opposed to medical model.

LYNDA CARPENITO: I would agree with [what you said about] the term "therapy." When I went to the dictionary and found the defini-

tion, it truly was a medical view of prescriptions. The term "action" from my standpoint sounds like an immediate kind of thing and I'm not so sure it denotes, or connotes a plan, but that just may be semantics.

KRISTINE GEBBIE: I'd like some clarification on that inclusion about the basis for definitive "action" or "therapy." The diagnoses with which this organization has worked so far have primarily been ones that have been treated by nurses for a long time, so that the label and intervention connection is very clear. As we move forward as a profession, it seems very likely that we will, in fact, be able to identify, label, and reach a common understanding of conditions for which a therapy has yet to be invented. That is true in our related disciplines. If you needed a definitive therapy, AIDS still wouldn't be a proper diagnosis. How do we interpret that word, it is limiting or is it opening for that?

LYNDA CARPENITO: Your example of AIDS, I think, is a good one. I think that we have to assume that right now the therapy provided by medicine is the most definitive that they can provide. I question the value of placing situations on a list called Nursing Diagnoses for which we have no treatment. I'm not saying that necessarily we have closed the house on the treatment for that set, and when we look at proposed guidelines for developing nursing diagnoses, you will see we have asked for a sample for a particular diagnosis that is being submitted. But from a legal standpoint, do we define nursing accountable to something called a nursing diagnosis, then label something for which we have no treatment? But [we] use the word "definitive" from the standpoint of most authoritative discipline for that situation.

LAURA ROSSI: I'm wondering if there was any discussion about the use of nursing diagnoses by other disciplines. And I think it's particularly important to hear some comment about that with the introduction of it into the ICD-10. It would seem as though then it is truly in the public domain.

LYNDA CARPENITO: I am aware, and certainly the Board and the two Committees are aware, of other disciplines using nursing diagnosis, for example, my paper "Diversional Activity Deficit, Impaired Physical Mobility." It's problematic; it would be problematic to say to a physical therapist or an occupational therapist, you cannot use this term when, as nurses, we have used the term diabetes mellitus on our care plans for at least the first 15 years that I have been a nurse. I'm not opposed to entering into that discussion. In fact, I would be very interested in how we could as an association address that issue. But I think we have also walked in those moccasins as nurses, using the terminology of physicians.

LAURA ROSSI: I only bring it up because I think it also has an issue in terms of how we define non-nursing diagnoses, are they really collaborative problems or are they really medical diagnoses, because we're collaborating on everything.

LYNDA CARPENITO: Well, if insurance companies will not reimburse your hospital for an overnight stay unless nursing is there, then I would not call them medical diagnoses since by law a physician treats them officially. Insurance companies are clear you need to defend, if someone is to stay overnight after surgery, why nursing care is needed, not why the surgeon is needed. If the surgeon is needed and nursing is not, the patient leaves at five o'clock. That's my personal opposition to

calling them medical diagnoses. We *are* required for the treatment of these.

JACKIE THORNTON: I'm particularly concerned about looking at actual treatment for our diagnoses on two levels. The first is that actual treatment is going to vary considerably across different areas of our discipline and that will bring the level of abstraction of any diagnosis down to some real humble meaning. And the second is that it's going to imply some legal accountability. Once we start saying what the treatment is supposed to be, then people are going to have a right to say they didn't receive that treatment and, therefore, there will be legal accountability along with that. I think we're putting the cart before the horse because I think we need more research to guide us in making those kinds of decisions. I hope that we don't prematurely start trying to link treatments up to concepts that are [not fully developed].

JAN RADOSLOVICH: Are there any approved NANDA diagnoses specifically related to community response?

LYNDA CARPENITO: Are there any? No, there aren't.

MARJORY GORDON: I'd certainly like to congratulate the Committee for attempting to deal with the conceptual focus of nursing and the courage to do that, because it certainly is a task that is very difficult. I was also pleased to see that it remains not tied to a particular model, which I think is very advantageous for the profession at this point. We were reminded by James and Dickoff at the last convention that perhaps conceptual pluralism is something we should work with, for certainly the time being if not forever. I was wondering if the term "response" could possibly ever be "responses" and would say as an argument, but not a very strong one, that the American Nurses' Association uses the term "human responses" because that would open very interesting ideas. Then it would be a nursing diagnosis is responses to actual or potential health problems/life processes. What I find interesting is thinking about that in terms of the responses being the observables, that which we see, the behaviors that indeed we say in our heads are responses to actual or potential health problems or life processes which are to be defined and possibly labeled by nursing diagnoses. So the human responses would be the cluster of the signs and symptoms, behaviors, the observables, that indeed are from our own construction of, and putting our own constructions on the data, they are, we are saying, responses to actual or potential health problems/life processes. Which is another way of thinking about it; rather than saying the nursing diagnoses are the responses, but rather saying the database for the nursing diagnoses are the responses.

BRENDA LYON: I need clarification about the last phrase "definitive therapy toward achievement of outcomes for which the nurse is accountable." One of the things that comes to mind right away is obviously we are accountable for implementing medical treatments and doing that safely. Physicians must authorize that treatment but [nurses] are accountable for implementing it. How will we differentiate medical versus nursing diagnoses?

LYNDA CARPENITO: It was the unanimous agreement by the Board that every situation that a nurse intervenes in is not a nursing diagnosis. What we have attempted to do with the second part of the definition was to retrieve from the nursing literature what is an outcome. If you write "the patient will demonstrate normal sinus rhythm" as an outcome, and the patient proceeds to have an event of ventricular fibrillation, and you defibrillate that patient under protocols, if that patient dies, do you measure the effectiveness of nursing care because he is not in normal sinus rhythm? The answer is no. The Board did not define outcome criteria, and I am very pleased that it was not defined by the Board. We went to the nursing literature and examined the definitions of outcome criteria. I shared three or four with you, but they are all pretty consistent: outcome criteria for nursing diagnoses measure the effectiveness of nursing care. If anyone should be writing outcomes for cardiac rhythm it should be medicine. Certainly nurses can intervene with other interventions for cardiac dysrhythmias, and if they are definitive, then that is a nursing diagnoses. Nursing continues to monitor. Nursing continues to be instrumental in preventing morbidity and mortality. But when people die or get worse because of increased intracranial pressure, an expected outcome that the patient will be alert oriented, PERLA, vital signs within normal, etc., truly is not what nurses use to determine what nursing-prescribed interventions they will order.

WINNIFRED MILLS: To the person who was inquiring about community-related nursing diagnoses: I think the question was, are there any community nursing diagnoses at this time. It might be helpful to that person to know that the Taxonomy Committee has been doing some critical thinking about that whole issue and we did go through one exercise briefly that looked at the existing nursing diagnoses. It seems to me that you might want to think about, for example, *altered nutrition, less than*—it seems to me that in many instances we have practitioners in nursing working in the community who might well recognize that as a nursing diagnosis based on the epidemiological information that they have for that community. So, certainly when you hear about axes you might want to think back to that idea because that is an exercise that we've gone through although it's certainly not finished as yet. The second comment had to do with our responsibility for making nursing diagnoses. It seems to me in the world of nursing where my practice exists, I see all kinds of practitioners who may have the knowledge and some expertise that allows them to make clinical decisions about *ineffective family coping*. They may not, however, have the knowledge base nor the expertise to treat. That does not say that they should not identify that need, but certainly in our small institutions and rural facilities, that has to be a referral to a non-nurse very often for treatment. I think that probably it is important that the diagnosis be called nursing diagnosis, but that evidence be clearly documented that says that it is then referred to whatever other helping profession is available—social worker, pastoral careperson, whatever.

Issues of Diagnosis Review

DONNA VER STEEG: I think some of the problems that we're facing in naming nursing diagnoses have to do with some difficulties that we have with the basic taxonomy. And having had those difficulties working with my own students, we put together what we called a model neutral taxonomy which is published in the August and December *Western Journal of Nursing Research.* The whole issue of modifiers in the taxonomy or what are being called axes at this point, I think with development will help us considerably in the process of dealing with how we name nursing diagnoses. It has to do with the fact that we're trying to do Level 1, Level 2, and Level 3 things all in the same title. I really believe that's where the difficulty lies. If we can put together a taxonomy which deals with areas of phenomena of concern in nursing in a way which allows average nurses to deal with those phenomena in an understandable fashion, I think we're going to make a great deal of progress. Finally, I would suggest to you that one of the functions of the regional districts might be as a resource to clinicians. And I think that really needs to be looked into. The alternative to that is a colleague of mine, a geriatric physician, who was enamored of the idea of nursing diagnoses in nursing homes. He was totally turned off by what he saw in the literature on nursing diagnoses. So he was funded to allow the nurses in his facility to make up their own nursing diagnoses.

LYNDA CARPENITO: [With regard to] the comment about the regional groups or district groups: a suggestion came out of the New England group, who, in a very formal way, make a deliberate effort to meet specifically to review diagnoses that are in review. The March 1st deadline is going to open up many more possibilities for us. We can immediately put [the submitted diagnoses] in our new journal and, I would venture to say, that a review by a regional group—and of course individuals—would be considered in addition to the secondary reviewers. The danger in considering individual reviewers is, of course, that friend of a submitter, or faculty of a submitter, or student of a submitter. If we could organize regular sessions in each district for the purpose of reviewing diagnoses in this cycle and have you complete the same review forms that the expert panel members will complete, that should represent a review and be weighted the same as the expert panel reviews.

LINDA MIERS: I appreciated and enjoyed Dr. Randall's presentation and it may have accomplished something for me at least that you didn't intend to accomplish which was to point out some of the lack of clarity once again. Yesterday or two days ago, we defined a nursing diagnosis, which is what I think is our definition for the taxonomy purposes, as a clinical judgment. Today you defined actual and high-risk nursing diagnoses as three-part statements which we are not putting into a taxonomy according to this definition. So, in my mind it brings to forefront the idea that I have proposed for some work I'm doing in my doctoral studies that perhaps we need to know at what level we are working with the nursing diagnosis. The labels that you gave, I believe, are at the fourth level of theory development. They are truly prescriptive definitions. They allow the clinician to know what to do for the patient because she has all the information, the label, the etiology or the stimulus, as well as the signs and symptoms of both the response and the etiology. On the other hand, the level that we're working at in this organization, I believe, is at the first level of theory development which is to name. And the name is just that, the name of the response. According to the ANA all human responses are within the context and domain of nursing as phenomena of concern. At what point they become a concern and to what level they're a concern will probably depend upon the context, the relationships, the situations that then guide our prescriptive activities. So if I were one to submit a label, once again I wouldn't know what to submit—a label that is three parts, that's a statement, or a label that is actually what's being put into the taxonomy which is a one- or two-word statement.

Liz Hiltunen: I need some clarification on the language. The example was given of how to make a diagnostic statement of a potential or a newly named high-risk diagnosis, and it stated *high-risk impaired skin integrity* related to immobility and incontinence. Is that the way that we are now going to be stating high-risk diagnoses? In the past, my understanding was that high-risk diagnoses had risk factors and when I document those, I usually put the risk factors in the subjective and objective information, as opposed to an actual diagnosis when I state the label and then add the related to statement with the etiology. My understanding is with potential or high-risk diagnoses that the risk factors only become etiologies when [the diagnosis] becomes an actual.

Joe Davie: Potential or high-risk nursing diagnoses are two-part statements. The problem at risk, the high risk, and the risk factors which exist as defining characteristics but defining characteristics are risk factors. Actual nursing diagnosis statements consist of the problem, the etiological related factors, and the signs and symptoms.

Liz Hiltunen: So with the high-risk diagnosis, I would not continue that statement with a related to.

Joe Davie: You can say related to implying the risk factors, or you can say "risk factors."

Liz Hiltunen: My recommendation would be that we not say "related to" for a high-risk diagnosis because that confuses the staff and implies an etiology.

Lynda Carpenito: How would you phrase that diagnosis?

Liz Hiltunen: I would simply call it *high risk for impaired skin integrity.* I use a problem-oriented format, so in my "S" and my "O," I would include the signs and symptoms or the risk factors.

Lynda Carpenito: That's probably an agency designation. If you don't use problem-oriented charting, your validation of your diagnosis wouldn't be there. Both are right. And let me correct the term "problem." We are not only looking at problems, according to our definition of nursing diagnosis, so if any of us say the word problem, it's just for ease and please forgive that.

Liz Hiltunen: I think you include the risk factors in a narrative if you weren't using a problem-oriented approach.

Cecile Lambert: When you said, "I am what I say," and then, "I need to say what I mean," I think as long as we're insiders and we're talking to one another and we're doing inside networking, "I am what I say" is OK. But as soon as we're going to want to speak to other people—and I don't mean just other countries, I mean social workers, doctors—we're going to have to say what we mean, and that is very important. There is a sentence written in the 17th century which goes something like this: "What is well conceived can be spoken with clarity and the words to say it come easily." I think that phrase is something that we can remind ourself quite easily, just simply have it as a little label when we're writing diagnoses, just to say, "How is this being conceived?" and it will help a great deal.

[I can add that] What I know is that once we've named something, we become emotionally identified with it. What I'm hearing at this conference is this loss and I think we're going to have to be careful of that, because as soon as we name something, the identification is there and we have to deal with the loss after that. In the naming process [we must] be attentive to that.

Margaret Lunney: When we were discussing the previous papers, I thought that the problem, etiology, signs and symptoms were for submission of diagnoses. I didn't interpret that at the time that we were required to have in a nursing diagnosis statement, the three parts. Is this a change in policy?

LYNDA CARPENITO: In the [submission] guidelines that you have in your packet, we're asking for a sample diagnosis with a goal and an intervention.

MARGARET LUNNEY: Are you interpreting that also that it have meaning for hospitals and agencies that in order to be a nursing diagnosis it has to have the three parts in the statement or can the cues or signs and symptoms be in the database rather than in the diagnosis itself?

LYNDA CARPENITO: We'll take into consideration that if the three-part statement is not how you normally record your data, and we have to discuss this because this is a new issue, then we'll have to look at an alternative for validation. We're thinking that if the submitter was asked to give us clinically how they would use it, then perhaps some of the issues that were raised by us could be raised before submission. We are by no means asking for research or even literature validation for your sample. We're saying "Give us a sample of how this would appear in a clinical area."

MARGARET LUNNEY: So then, in other words, this is not a directive to clinical agencies that they need to have the three parts in a diagnostic statement.

LYNDA CARPENITO: That's up for discussion. It *may* be a directive. That's all I can say because this is the first time we've heard this and we need to discuss this. I appreciate your feedback about the different agencies not using the three-part statement, not using the two-part statement. That's new information for us and we will look at that and consider that tomorrow.

EMMY MILLER: I first would like to say how pleased I was when I saw the program to see the concept of etiology included as a formal component of something because over the years, etiology has not been a popular concept at these meetings. I think that the concept of etiology as probable cause, though, is very useful in working with actual responses and probable cause as a two-part statement, or high-risk condition response and risk factor as a probable cause, in a situation where you may have multiple risk factors identified in your subjective and objective data. But there's one particular one that, linked with that high-risk condition, really gives direction for nursing care. That, I think, is the crux of the matter here. It's the combination of response and probable cause that makes the diagnostic label both descriptive and prescriptive. So I would encourage people to continue working with etiology as probable cause and I am very pleased to see that included in the DRC's work.

AUDREY MCLANE: I want to address the issue of risk factors. On two occasions, a presenter has referred to risk factors as the defining characteristics of a potential or a high-risk diagnosis and conceptually that is incorrect. The risk factors are more conceptually aligned with the related factors rather than defining characteristics. So to say risk factors are the defining characteristics for potential diagnosis is both incorrect and conceptually confusing.

LYNDA CARPENITO: What would you call those defining characteristics for high-risk problems?

AUDREY MCLANE: They are just risk factors. I don't think we should call them defining characteristics because that's not what they are. They are risk factors and they are conceptually aligned with the related factors in a regular diagnosis.

LYNDA CARPENITO: Right, but if you look at NANDA's definition of defining characteristics which, pardon me if my history is in error, was a made-up word by NANDA, defining characteristics was a concept made up by this organization and that concept can be defined by this organization. The definitions of that came from this group.

Audrey McLane: But I still think we should move toward more conceptual clarity. That's all I'm asking.

Joe Davie: You know, I actually stood up and made that very comment a couple of conferences ago. I agree that risk factors are etiologic if anything. They are not symptoms. There *are* no symptoms if the problem hasn't become manifest. But I have learned to go with the NANDA terminology which lists risk factors as defining characteristics. That's the way it is in the literature. But I agree, I find that conflicting conceptually or inconsistent conceptually.

Jan Radoslovich: In our institution we're still grappling with the issue of incorporating medical diagnoses into etiologies and [I] wondered if the DRC has any comment about that.

Joe Davie: We haven't taken an official position on this, but if you think of etiologic factors as being the focus of nursing intervention, then it would probably be conceptually inadvisable to cite a medical diagnosis as an etiology because it becomes a focus of nursing treatment.

Lynda Carpenito: If you want to talk about inconsistencies when you start putting etiologies in statements, then you start talking about pathophysiology as the etiology for stress incontinence. You talk about pathophysiology being the etiology for reflex incontinence. When you start putting etiology in a statement, and please don't hear this as "it can't happen," but it becomes problematic for your "related tos." I think it's easier to say no pathophysiology or medical diagnoses in your related tos, [otherwise] what do you do with something like "reflex incontinence related to spinal cord injury," which is really a redundancy of how reflex incontinence is defined. Those are some of the issues we grapple with.

Marguerite Kinney: I need help, Lynda. Perhaps it's the editor in me who begs for clarity. But just when I think I have it, you throw in a new wrinkle. How am I to reconcile risk factors with normal life processes? If these characteristics are to be called risk factors, I cannot imagine having a risk factor for a normal life process.

Brooke Randell: I think your question relates to some of the issues that I was trying to raise and that have been raised from the floor repeatedly—the-what-comes-first-the-chicken-or-the-egg phenomenon. We are looking for human responses to life processes, but from my way of thinking life processes may put some people at risk. And I think it has to do though with other etiological factors or other risk factors that are present that make the life process. Lynda's example that all of us who are parents are at risk for child abuse or being abusers, and yet that's the life process of becoming a parent that got you there. It gets very complicated and the more you talk about it, I think the more confused you get. And I would agree with you that it gets very wrinkly.

Lynda Carpenito: At this point, it probably is going to continue to be, until we have better data, the judgment of the diagnostician. I don't think at this point anyone can tell you that you can't designate someone, and hopefully perhaps in some cases in contract with that person, as high risk. Someone else may see that person as not high risk, but at some point it comes down to that relationship of the patient and that particular diagnostician who is that nurse. And at the stage we're at, that's something I think we need to be comfortable with, so we have to be careful with students when we say "No, that's not right."

Marguerite Kinney: I do have a suggestion. I would like to charge the DRC Committee to take a look at these terms again now that some changes have been made at this meeting and see if there is clarity.

Winnifred Mills: I wanted to make a comment about the three-part statement. When I put my quality-assurance hat on, I feel I need to encourage this organization to encourage the use of the three-part statement. Whether you mandate it or not is another whole issue.

Certainly in clinical situations there are clinicians who rail against having to do all that writing. Nevertheless it leaves a marvelous track for quality assurance audit if you have a three-part statement to begin with because you can go back and look at the related factors and determine whether the interventions were appropriate and also whether the outcomes were appropriate as they refer to the defining characteristics that were identified. May I make one point? It has to do with the question of a medical diagnosis in etiology. A number of years ago we had in our newsletter an interesting article. I can't remember the author's name; I can certainly track that down for you. But the pithiness of it was that if you're dealing with what looks like a medical diagnosis in etiology, you move your label to the etiology and ask the question "Why do I treat?" and this gets away from a whole lot of the problems in having a medical diagnosis in the etiology.

DOROTHY JONES: I have two comments. One is in relation to these high-risk diagnoses. I think some of the issue around that has to do with people's definition of wellness and looking at the life processes in terms of parameters of norm. Which kind of go into the discussion that Karen had around general versus specific, because the variance of the parameters within which you interpret each of those life processes include age and the situation the person is involved with as well as culture and other dimensions. I think that discussion and the understanding of those parameters and the breadth of those parameters help you become more refined in the diagnosis piece, and [in] looking at those things that critically differentiate. Age becomes a variable or a context or a situation that you will get the diagnosis or the response within, and it may in fact help refine the knowledge that we're dealing with and refine the diagnoses. I think that a lot of this discussion around what is wellness and what is not wellness may in fact be much more complex, much more abstract, and have to do with those life processes in a much more complicated way. But defining that also helps you to look at the problematic piece. I look at wellness and the aspects of that and look at that as being the guiding force, and look at the differentiation or the alterations or the diagnosis, if you will, as being those things that are different from, and maybe you look at diagnosis in relation to wellness as opposed to wellness in relation to diagnosis.

DONNA VER STEEG: Brooke told you yesterday she's a Johnsonian. I'm a Newman person. And because Newman concludes the concept of primary prevention, one of the modifiers that we developed was the term "unstable" so that we could attach unstable to a normal life process event and indicate the need for some nursing intervention to support and strengthen that. I would commend that term to your consideration. Not everybody who is breast-feeding, for example, has already had three children and is quite comfortable with it. They may be committed to it, they may be functionally capable and all those kinds of things, but if you add the term "unstable" as a modifier in terms of dealing with it, then you've got a clear direction for some primary preventive activities.

LOUETTE LUTJENS: At some time did we define high risk and differentiate it from medium risk, low risk, and I missed that?

LYNDA CARPENITO: Probably you didn't miss it. Again, I think at the stage we're at that it would be very difficult for us to tell the diagnostician what is the difference between medium or high. I think again in that relationship with that patient with those factors that you have as risk factors, you may choose to put someone at high risk because they have one of those risk factors whereby [another nurse] may choose to use it with two. Maybe in the future we will say "this combination increases it" or maybe we will only have as our risk factors those that represent the high [risk], but I don't think we're there yet. If you have suggestions for definitions, we'd welcome them to consider.

LOUETTE LUTJENS: Obviously my concern is the value-laden terms and consistency within our diagnoses. The comment I had was in regard to the risk factors. My recall is that Gordon said that risk factors are those factors that put the individual at risk because those factors are different than the normative population. That brings me back to Brooke's comment. Certainly as parents we are all at risk to be abusers. But I would only be considered "at risk" if perhaps I had some other kinds of factors that differentiated me from the population, such as a family history of perhaps being an abused child myself.

BROOKE RANDELL: I think that what I was trying to say, Louette, was that the life process, the fact that an active substance abuser becomes a parent, that puts them at risk for abuse. It's the combination of the substance abuse and the life process change, so it does seem that life processes as such can be etiological; however, they are not so necessarily by themselves. I think the whole issue of etiology is an enormous can of worms that we haven't actively addressed in this group. I know for myself that one of the ways that you define what counts as etiology is by whatever conceptual structure you operate from. I think that we sometimes get into a bind, in the sense that a lot of us operate from a variety of structures and what counts as etiology for one of us may not count as etiology for another. NANDA per se has not taken a stance on what that is. Therefore, until we say "we," meaning NANDA, not DRC, what it is, coming up with examples of it get very confounded, I think.

Syndromes

KATHLEEN POWERS: The example that you put on the slide was a sample of different nursing diagnoses that made a cluster. The definition that you were using for a syndrome had to do with symptoms and I was wondering how we're going to differentiate that from, say, in

syndromes in genetics, [where] they pick out different signs and symptoms that a child exhibits.

ANN McCOURT: That is exactly what I said and this is why it is terribly confusing. It is also why I have a list and a half of references. I kept trying to find somewhere that a syndrome isn't just signs and symptoms. But, in fact, that's what the literature says. But in reality that is not the way medical has reacted. Many medical syndromes are combinations of all kinds of things.

KATHLEEN POWERS: With that response, then, I have another question. Are we looking at clustering diagnoses because they have similar interventions?

ANN McCOURT: I'm saying that in my own practice, I found it expedient to cluster diagnoses that have the same etiology and the cluster continually occurs together. In so doing, we found we also cut down on the documentation for the interventions because they were related, too.

KATHLEEN POWERS: If we're going to do that, are we going to actually be writing protocols?

ANN McCOURT: Well, what does medicine do? I guess I'd have to ask, does medicine have protocols for their syndromes or are they just considered another diagnosis?

KATHLEEN POWERS: I'm not sure that they always do anything about the syndromes that they identify.

ANN McCOURT: It is a good question. We are not trying to write protocols, but your point is well taken.

LYNDA CARPENITO: I'm not so sure that we would have the requirement to write a protocol for that as we would have for writing for any other diagnosis we have on the list. What we'd have to be clear about is if we are embellishing a set of nursing diagnoses under a syndrome, that we want to be confident that when you call it that, that you are contracting or committing yourself to manage that set underneath it. So when you have alcohol abuse syndrome, if the ANA document is correct, there are 22 nursing diagnoses under that. That doesn't mean that you couldn't develop alcohol abuse syndrome and imply in that five nursing diagnoses, that you're saying this is what *this* syndrome means. I don't know, but it's all brand new, virgin territory for nursing. It's exciting.

JOYCE DUNGEN: I think that a lot of us are converging to a point where we're recognizing the function of nursing in strategic management of people who are translocated, sometimes in time, sometimes situationally, into vulnerable groups. Barbara Lamb worked with chronic disease populations, and she submitted a diagnosis. I can't remember now just what she called it, but I think it was something like *potential for compromised life-style management related to chronicity.* She saw the approach as very similar to those that are used in trauma syndrome where she talked about strategies for managing the physical [problems] that have developed from these conditions, the emotional displacement in role and body image, and the social support that's needed in order to help people manage in those conditions. So I think we are converging in our professional growth on the acknowledgement of strategic management as a very real part of the domain of nursing.

DONNA VER STEEG: I want to assure you that there is light at the end of the tunnel. Number one, I strongly support the syndrome approach. Number two, I think it's important that they be phased. I think the phasing is a far better approach than the acute/chronic idea that was being suggested earlier in this conference. Number three, I think one of the things that we've not looked at as closely as we should is that when you look at client needs and response to nursing diagnosis, which is part of what my practitioners were doing, you find a lot of overlapping interventions. I think we're looking to the point where we can maybe find the intervention equivalent of syndromes on the other end, so that a person may have five different needs but the nursing responses to those are maybe

only two or three. I don't think we should feel uncomfortable with this. I think it's a sign of considerable growth that we're really beginning to figure out what it is we're doing. And when we can move it to a computer, we can even get paid for it.

LAURA ROSSI: I'm wondering, Ann, if at this point it may be a little bit premature to sort of decide that [syndromes] can be diagnoses or signs and symptoms. I wonder if, as people propose the use of syndromes, we might not learn more about what is really a nursing diagnosis. For example, is *ineffective coping* the diagnosis or is it a sign or a symptom of something bigger? We've been looking at this in sort of a clinical ground setting where nurses are dealing with the timeframe in terms of documentation, and [we're] also looking at how frequently some of their interventions are similar for different nursing diagnoses. What we've started discussing is, is there a theme emerging from the diagnoses that you have identified? Maybe the diagnosis is at a higher level of abstraction. To what extent in the literature did you see that the treatment for the syndrome almost suggested which things could be clustered?

ANN MCCOURT: I didn't notice. I think it's a difficult question, but it does bring up something else I would comment on. One of the things I think we have to look at in terms of these defining characteristics or diagnoses or signs and symptoms is the populations. That would appear to be more key than trying to be more definitive on the etiology is what I found from the literature. If you had a spinal cord injury population versus a severely burned population versus somebody in skeletal traction, what then are the different defining characteristics, and is it the same cluster? I think *that's* what we've really got to look at.

KATHLEEN MCMILLAN: Quite serendipitously I happened to come across this article called "An N of One" which is addressing syndrome letters in the *New England Journal of Medicine*. It was published in *Perspectives* *and Biology in Medicine,* and beside it is this wonderful little poem called "After A Lecture By A Noted Biochemist," which I thought was kind of a propos. And if you'll bear with me, I think I'll share it with the audience.

*So what today do we erect upon our
   predecessors' fractured backs
And dazzle into vacillation our bewildered
   youth.
And what tomorrow now project this vast, yes,
   staggering pyramid of facts, base heavenward,
   still in the name of truth.
To make us free! In fact, we number
   scintillating atoms on the head of any pin,
   say, even more precisely on its point.
Infinity and nothingness become inseparable.
What have we done with our new toys!
What games we play with more sophistication!
Have we rejoined a separated world!
What language in the same time do we all
   speak so incomprehensibly in this new age as
   old as any other,
As we still seek enlightenment in crypts and
   caverns, pretend to understand what we can
   never comprehend.*

JEAN JENNEY: I have two points I'd like to bring out. One, the question [was] asked, are there potential nursing syndromes? Second, I'd like to speak to placement in the taxonomy. [For] the first point, I suspect the answer is affirmative. If a syndrome represents a human condition needing nursing intervention, I think we will find in the future that there will be ways to identify potential situations or populations which, if unchecked, will lead to a syndrome. I suspect also that there is going to be a heavy situational factor defining "syndrome." It will be the influence or response to the situation which generates a repeated complex of diagnoses, and we might if we look situationally find that a key

to some of our future syndromes will be in the situational or contextual where all this usually takes place. I think some of us are acutely aware that during this marvelous session this week, people have repeatedly demonstrated the various dissatisfactions with the elements of Taxonomy I, which seem to focus on the logical fallacy which has been compounded by attempting to categorize human responses within a taxonomy of human responses. Now, there is a philosophic and a logical inconsistency here which I would just end my dissertation with, because it's so critical to us as nurses. Philosophically, nursing have traditionally espoused holism as a major ethical plank in validating nursing, so that any taxonomy which divides people into nine sections or categories immediately violates our primary ethical premise which is to view the person as an integrated whole response. My second problem is the logical fallacy. Rules of taxonomy have frequently been specified, but one does not use the same generic phenomena to categorize phenomena. And that's the problem, particularly with behavior because I don't just believe in holism, I demonstrate it and I see it demonstrated every moment in my life. Human responses are so complex, they require responses from at least four out of the nine categories in our taxonomy. I think a good example clear to all of us is *noncompliance. Noncompliance* may be filed under Choosing or it may be filed under Moving, but compliance as an act requires Knowing, Valuing, Choosing, and Moving. So, there is the dilemma which has been so delightfully demonstrated during this wonderful session. Let's not hesitate in considering the utility of syndromes because we can't plunk it under one pattern, because we have been unable to satisfactorily locate a lot of our nursing diagnoses under one pattern.

III

Scientific Papers

Validation of the Nursing Diagnosis *Hypothermia*

Sharon Summers, PhD, RN
Nancy Dudgeon, BSN, RN, CPAN
Kitty Byram, RN, CCRN, CPAN
Kay Zingsheim, RN, CPAN

Although nursing diagnosis-based charting is not a current postanesthesia care unit (PACU) practice, institution accreditation criteria are moving in this direction. Although warmed blankets are frequently applied to hypothermic postanesthesia patients, PACU nurses do not usually conceive of this nursing intervention in the context of outcomes derived from assessment and nursing diagnosis-based care. Although standards of practice advocate the use of nursing diagnosis, nurses must be introduced to *valid* nursing diagnosis statements to promote acceptance into charting documentation. The validation of the nursing diagnosis *hypothermia* was conducted to (1) validate the nursing diagnosis in a clinical setting where this patient problem is encountered daily, (2) determine if the medical term, hypothermia, is appropriate as a nursing diagnosis, and (3) evaluate nursing interventions to promote patient thermal comfort while reducing physiologic stressors associated with hypothermia.

Current standards of PACU nursing practice advocate the use of nursing diagnosis, yet few PACU nurses know how to implement these standards. Validation of a nursing diagnosis in the PACU was undertaken to educate these nurses in the language of nursing diagnosis, the advantages of using nursing diagnosis, and the research process used to test nursing diagnosis in the clinical setting.

When patients are assessed using validated nursing diagnosis criteria, such as the defining characteristics of *hypothermia*, which includes physiologic stressors, then postanesthesia nurses may view nursing interventions as logically derived from the antecedents or major and minor criteria. When patient care is evaluated using validated nursing diagnosis criteria, the postanesthesia nurse may view the evaluation phase of the nursing process as the consequence of nursing interventions.

Theoretical Framework

This study was guided by Selye's (1936) stress theory, where stress was defined as the "non-specific response of the body to any demand"

(p. 7). The stress theory contains two components—the General Adaptation Syndrome (GAS) and the Local Adaptation Syndrome (LAS).

The GAS response consists of the stage of alarm, the stage of resistance, and the stage of exhaustion. The stage of alarm is elicited when the individual is suddenly exposed to unexpected stressors that stimulate autonomic nervous system responses of tachycardia, decreased muscle tone, and decreased body temperature. These events are frequently accompanied by adrenal cortical enlargement and increased secretion of corticoid hormones. If the alarm-stage responses are incompatible with life, then death may ensue. If the alarm-stage stimuli are compatible with life, then the patient may progress to the stage of resistance.

The stage of resistance is an anabolic event where metabolic homeostasis is restored following the catabolic alarm stage. At this time, the patient is considered to be fully adapted. The patient who is confronted with another alarm-stage stressor may experience the exhaustion stage (Selye, 1982).

The exhaustion stage signifies that catabolism has exceeded anabolism and that further adaptation is no longer capable of sustaining life (Selye, 1976). Selye (1982) indicated that the stages of GAS occur in addition to normal, life-sustaining, physiologic processes. Events that evoke GAS are known as stressors; these stressors may be either pleasant or unpleasant, physical or psychologic. Regardless of the source of the stressor, the outcome is a series of events known as the stress mechanism.

During anesthesia, the patient stressors that are evoked are at the hypothalamic level (Levy, 1982; Salo, 1982). Hypothalamic stress results in both a rapid response and a slow response. The rapid response is mediated through the sympathetic-adrenal medulla mechanism. The sympathetic-adrenal medulla mechanism results in the release of catecholamines that may have a deleterious effect on the cardiovascular system, where tachycardia and hypertension may occur as well as compromised myocardial oxygen consumption (Blitt, 1985). During this catabolic event adrenocorticotropic and growth-hormone secretion are increased, resulting in increased heat production and utilization of cellular nutrients (Wilmore, Long, Mason, & Pruitt, 1976). Anesthesia and various intraoperative medications, however, may block the neuroendocrine responses that may alter thermoregulation, oxygen consumption, and energy utilization (Wilmore et al., 1976). As levels of anesthesia and medications diminish, the neuroendocrine responses may result in shivering for increased heat production, which has been cited as uncomfortable (Fraulini, 1986; Wilmore et al., 1976).

The slow response is mediated through the pituitary-adrenal cortex mechanism. Delayed responses of the pituitary-adrenal cortex mechanism may elicit responses including the release of antidiuretic hormone (ADH). ADH is believed to be elevated by circulating catecholamines and results in fluid retention. Increased fluid retention is believed to cause an increase in cardiac work load and variations in blood pressures (Blitt, 1985).

In contrast to the GAS, the LAS pertains to a local tissue response that includes inflammation, proliferation of fibrous connective tissue to prevent the spread of pathogens, granulation of new tissue to replace damaged tissue, and chemotaxis to neutralize waste and toxins and to kill bacteria (Blitt, 1985). It is assumed that the neuroendocrine responses related to surgery, anesthesia, and medications will elicit both the GAS and the LAS stress responses. Therefore, the stress theory was used to describe and to explain the defining characteristics of *hypothermia* in postanesthesia patients.

Literature Review

Perioperative Hypothermia

Augustine (1989) reported that the incidence of perioperative hypothermia may be as great as 60% to 80% or 12 to 16 million patients nationwide per year. Gewolb, Hines, and Barash (1987) stated that the length of stay in the postanesthesia care unit is directly related to the patient's admission temperature. A pilot study identified a mean body temperature of 36.8°C (range 35° to 38°C) as a significant correlate ($r = .39$, $p < .05$) of postanesthesia hypertension in normotensive young adult males (Summers, Dudgeon, & Dubin, 1988). Other physiologic effects of hypothermia include precipitation of respiratory acidosis, circulatory insufficiency, increased metabolism attributed to shivering, inhibition of ADH, and resultant increase in urinary output (Hudak, Lohr, & Gallo, 1977). The length of stay for patients with temperatures less than 36°C ranged from 82 to 222 minutes, and for patients with temperatures greater than 36°C ranged from 45 to 163 minutes (Gewolb et al., 1987).

A key contributor to postanesthesia hypothermia is heat loss by conduction, radiation, convection, and evaporation. Heat loss by conduction occurs when patients are exposed to cold skin-preparation solutions, room-temperature irrigation solutions, and refrigerated blood transfusions (Augustine, 1989). Conduction heat loss as great as 50% also occurs when the patient's uncovered head is exposed to the cold room (Carlson, 1988). Heat is also lost by radiation during surgery from patient exposure to cold ambient operating room temperatures, from open wounds resulting in lowering of visceral temperatures, and from lying on wet surfaces. Lewis and Cressey (1980) suggested the possible temperature gradient while the patient is in the operating room may be as great as 12° to 17°C. Heat loss by convection can

also occur as cool air moves across the patient's body surface (Augustine, 1989). Heat loss by evaporation may occur through general water evaporation, from the respiratory tract, and from exposed viscera (Augustine, 1989).

Guyton (1986) indicated that surface skin temperatures could fluctuate quickly depending on ambient temperatures. In contrast, core temperatures remain fairly constant at 37.1°C ($\pm 1°$). Maintenance of the constant core temperature is possible through a set-point feedback mechanism mediated between surface receptors in the skin, temperature of the blood, and central thermic receptors in the hypothalamus. In addition, there are deep thermoreceptors in the spinal cord, abdominal viscera, and great veins that respond to cold stimuli. When humans are exposed to cold, a sequence of short-term events leads to heat generation: (1) generalized vasoconstriction to the skin as a result of stimulation of posterior hypothalamic sympathetic centers, (2) sympathetic stimulation to piloerector muscles resulting in piloerection (goosebumps), and (3) sympathetic stimulation for heat production as a result of cold stimuli from skin and spinal receptors (shivering) (Guyton, 1986).

Shivering is frequently seen in postanesthesia patients in response to gradients between core and surface temperatures (Ganong, 1985). Guyton (1986) stated that shivering can occur when the hypothalamic temperature is near normal values but the skin temperature is lowered, and is possibly a defense in maintaining core-temperature consistency. Also central to the hypothalamic stimulation for heat regulation is the control of appetite, food intake, and generalized metabolism. Fraulini (1987) and Lewis and Cressey (1980) indicated that shivering can increase an adult's heat production and metabolism 20% to 50% and the rhythmic muscle contractions are reported by patients to be uncomfortable. Guyton (1986) stated that exposure to cold can result in increased metabolism where shivering may increase oxygen consumption 300% to 400% because of the intense muscle contraction efforts to produce heat. Vaughn, Vaughn, and Cork (1981) and Augustine (1989) indicated that oxygen consumption during shivering may be increased as much as 700%. When patients enter surgery in the fasted state and with fluid restrictions, alterations in metabolism are more pronounced where hepatic glucose stores of approximately 75 grams are insufficient to meet patient needs and result in gluconeogenesis (Davis, Drucker, Gann, Foster, Pruitt, Gamelli, & Sheldon, 1987).

General anesthetics (e.g., halothane) and neuromuscular blocking agents can precipitate heat loss through vasodilatation, lack of muscle contraction, and inhibition of temperature regulation resulting in shivering (Augustine, 1989; Drain & Christoph, 1987; Fraulini, 1878; Lloyd, 1986). Wilmore (1977) indicated that general anesthesia results in redistribution of body heat where core temperatures fall during the first 15 to 30 minutes postinduction, resulting in an increased surface temperature and thus promoting further heat loss. Lloyd (1986) indicated that anesthetic agents interfere with the surface-to-core-temperature feedback regulation as well as with metabolism. Decreased anesthetic depth toward the completion of surgery results in increased heat production through muscle activity and overall increase in core temperatures.

Lloyd (1986) supports the recommendation that comfort for the postanesthesia patient can be enhanced and shivering suppressed if hypothermia is quickly reversed. Quick rewarming by water baths with water temperatures that range from 40° to 45°C are recommended. Because surgical patients cannot be immersed in water baths, it is frequently recommended that warmed blankets be used to comfort and rewarm postanesthesia patients.

Ackley (1984) studied the effect of intraoperative hypothermia in elderly (n = 20) and young adult (n = 20) patients. Hypothermia was defined as core temperatures of less than 36°C as measured by tympanic temperatures. During surgery elderly subjects had a greater decrease in mean temperatures from 36.37°C (SD ±0.48) postinduction to 35.12°C (SD ±0.62). The young adults' mean temperatures during surgery ranged from 36.89°C (SD ±0.42) to 35.96°C (SD ±0.74). On admission to the recovery room both groups had additional decreases in body temperature. Of the young adult group, 60% (n = 20) were hypothermic (X̄ = 35.11°C, SD ±0.72) and 90% (n = 20) of the elderly were hypothermic (X̄ = 35.88°C, SD ±0.78) on admission to the recovery room. The greatest degree of heat loss occurred in a patient who underwent an aortofemoral bypass graft resulting in a large amount of surface area being exposed to cold ambient temperatures.

Hypothermia is frequently discussed in postanesthesia literature as *inadvertent hypothermia* because the loss of body heat by patients is considered a side effect of the surgical experience (Burkle, 1988; Lilly, 1987; Wehmer & Baldwin, 1986). Thus, support was found that hypothermia, defined as body temperature less than 36.0°C, is an actual postanesthesia patient stressor, and that the PACU is a pertinent place to validate the defining characteristics of *hypothermia* as it is a common postanesthesia problem.

The Nursing Diagnosis *Hypothermia*

Carpenito (1987) defined *hypothermia* as a "sustained reduction of body temperature of below 35°C (95°F) orally or 35.5°C (96°F) rectally" (p. 135). This definition also provides the major defining characteristic for this diagnosis. Minor defining characteristics include skin changes (e.g., coolness, pallor, redness, blanching); mental changes (e.g., drowsiness, confusion, restlessness); decreased pulse or respiration; and shivering, malnutrition, or cachexia (Carpenito, 1987). Situational factors also cited by Carpenito include exposure to snow, sun, wind, or cold; inappropriate clothing, poverty; extremes in body weight; dehydration or malnutrition; and inactivity.

The North American Nursing Diagnosis Association (NANDA) (1989) defined hypothermia as "a state in which an individual's body temperature is reduced below normal temperature" (p. 16). Major defining characteristics are listed as body temperature below normal range, shivering (mild), cool skin, and minor pallor. Minor defining characteristics include slow capillary refill, tachycardia, cyanotic nail beds, hypertension, and piloerection. Related factors are exposure to cool or cold environment, illness or trauma, damage to the hypothalamus, inability or decreased ability to shiver, malnutrition, inadequate clothing, consumption of alcohol, medications causing vasodilation, evaporation from skin in environment, decreased metabolic rate, inactivity, and aging.

Kim, McFarland, and McLane (1989) defined hypothermia as "the state in which an individual's body temperature is reduced below his/her normal range but not below 35.6°C (rectal)/36.4°C (rectal) in newborns" (p. 33). Related factors are exposure to cool or cold environment, illness or trauma, inability or decreased ability to shiver, malnutrition, inadequate clothing, consumption of alcohol, medications causing vasodilation, evaporation from skin in cool environment, decreased metabolic rate, inactivity, and aging. Defining characteristics include shivering (mild), cool skin, pallor (moderate), slow capillary refill, tachycardia, cyanotic nail beds, hypertension, and piloerection.

Miller-Carroll (1989) suggested the separation of hypothermia into mild, moderate, and severe, however temperature ranges for these categories were not given. Defining characteristics for hypothermia include shivering, cool skin, pallor, slow capillary refill, tachycardia, normal urine output, altered nail-bed color, hypertension, and piloerection.

Method

Sample and Settings

A sample of 91 adult patients was studied in two PACUs in the midwest. Adult patients were defined as being at least 18 years old and of either sex. All subject data were coded and analyzed as grouped data, thereby protecting subjects' anonymity and confidentiality. Taking temperatures and observing for defining characteristics of *hypothermia* are routine nursing care procedures. None of the procedures for data collection were invasive or in any way harmful to the patient. The human subjects review committee of both hospitals approved the study and determined that taking temperatures and observing patients qualified as routine nursing care and were exempt from written patient consent.

Research Design and Instruments

A descriptive design was used to validate the defining characteristics of *hypothermia*. The patients studied were selected based on an admission core temperature of less than or equal to 36.0°C (Ackley, 1984; Fraulini, 1987; Gewolb et al., 1987; and Lilly, 1987). Core temperatures were measured by a FirstTemp thermistor thermometer that read infrared rays from the tympanic membrane as an indirect measure of the hypothalamic temperature.

A data-collection sheet was developed that listed major and minor defining characteristics of *hypothermia* as described by Carpenito (1987). A core temperature of less than or equal to 36°C (rather than 35°C) was used as the criterion for inclusion in the study. After admission to the PACU patients' temperatures were taken. Patients with temperatures less than or equal to 36°C were assessed for the major and minor defining characteristics of *hypothermia*. Data were recorded as present (yes) or absent (no) on all defining characteristics.

Table 1: Varied Defining Characteristics of the Nursing Diagnosis *Hypothermia*

	NANDA	Carpenito	Miller-Carroll	Kim et al.	Summers	
Temperature °C	Below normal	≤35.0[a] ≤35.5[b]	N/A	not <35.6 not <36.4	≤36	
					Yes	No
Shivering	Yes	Yes	Yes	Mild	29	62
Decreased ability to shiver	Yes	No	N/A	Yes	Rx	
Cool skin	Yes	Yes	Yes	Yes	91	0
Pallor	Yes	Yes; blanching, redness	Yes	Yes	88	3
Piloerection	Yes	Yes	Yes	Yes	0	91
Slow capillary refill	Yes	No	Yes	Yes	45	46
Cyanotic nail beds	Yes	No	Altered color	Yes	16	75
Exposure to cool/ cold environment	Yes	Yes; also sun, wind, snow	N/A	Yes	88	3
Illness/trauma	Yes	No	N/A	Yes	91	0
Damage to hypo- thalamus	Yes	No	N/A	N/A	N/A	
Malnutrition	Yes	Yes, plus cachexia	N/A	Yes	3	88
Dehydration	Yes	Yes	N/A	N/A	91	0
Extremes in weight	No	Yes	N/A	N/A	3	88
Inadequate clothing	Yes	Yes	N/A	Yes	91	0
Alcohol consump- tion	Yes	No	N/A	N/A	N/A	
Vasodilatation	Yes	No	N/A	Yes	91	0
Evaporation from skin	Yes	No	N/A	Yes	N/A	
Decreased metabolic rate	Yes	No	N/A	Yes	Not measured but known to increase with OR patients	
Inactivity	Yes	Yes	N/A	Yes	91	0
Aging	Yes	Yes, also very young	N/A	Yes	18–88	
Mental confusion	No	Yes	N/A	N/A	91	0
Drowsiness	No	Yes	N/A	N/A	91	0
Restlessness	No	Yes	N/A	N/A	0	91
Tachycardia	Yes	Yes	Yes	Yes	5	86
Hypertension	Yes	No	Yes	Yes	11	80
Decreased pulse	No	Yes	N/A	N/A	8	83
Decreased respira- tion	No	Yes	N/A	N/A	28	63
Cardiac arrhythmias	No	Yes	N/A	N/A	4	87
Poverty	No	Yes	N/A	N/A	N/A	

[a]Oral
[b]Rectal
Rx = prescribed drugs
N/A = information not available

Results

Descriptive statistics were used to analyze demographic data and the defining characteristics. The subjects, 45 males and 46 females aged between 18 and 88 years, had undergone major surgery lasting from 1 to 6 hours. The findings of this study differed from those of NANDA (1989), Carpenito (1988), Kim et al. (1989), and Miller-Carroll (1989) (see Table 1).

Discussion and Recommendations

There seems to be variation in the ways in which *hyperthermia* is defined and described in the nursing literature. This study of 91 postanesthesia patients documented defining characteristics that differed from those cited by Carpenito (1987), Kim et al. (1989), and Miller-Carroll (1989). Some of the characteristics (e.g., exposure to snow or wind, alcohol intake, inadequate clothing, poverty) suggest hypothermia that may exist in a homeless or indigent population, or those stranded by winter storms. Augustine (1989) stated that the incidence of postanesthesia hypothermia is estimated to be 12 to 16 million patients per year. It is concluded that with this high incidence of hypothermia, the nursing diagnosis criteria for *hypothermia* need to be revised to fit this commonly occurring stressor in postanesthesia patients, rather than in other groups of patients who may experience hypothermia less frequently.

As this study was conducted and data were gathered to validate the nursing diagnosis of *hypothermia*, it occurred to the researchers that data were being gathered to validate a medical diagnosis. The term *inadvertent hypothermia* has also been used by postanesthesia nurses; however, this is still a medical diagnosis (Burkle, 1988; Wehmer & Baldwin, 1986). Because hypothermia is a medical diagnosis, it is suggested that the nursing diagnosis *hypothermia* be replaced with *altera-*

tion in thermal comfort. Postanesthesia patients who arrive in the PACU with temperatures less than or equal to 36°C are treated by nurses with nursing interventions such as warmed blankets to cover the head and body. There is an electric warming device, the Bair Hugger, that is also used by some PACUs on an as-needed basis. *Alteration in thermal comfort* and nursing interventions to monitor and warm the postanesthesia patient describe routine postanesthesia nursing care. Therefore, these researchers strongly urge consideration for the replacement of the nursing diagnosis of *hypothermia* with *alteration in thermal comfort* to describe more accurately this postanesthesia patient problem and subsequent nursing interventions.

If nursing diagnoses are to be useful for practicing nurses they must fit commonly encountered patient problems and represent the reality of nursing practice. The sample size in this study was small and data were collected from only two PACUs. Further studies are needed to validate these findings. Further studies are also needed to support the suggestion of changing the nursing diagnosis of *hypothermia* to *alteration in thermal comfort.*

References

Ackley, R. E. (1984). *A comparison of the incidence of perioperative hypothermia and postoperative confusion in the elderly and younger adult perioperative patients.* Unpublished master's thesis, University of Kansas.

Augustine, S. D. (1989, April). *Perioperative hypothermia—PACU considerations.* Presentation at ASPAN 8th Annual National Conference, Orlando, FL.

Blitt, C. D. (1985). *Monitoring in anesthesia and critical care medicine.* New York: Churchill Livingstone.

Burkle, N. L. (1988). Inadvertent hypothermia. *Today's OR Nurse 10*(7), 27–31.

Carlson, K. (1988, November). Hypothermia: An insidious imbalance. *Breathline, 8*(3), 3.

Carpenito, L. J. (1987). *Nursing diagnosis: Application to clinical practice* (2nd ed.). Philadelphia: Lippincott.

Davis, J. H., Drucker, W. R., Gann, D. S., Foster, R. S., Pruitt, B. A., Gamelli, R. L., & Sheldon, G. F. (1987). *Clinical surgery.* St. Louis, MO: Mosby.

Drain, C. B., & Christoph, S. (1987). *The recovery room.* Philadelphia: Saunders.

Fraulini, K. E. (1987). *After anesthesia: A guide for PACU, ICU, and medical-surgical nurses.* Norwalk, CT: Appleton & Lange.

Ganong, W. F. (1985). *Review of medical physiology.* Los Altos, CA: Lange.

Gewolb, J., Hines, R., & Barash, P. G. (1987). A survey of 3,244 admissions to the post anesthesia recovery room at a university teaching hospital. *Anesthesiology,* 67(3A), A471.

Guyton, A. C. (1986). *Textbook of medical physiology* (7th ed.). Philadelphia: Saunders.

Hudak, C. M., Lohr, T. S., & Gallo, B. M. (1977). *Critical care nursing.* Philadelphia: Lippincott.

Kim, M. J., McFarland, G. K., & McLane, A. M. (1989). *A pocket guide to nursing diagnosis* (3rd ed.). St. Louis, MO: Mosby.

Levy, C. J. (1982). Changes in plasma chemistry associated with stress. In J. Watkins & M. Salo (Eds.), *Trauma, stress, and immunity in anaesthesia and surgery* (pp. 141–160). London: Butterworth Scientific.

Lewis, K. P., & Cressey, I. (1980). Nursing care of postanesthesia shivering. *Breathline,* 1(2), 80–82.

Lilly, R. B. (1987). Inadvertent hypothermia: A real problem. *ASA Refresher Courses in Anesthesiology, 15,* 93–107.

Lloyd, E. L. (1986). *Hypothermia and cold stress.* Rockville, MD: Aspen.

Miller-Carroll, S. (1989). Nursing diagnosis: Hypother-mia. In R. M. Carroll-Johnson (Ed.), *Classification of nursing diagnoses: Proceedings of the eighth conference* (pp. 425–428). Philadelphia: Lippincott.

North American Nursing Diagnosis Association. (1989). *Taxonomy I revised.* St. Louis: Author.

Salo, M. (1982). Endocrine response to anaesthesia and surgery. In J. Watkins & M. Salo (Eds.), *Trauma, stress, and immunity in anaesthesia and surgery* (pp. 241–256). London: Butterworth Scientific.

Selye, H. (1936). A syndrome produced by diverse nocuous agents. *Nature, 138,* 32–48.

Selye, H. (1976). *Stresses of life.* New York: McGraw-Hill.

Selye, H. (1982). History and present status of the stress concept. In L. Goldberger & S. Breznitz (Eds.), *Handbook of stress theoretical and clinical aspects* (pp. 7–20). New York: Free Press.

Summers, S., Dudgeon, N., & Dubin, J. (1988). Postanesthesia care unit hypertension in normotensive young adult males: A pilot study. *Journal of Post Anesthesia Nursing, 3*(5), 324–331.

Vaughn, M. S., Vaughn, R. W., & Cork, R. C. (1981). Postoperative hypothermia in adults: Relationship of age, anesthesia, and shivering to rewarming. *Anesthesia and Analgesia, 60*(10), 746–751.

Wehmer, M. A., & Baldwin, B. J. (1986). Inadvertent hypothermia. *AORN, 44*(5), 788–796.

Wilmore, D. W. (1977). *The metabolic management of the critically ill.* New York: Plenum.

Wilmore, D. W., Long, J. M., Mason, A. D., & Pruitt, B. A. (1976). Stress in surgical patients as a neurophysiologic reflex response. *Surgery, Gynecology & Obstetrics, 142,* 257–269.

The Identification and Clinical Validation of the Defining Characteristics of *Alteration in Cardiac Tissue Perfusion*

David J. Kelly, MS, RN

Introduction

The human heart responds to a compromise in tissue perfusion with the manifestation of cardiac tissue ischemia, necrosis, and a variety of electrical conduction problems. Today almost five million people have a medical history of cardiac tissue ischemia, necrosis, or both (American Heart Association, 1989). The North American Nursing Diagnosis Association (NANDA) developed the Nursing Diagnosis Taxonomy I in 1986, and Nursing Diagnosis Taxonomy I Revised in 1988. Both taxonomies included *alterations in tissue perfusion* under the human response pattern of Exchanging at Level IV, with subcomponents for the specific organs affected: (a) renal, (b) cerebral, (c) cardiopulmonary, (d) gastrointestinal, and (e) peripheral. Further developmental work was recommended for all the subcomponents.

The cardiac and pulmonary systems are separate systems with distinct functions and subject to different responses to the pathophysiologic phenomenon of altered tissue perfusion. It is difficult to develop defining characteristics, related factors, and nursing interventions that encompass both systems. There is, therefore, a need to develop and validate subcategories for both the cardiac and pulmonary systems. In this study the identification and clinical validation of the defining characteristics for the nursing diagnosis *alteration in tissue perfusion: cardiac* was investigated.

A definition of *alteration in cardiac tissue perfusion* was needed to establish a basis for development of a content-validated assessment tool to identify and test the clinical validity of defining characteristics as well. The following definition was developed within the NANDA definition for *alteration in tissue perfusion* but is differentiated for cardiac tissue perfusion:

Alteration in Tissue Perfusion: Cardiac is a state in which an individual experiences at the cellular level, decrease in the nutrition and oxygenation with a concomitant increase in carbon dioxide due to an imbalance in cardiac oxygen supply and demand (Kelly, 1989).

Literature Review

Rossi and Haines (1979) were two of the first diagnosticians to identify nursing diagnoses to be used with cardiovascular patients. They used their prior clinical experiences with cardiovascular patients to match existing nursing diagnoses developed by NANDA to human response patterns experienced by their collective patients. The diagnoses identified were (a) alteration in comfort level: pain, (b) alteration in cardiac output/activity intolerance, (c) altered sleep patterns, (d) knowledge deficit, (e) noncompliance, (f) alteration in self-concept/body image, and (g) maladaptive coping patterns (Rossi & Haines, 1979).

Kim et al. (1980) used 18 staff nurses and four clinical nurse specialists to identify nursing diagnoses in adult hospitalized patients with cardiovascular diseases. *Decreased cardiac output* and *alteration in cardiac circulation* were the most frequently identified nursing diagnoses.

In 1984 this same group of researchers replicated their 1980 study with a sample of 158 cardiovascular patients. The most frequently reported nursing diagnosis was *alteration in coronary circulation*. The most frequent defining characteristic associated with *alteration in coronary circulation* was ischemic pain. Ischemic pain was defined as (a) pain, (b) angina, (c) neck pain, and (d) hand–arm pain. The most frequently identified etiologies for nursing diagnoses formulated for patients with cardiac problems included (a) coronary artery disease, (b) atherosclerotic heart disease, (c) ischemic heart disease, and (d) heart disease (Kim et al., 1984). Therefore, Kim et al. were the first to identify and relate the human response, that is *alteration in coronary circulation*, to the pathophysiologic phenomenon of compromised cardiac circulation.

In recent years, NANDA adopted the label of *altered tissue perfusion* to address the phenomenon of compromised circulation (Kritek, 1986; NANDA, 1988, 1989). Five subcategories of *alteration in tissue perfusion* were identified, one of which was cardiopulmonary. The cardiopulmonary subcategory needs to be further separated into cardiac and pulmonary. A search of the literature revealed no studies to validate the existence of the label *alteration in tissue perfusion: cardiac*, nor of its associated defining characteristics, related factors, or nursing interventions.

Research Design and Methods

This study used an exploratory, descriptive research design. Fehring's (1986) Diagnostic Content Validity (DCV) model was used to validate the content of the Kelly Cardiac Assessment Tool (KCAT). Fehring's (1986) Clinical Diagnostic Validity (CDV) model was used in conjunction with the content validation of the KCAT.

Sample

The sample was composed of 20 adult patients experiencing cardiac problems in a southwestern university medical center. The subjects for this study met the following criteria:

1. Were 18 years of age or older
2. Had a medical diagnosis of angina, unstable angina, rule out myocardial infarction, or myocardial infarction
3. Did not exhibit signs and symptoms of cardiac failure
4. Remained in the hospital for at least 48 hours or until three blood samples of CPK-MB cardiac enzymes were drawn.

Instrument

Tool Development

The literature-based KCAT was developed to be used in conjunction with Fehring's CDV model to test the clinical validity of subjective and objective defining characteristics frequently seen in patients with a compromise in cardiac tissue perfusion. In addition, the KCAT was designed to assess the relevance of each defining characteristic by having expert nurse raters judge the degree of importance of each characteristic in making the diagnosis.

Content Validity Testing

Using Fehring's DCV model, the content validity of the KCAT was assessed in two steps by a panel of seven cardiovascular nursing experts who were either master's or doctorally prepared. The definition of *alteration in tissue perfusion: cardiac* and directions were provided to the panel. Each member of the panel independently used a dichotomous scale of "yes" or "no" to judge if each defining characteristic was clear. If a major revision was needed to make a defining characteristic clear, the revision was resubmitted to the panel for examination. The panel then used a five-point Likert-type scale to rate the relevance of the defining characteristics to the nursing diagnosis. The computation of the DCV was performed in four steps:

1. Numerical ratings were assigned: 1 = not at all characteristic, 2 = very little characteristic, 3 = somewhat characteristic, 4 = quite characteristic, 5 = very characteristic.
2. Weights were assigned to each of the ratings: 1 = 0, 2 = 0.25, 3 = 0.50, 4 = 0.75, and 5 = 1.00.
3. The weighted ratio for each characteristic was calculated by summing the weights assigned to each response and dividing by the total number of responses.
4. Defining characteristics with a weighted ratio of less than 0.50 were discarded.

The overall DCV score of the entire KCAT was determined by obtaining the mean of the sum of the weighted individual defining characteristic ratings.

Interrater Reliability

To establish interrater reliability prior to data collection, the nurse raters independently assessed three patients. To attain interrater reliability, the nurse raters had to be in agreement at least 90% of the time on both the dichotomous scale and the degree-of-importance scale. An acceptable level of interrater reliability was not attained on the assessment of the first three patients. Together the nurse raters reviewed and discussed the KCAT. Independent assessment of subjects continued until the 90% interrater reliability level was attained. Assessment of six patients was required to attain acceptable interrater reliability levels.

Data Collection

Once the content validity of the KCAT was determined, the clinical data-collection phase began. Each subject and the medical record were independently examined by two nurse raters. The two designated nurse raters were the principal investigator and a master's-prepared nurse with cardiovascular experience.

The subjective data were obtained from independent patient interviews. The subjective concepts of pain, discomfort, chest pressure, and chest tightness were examined separately. Objective data were obtained from independent nurse assessment of the subject, review of the medical record, laboratory data, and 12-lead ECG data.

The data generated from the independent nurse assessments were examined in two phases. The first phase was to determine the clinical diagnostic validity of each characteristic by inserting into Fehring's CDV formula the frequency with which the defining characteristic was observed:

$$R = [A/A + D] \times [(F_1/N + F_2/N)/2]$$

where

A = number of agreements
D = number of disagreements
F_1 = frequency of characteristics observed by the first observer
F_2 = frequency of characteristics observed by the second observer
N = number of subjects observed
R = mean individual CDV score.

The second phase was to determine the degree of importance of each characteristic to making the diagnosis. For this, each nurse rater used a five-point Likert-type scale where 1 = not at all characteristic, 2 = very little characteristic, 3 = somewhat characteristic, 4 = quite characteristic, and 5 = very characteristic. Weights were assigned to each of the ratings, so that 1 = 0, 2 = 0.25, 3 = 0.50, 4 = 0.75, and 5 = 1.00. The degree of importance was determined by averaging the sum of the ratings of each nurse rater.

Results

Eighty percent of the sample (n = 16) were admitted with the medical diagnoses of myocardial infarction (50%, n = 10) or rule out myocardial infarction (30%, n = 6). The remaining subjects were admitted with angina (5%, n = 1) or unstable angina (15%, n = 3). Seventy percent (n = 14) of the sample were either married or widowed, 20% (n = 4) were divorced, while 10% (n = 2) were separated. Although the mean age of the sample was 66 years, 40% (n = 8) were 60 years old or younger. Interestingly, the majority (65%, n = 13) of this sample were women, which does not conform to the national norms for a cardiac population.

Content Validity

All the defining characteristics on the KCAT attained DCV scores of greater than 0.50 and were retained for clinical testing. The mean DCV score for the total KCAT was 0.70. This value exceeds the 0.60 criterion recommended by Fehring (1986) for validation of a nursing diagnosis.

The clinical testing of the presence/absence of the 43 subjective and objective defining characteristics contained in the KCAT resulted in the clinical validation of 14 defining characteristics (see Table 1). The overall CDV score for the entire KCAT was 0.62, which exceeds Fehring's 0.60 criterion.

The degree of importance of each defining characteristic to making the diagnosis was also assessed. Table 1 displays the mean of each nurse rater's rating of the degree of importance calculated for each defining characteristic. These means were then averaged to obtain the overall mean of the degree of importance for each defining characteristic. The second column of Table 1 displays the average mean rating of the degree of importance by the nurse raters. All but one characteristic was rated as important.

Additional characteristics were identified in field notes of subjective defining characteristics recorded during the clinical data-collection phase. These subjective characteristics were categorized and analyzed and are shown in Table 2.

Nurse raters also observed the presence of four objective signs and symptoms that were not included in the KCAT. These were (1) T-wave with an opposite polarity of a normal sinus rhythm QRS complex on an ECG, (2) bundle branch block on ECG, (3) coronary artery lesions documented in the medical records by a physician who performed a cardiac catheterization, and (4) reperfusion ventricular tachycardia following infusion of streptokinase or tissue plasminogen activator. The frequency of occurrence of these signs and symptoms was not measured.

Table 1: Degree of Importance of Clinically Validated Defining Characteristics (CVD) for *Alteration in Tissue Perfusion: Cardiac*

Defining Characteristic	Individual CVD Score	Mean Degree of Importance
1. Presence of CPK-MB or CPK_2 in 1st 3 blood samples drawn within 1st 48 hours of admission	0.84	0.99
2. Verbalizes chest discomfort	0.78	1.00
3. Verbalizes relief from chest pain with administration of nitrates	0.78	0.98
4. Verbalizes arm discomfort	0.70	0.59
5. Verbalizes shortness of breath	0.65	0.59
6. Verbalizes chest pain	0.63	0.98
7. Verbalizes arm pain	0.62	0.67
8. Verbalizes chest pressure	0.59	1.00
9. Verbalizes history of chest pain	0.55	0.99
10. Diaphoresis	0.55	0.55
11. Verbalizes history of chest discomfort	0.54	0.99
12. Verbalizes shoulder discomfort	0.50	0.56
13. Verbalizes shoulder pain	0.50	0.61
14. Verbalizes nausea	0.50	0.37

NOTE: 0.00 = not at all important
0.25 = not very important
0.50 = somewhat important
0.75 = quite important
1.00 = very important

Discussion

Sixty-five percent of this study sample of 20 adults were women (n = 13), which is not representative of the normal cardiac patient

Table 2: Summary of Subjective Field Note Characteristics

Characteristic	Frequency	Percentage[a]
1. Verbalized experiencing diffuse perspiration	6	30
2. Numbness of arm or fingers	5	25
3. Burning pain: chest or substernal	4	20
4. Chest aching	2	10
5. Burning pain: throat or mouth	2	10
6. Arm heaviness	2	10

[a]Subjects reported more than one subjective complaint

population. In a report reviewing women and heart disease, Murdaugh and O'Rourke (1988) reported that women under the age of 60 with coronary heart disease had angina as the initial clinical symptom substantially more than men—56% compared to approximately 33%. Women also have an increased incidence of coronary artery spasm producing an imbalance of cardiac oxygen supply and demand. Alternatively, women tend to have more atypical chest pain and a higher incidence of silent myocardial infarctions than men (Murdaugh & O'Rourke, 1988). The findings of the current study need to be viewed in the light of the skewed sample.

According to Fehring (1986), the criterion for validation as a major defining characteristic is an individual CDV score of ≤0.80. One characteristic, "the presence of CPK-MB or CPK_2 within the first three blood samples drawn within the first 48 hours," qualified as a *major* defining characteristic (CDV score =

0.84). Two minor subjective defining characteristics, "verbalizes chest discomfort" and "verbalizes relief of chest pain with administration of nitrates," each had individual CDV scores of 0.78 and thus were very close to qualifying as major defining characteristics.

Because of the physiologic nature of the phenomenon examined, it is surprising that only two objective characteristics were clinically validated as minor defining characteristics. A larger sample more representative of a normal cardiac population may have resulted in a larger cluster of major and minor *objective* defining characteristics.

Thirteen characteristics had individual CDV scores between 0.50 and 0.79. They were clinically validated as *minor* defining characteristics, of which 12 were subjective. If the data from the subjective concepts of pain and discomfort were collapsed, the result might yield an increase in minor defining characteristics particularly when testing a larger sample.

Recommendations

The KCAT needs to be revised to reflect the findings of this study. The subjective defining characteristics of pain and discomfort need to be combined. The retained defining characteristics with individual CDV scores between 0.25 and 0.49 need to be subjected to additional clinical testing. The four additional objective characteristics observed by the nurse raters need to be included in the KCAT and clinically tested. The six subjective signs and symptoms that were identified in the field notes need to be examined for possible inclusion into the KCAT for testing. Future testing of KCAT needs to be done with a sample that is more representative of a normal cardiac population.

To achieve a geographic representation, the content validity of the revised KCAT needs to be retested using Fehring's DCV model by having cardiovascular nurse experts across the country rate the items for content validity. Clinical testing using Fehring's CDV model with a larger sample using multiple settings can then be done. The number of nurse raters using the KCAT to evaluate subjects needs to be expanded to include staff nurses caring for the cardiovascular patient.

Fehring (1986) proposed three types of standardized tests of validity to be provided for each nursing diagnosis: (1) the diagnostic content validity (DCV), (2) the clinical diagnostic validity (CDV), and (3) etiologic correlation ratings (ECR). The ECR is used to rate the etiology's ability to predict the existence of a nursing diagnosis (Fehring, 1986). Etiologies for *alteration in tissue perfusion: cardiac* need to be identified and tested to complete the three validation tests for the nursing diagnosis.

Fehring's DCV or ECR models could be modified to validate independent, collaborative, and dependent nursing interventions for the nursing diagnosis *alteration in tissue perfusion: cardiac*. Evidence provided by such testing would complete the nursing diagnosis circle: that is, the existence of a patient response pattern to a state of altered cardiac tissue perfusion, the presence of relating factors, defining characteristics, and the direction for nursing interventions for *alteration in tissue perfusion: cardiac*. Modification of Fehring's ECR or DCV models for testing nursing interventions may provide nurses with a valid and reliable tool to measure the relationship of nursing interventions to the proposed diagnostic category.

Summary

Nursing diagnoses provide the nomenclature that reflects the body of scientific knowledge unique to nursing. This study used two previously tested validation models to provide evidence to support the clinical validation of *alteration in tissue perfusion: cardiac*. In the validation process a new diagnostic tool, the KCAT, was designed, content validated, and clinically tested. The clinical validation of *alteration in tissue perfusion: cardiac* will assist nurses to identify defining characteristics associated with patients' response to altered cardiac tissue perfusion and to communicate their findings in a consistent manner. In addition, nurses will have empirically based data on which to direct, document, and evaluate care of patients with this diagnosis.

NOTE: Queries regarding the KCAT and its use should be directed to the author at the University of Arizona, College of Nursing, Tucson, Arizona.

References

American Heart Association. (1989). *Heart facts.* Dallas, TX: Author.

Fehring, R. J. (1986). Validating diagnostic labels: Standardized methodology. In M. A. Hurley (Ed.), *Classification of nursing diagnoses: Proceedings of the sixth national conference* (pp. 183–190). St. Louis, MO: Mosby.

Kelly, D. J. (1989). *The identification and clinical validation of the defining characteristics of the nursing diagnosis alteration in tissue perfusion: Cardiac.* Unpublished master's thesis, University of Arizona, Tucson.

Kim, M. J., Amoroso, R., Gulanick, M., Moyer, K., Parsons, E., Scherubel, J., Stafford, M. J., Suhayda, R., & Yocum, C. (1980). Clinical use of nursing diagnosis in cardiovascular nursing. In M. J. Kim & D. A. Moritz (Eds.), *Classification of nursing diagnoses: Proceedings of the third and fourth national conferences* (pp. 184–190). New York: McGraw-Hill.

Kim, M. J., Amoroso-Seritella, R., Gulanick, M., Moyer, K., Parsons, E., Scherubel, J., Stafford, M. J., Suhayda, R., & Yocum, C. (1984). Clinical validation of cardiovascular nursing diagnoses. In M. J. Kim, G. K. McFarland, & A. M. McLane (Eds.), *Classification of nursing diagnoses: Proceedings of the fifth national conference* (pp. 128–137). St. Louis, MO: Mosby.

Kritek, P. B. (1986). Development of a taxonomic structure for nursing diagnoses: A review and an update. In M. A. Hurley (Ed.), *Classification of nursing diagnoses: Proceedings of the sixth national conference* (pp. 23–38). St. Louis. MO: Mosby.

Murdaugh, C. L., & O'Rourke, R. A. (1988). Coronary heart disease in women: Special considerations. *Current Problems in Cardiology, 13*(2), 73–156.

NANDA. (1988). NANDA approved nursing diagnostic categories. *Nursing Diagnosis Newsletter, 15*(1), 3.

NANDA. (1989). *Taxonomy I revised (1989).* St. Louis, MO: Author.

Rossi, L. P., & Haines, V. M. (1979). Nursing diagnosis related to acute myocardial infarction. *Cardiovascular Nursing, 15*(3), 11–15.

A Nursing Diagnosis Validation Study: Defining Characteristics of Spiritual Distress

Frances A. McHolm, MSN, RN

Despite the fact that the origins of organized nursing were nurtured by religious orders (Dolan, Fitzpatrick, & Herrmann, 1983; Kalisch & Kalisch, 1978) and that Florence Nightingale viewed nursing as a calling from God (Nightingale, 1859/1969), spiritual perspectives in modern nursing practice have been largely ignored as a result of an emphasis on scientific empiricism, a lack of educational preparation in regard to spiritual issues, and a discomfort on the part of many nurses about how to deal with spiritual issues (Ellis, 1980; Fish & Shelly, 1983; Hubert, 1963). Chadwick (1973) and Miaskowski and Garofallow (1986) demonstrated that nurses were hesitant to identify and deal with spiritual distress in their nursing practice; Highfield and Cason (1983) found that nurses were unable to differentiate spiritual distress from psychologic distress.

Recent holistic and phenomenologic trends in nursing have reawakened awareness of nursing's responsibility to address the spiritual as well as mental, emotional, and physical needs of patients (Clemence, 1966; Colliton, 1981; Dickinson, 1975; Ellis, 1980; Stallwood & Stoll, 1975). This is especially pertinent in light of the fact that many researchers have shown that meeting spiritual needs helps people cope with life-threatening diseases such as cancer (Brandt, 1987; Carey, 1974; Gibbs & Acterberg-Lawlis, 1978; Miller, 1983; Slaughter, 1979; and Sodestrom & Martinson, 1987). Nurses who are more aware of cues indicating that an individual is experiencing spiritual distress would be more confident in addressing spiritual issues. They could then plan appropriate interventions to facilitate coping.

The nursing diagnosis *spiritual distress*, together with 13 defining characteristics, was accepted for further testing by the North American Nursing Diagnosis Association (NANDA) in 1980 (Kim & Moritz, 1982) (see Table 1). Since that time only one study by Weatherall and Creason (1987), who triangulated the NANDA characteristics of *spiritual distress* with cues found in the literature and a small sample of patient data, has sought to validate behaviors observed in patients with spiritual concerns. If nurses are going to intervene on behalf of a patient's spiritual

Table 1: Defining Characteristics of *Spiritual Distress* Accepted for Testing by NANDA in 1980

Expressed concern with meaning of life/death or be-
  lief system*
Anger toward God
Questions meaning of suffering
Verbalizes inner conflict about beliefs
Verbalizes concern about relationship with deity
Questions moral/ethical implications of therapeutic
  regimen
Gallows humor
Displacement of anger toward religious
  representatives
Description of nightmares/sleep disturbance
Alteration in behavior/mood evidenced by anger, cry-
  ing, withdrawal, preoccupation, anxiety, hostility,
  apathy, etc.

---

*Critical defining characteristic
SOURCE: Gordon, M. (1985). *Manual of Nursing Diagnosis.*
  New York: McGraw-Hill.

needs, the cluster of signs and symptoms that point to the diagnosis of *spiritual distress* need to be further clarified.

Purpose

The purpose of this descriptive study was to identify the defining characteristics of *spiritual distress* observed by nurses in oncology patients whom they perceived to be experiencing *spiritual distress,* and to compare those characteristics with the list presently approved by NANDA. Further, the intent of the study was to determine the level of confidence with which those characteristics might be used in clinical practice as indicators of *spiritual distress.*

Theoretical Assumptions

The basic assumption of this study was that people are spiritual as well as biologic and psychosocial beings. The spiritual dimension involves the core of being where the search for personal meaning occurs (Colliton, 1981; Fish & Shelly, 1983; Frankl, 1963).

Stallwood and Stoll (1975) have suggested a model of the dimensions of the person that is helpful in understanding the dynamics of *spiritual distress.* This model presents the biologic and psychologic dimensions of the whole person as concentric rings around the innermost circle of the spirit. The dotted lines that define the circles suggest the interrelatedness of these three dimensions. Arrows extending from the outer circles into the circle of the spirit represent the penetrating effect of life experiences and crises on the inner being; arrows pointing outward from the spirit circle demonstrate that experiences affecting the spirit are expressed through the emotional and physical aspects of the person. The model suggests that when life events cause disruption in spiritual equilibrium, the spiritual distress that results may be expressed in the psychosocial realm of the moral sense (guilt); emotion (crying, anger, depression); intellect (denial); or will (withdrawal). *Spiritual distress* may be further manifested in physical symptoms of stress illnesses such as peptic ulcer, headache, or fatigue (Selye, 1976; Stallwood & Stoll, 1975).

The conceptual definition of spiritual distress used in this study, adapted from the suggestion by Carpenito (1983), is that *spiritual distress* is the state of experiencing or being at risk of experiencing a disturbance in the relationships or in the belief/value system that is the person's source of strength, hope, and meaning in life.

Methods

Data-Collection Procedure

Randomly selected mailing labels of 300 Oncology Nursing Society members from all over the United States who had at least a BSN or nursing doctorate degree were obtained. A single-folded form that included a letter to participants, the Spiritual Distress Defining Characteristic Tool (SDDCT), and a demographic data form was sent to each nurse with a request to return the completed form by a specified date. To be included in the sample, the subjects had to have at least 6 months' experience as a registered nurse, and at least 6 months' experience working with oncology patients in the previous 2 years.

Instrument

The SDDCT was a Likert-type tool developed for this study. It listed 41 characteristics of *spiritual distress* identified in the nursing literature. Items selected for the tool included the 13 characteristics approved for testing by NANDA and six additional characteristics suggested at NANDA's Fifth Conference in 1982 (Kim, McFarland, & McLane, 1984). Also included were 17 characteristics not on the NANDA-approved list, but which were validated by Weatherall (1986). The seven subcategories listed under the NANDA characteristic "alteration in behavior/mood" were listed as separate items. Two items, "gallows humor" (Kim & Moritz, 1982) and "use of humor to indicate spiritual need" (Weatherall, 1986), were combined into one item because of their similarity.

According to the validation method suggested by Fehring (1986) and implemented by Vincent (1986), respondents were asked to use a five-point Likert scale ranging from "nearly always present" to "rarely present" to indicate how frequently they observed each characteristic in patients whom they perceived to be experiencing *spiritual distress*. In addition to demographic data questions, the subjects were asked to indicate how often they perceived that patients experience *spiritual distress*, and whether they used this diagnosis in their clinical practice.

Analysis

To compute diagnostic content validity (DCV) ratings for each characteristic, weights were assigned to each response so that $5 = 1$, $4 = 0.75$, $3 = 0.50$, $2 = 0.25$, and $1 = 0$. The ratings given by respondents to each cue were added together and divided by the total number of nurses who evaluated that cue (Fehring, 1986). The closer the resulting ratio was to 1.0, the more valid the item was considered to be. Characteristics with ratios greater than 0.75 were considered to be critical supporting characteristics, and those with ratios greater than 0.50 but less than 0.75 were labeled as supporting characteristics. Cues with ratios 0.50 and lower were discarded from the final list.

To compute overall DCV ratios for lists of characteristics identified by groups of nurses in the study, the individual DCV scores of each characteristic on the list were added together and divided by the total number of items in that list. Statistical computation was accomplished by means of a computer program developed specifically for this study. Accuracy of results was verified by corresponding manual calculation of selected items.

Findings and Discussion

Ninety-seven Oncology Nursing Society members from 31 different states returned questionnaires and met criteria for the study. Most of the nurses ranged in age from 20 to 39 years (71.2%), and had an average of 11.1 years' experience in nursing and 5.8 years' experience in oncology nursing.

While 51 (52.6%) of the respondents indicated they were familiar with the NANDA list of nursing diagnoses, only 28 (28.9%) indicated that they utilized the nursing diagnosis of *spiritual distress* in their clinical practice. The latter subset of 28 nurses was designated as the "diagnosis users" in the data analysis because they represented a group of experts. Forty-four respondents who indicated that their patients experienced *spiritual distress* "frequently" to "nearly always" were identified as the "clinical identifiers" in the data analysis because they recognized that the state occurred on a regular basis. These two subgroups were not mutually exclusive: all but 2 of the 28 diagnosis users were also included in the group of 44 clinical identifiers. The results of the sample as a whole were also included in the data analysis designated as the "total nurses" group.

The three groups of nurses in the study identified a range of 1 to 6 critical, and 25 to 28 supporting defining characteristics (see Tables 2 and 3).

Similarities were noted among groups. For example, all groups identified anxiety as a critical defining characteristic. Most of the other critical defining characteristics identified by the nurses in the study were also alterations of mood or affect and included fear, depression, helplessness, discouragement, and crying. Only one critical defining characteristic, "cues that religious/spiritual needs are important," more specifically pointed to spiritual concerns.

Table 2: Critical Defining Characteristics of Spiritual Distress (>0.75) as Identified by Groups of Oncology Nurses

Total Sample (*n* = 97)	Diagnosis Users (*n* = 28)	Clinical Identifiers (*n* = 44)
Anxiety (0.78)	Anxiety (0.81)	Anxiety (0.85)
	Helplessness (0.78)	Crying (0.78)
	Crying (0.77)	Helplessness (0.78)
	Cues that religious/ spiritual needs are important (0.76)	Depression (0.78)
		Fear (0.78)
	Fear (0.76)	Discouragement (0.76)

As seen in Table 3, nurses in the study also identified many supporting defining characteristics that were cues of distress not specifically related to spiritual issues. Examples of these cues were withdrawal, preoccupation, sighing, and description of somatic complaints. Additional cues relating specifically to religious/spiritual issues, such as "questions meaning of suffering," "seeks spiritual assistance," and "verbalized inner conflict about beliefs," were validated but generally did not have higher DCV scores than the more general characteristics.

These findings emphasize the nonspecific indicators of distress and are consistent with the model of the person presented by Stallwood and Stoll (1975) that suggests that experiences affecting the spirit are expressed through emotional and biologic responses. The finding that most of the critical cues involved alterations in mood or affect also suggests that the reason nurses have difficulty differentiating spiritual from psychosocial distress (Highfield & Cason, 1983) is because of the similar manner in which these are outwardly expressed.

It is of interest that three of the nonspecific critical defining characteristics identified in the study are approved nursing diagnostic categories in themselves, namely *anxiety, fear,* and *depression*. This result does not mean that these characteristics cannot be valid cues for *spiritual distress*. It does mean, however, that the diagnosis of *spiritual distress* must also be considered when these cues are observed, or when these categories are selected as appropriate nursing diagnoses. It also suggests that *spiritual distress* can be considered as an etiologic factor for any of these, or other, diagnostic categories (e.g., *anxiety* related to spiritual distress).

Several similarities and differences were noted between the characteristics identified in the study and the NANDA-approved list. The critical cue on the NANDA list, "expresses concern with the meaning of life and

Table 3: Supporting Defining Characteristics of *Spiritual Distress* (>0.50) as Identified by Groups of Oncology Nurses

Total Sample (n = 97)	Diagnosis Users (n = 28)	Clinical Identifiers (n = 44)
Fear (0.74)	Depression (0.75)	Anorexia (0.75)
Helplessness (0.72)	Frustration/agitation (0.74)	Frustration/agitation (0.74)
Crying (0.71)	Discouragement (0.73)	Anger (0.72)
Discouragement (0.70)	Questions meaning of suffering (0.72)	Description of somatic complaints (0.70)
Cues that spiritual needs are important (0.69)	Preoccupation (0.69)	Questions meaning of suffering (0.69)
Anger (0.68)	Anorexia (0.69)	Cues having to do with relationships with others (0.69)
Frustration/agitation (0.68)	Anger (0.68)	Despair/hopelessness (0.69)
Anorexia (0.67)	Description of somatic complaints (0.66)	Cues that religious/spiritual needs are important (0.68)
Description of somatic complaints (0.66)	Cues having to do with relationships with others (0.66)	Inadequate coping (0.68)
Cues having to do with relationships with others (0.65)	Seeks spiritual assistance (0.65)	Preoccupation (0.66)
Questions meaning of suffering (0.65)	Despair/hopelessness (0.64)	Hostility (0.66)
Inadequate coping (0.64)	Silence (0.63)	Withdrawal (0.66)
Seeks spiritual assistance (0.62)	Withdrawal (0.63)	Sighing (0.64)
Preoccupation (0.62)	Inadequate coping (0.62)	Silence (0.64)
Despair/hopelessness (0.61)	Expresses concern with meaning of life and death or belief systems (0.62)	Expresses concern with meaning of life and death or belief systems (0.64)
Sighing (0.60)	Verbalizes inner conflict about beliefs (0.59)	Bitterness (0.63)
Talkativeness (0.59)	Cues having to do with guilt and forgiveness (0.59)	Seeks spiritual assistance (0.62)
Withdrawal (0.59)	Hostility (0.57)	Cues having to do with guilt and forgiveness (0.60)
Expresses concern with meaning of life and death or belief systems (0.59)	Bitterness (0.57)	Talkativeness (0.59)
Hostility (0.57)	Unable to accept self (0.54)	Apathy (0.56)
Bitterness (0.56)	Anger toward God (0.54)	Anger toward God (0.56)
Silence (0.55)	Questions meaning of own existence (0.53)	Verbalizes inner conflict about beliefs (0.55)
Cues having to do with guilt and forgiveness (0.55)	Engages in self-blame (0.52)	Questions meaning of own existence (0.59)
Apathy (0.51)	Use of humor to indicate spiritual need (0.51)	Unable to accept self (0.52)
Verbalizes conflict about beliefs (0.51)	Descriptions of nightmares or sleep disturbances (0.51)	Descriptions of nightmares or sleep disturbances (0.51)

death and/or belief system," was identified as a supporting characteristic, but not a critical characteristic, by each of the groups of nurses in the study. Of the 19 characteristics on the NANDA-approved list (with the alterations of mood and affect listed out separately), 14 were validated with scores greater than 0.50 by at least 2 groups of nurses in the study and 10 were validated by all 3 groups (see Table 4).

While a relatively high number of characteristics were validated by this study, more than 25% of the NANDA characteristics were not observed frequently enough to be considered usable indicators. Thirteen additional characteristics *not* included on the NANDA list were also validated with ratios greater than 0.50 by at least two groups of nurses in the study (see Table 5). These results indicate that the present list of charac-

Table 4: NANDA Characteristics of *Spiritual Distress* Validated by at Least Two Groups of Nurses with DCV Scores Greater Than 0.50

Expresses concern with meaning of life and death or belief system*
Anger toward God
Questions meaning of suffering*
Verbalizes inner conflict about beliefs*
Questions meaning for own existence
Seeks spiritual assistance*
Descriptions of nightmares and sleep disturbances
Anger*
Crying*
Withdrawal*
Preoccupation*
Anxiety*
Hostility*
Apathy

*Denotes characteristics validated with a DCV score greater than 0.50 by all three groups of nurses in the study and by NANDA.

teristics of *spiritual distress* approved for testing by NANDA may not be fully adequate to identify that state in patients. Further research studies similar to this one need to be conducted with various patient groups to develop a more usable approved list.

Overall standardized validity ratings for the lists of characteristics identified in the study were computed in order to determine how representative these lists are of the state of *spiritual distress,* and therefore how useful they would be in the clinical setting to identify that state. The list of characteristics identified by each group of nurses in the study received overall DCV ratings that ranged from 0.64 to 0.66 (see Table 6). While these ratings were of moderate level they do not indicate a strong consensus that the lists are highly representative of the state of *spiritual distress*. This finding indicates that the results of this study are not sufficient to validate the characteristics of *spiritual distress*. However, it is of interest to note that when the individual DCV scores for each characteristic as determined by the nurses were assigned to the present NANDA list, its ratings ranged from 0.55 to 0.59. This finding that the lists identified in this study were more highly representative of the state of spiritual distress than the present NANDA-approved list suggests that this study is at least one further step in validating a cluster of cues that point to the diagnosis.

Limitations

The limitations of this study included the assumption that oncology nurses were "ex-

Table 5: Characteristics of *Spiritual Distress* Given DCV Scores Greater than 0.50 by Two Groups of Nurses but Not on the NANDA-Approved List

Unable to accept self
Description of somatic complaints
Cues having to do with relationships with others
Cues having to do with guilt and forgiveness
Cues that religious/spiritual needs are important
Inadequate coping
Despair/hopelessness
Fear
Depression
Helplessness
Anorexia
Silence
Bitterness

Table 6: Overall DCV Scores of the Lists of Characteristics of *Spiritual Distress* as Identified by Oncology Nurses

Overall DCV	Total Group (*n* = 97)	Diagnosis Users (*n* = 28)	Clinical Identifiers (*n* = 44)
Characteristics identified in this study	0.64	0.66	0.64
Characteristics approved by NANDA	0.55	0.59	0.58

perts" in recognizing factors that indicate spiritual distress. Initially the researcher believed that because spiritual issues were sometimes acknowledged in oncology and specifically hospice nursing literature, a sample of oncology nurses would be more experienced in identifying *spiritual distress* than nurses in general. However, only a relatively small percentage of that sample reported that they identified *spiritual distress* regularly or that they used the diagnosis in their practice.

A second limitation involves the present lack of clarity within the healthcare field regarding the concept of *spiritual distress*. Formal research in this area is new and conceptual clarity has not yet been achieved. This lack of clarity has perhaps been a major restraining factor in the willingness of nurses to tackle the problems of dealing with spiritual aspects of practice. While it is necessary to tolerate some vagueness while further work in this area is pursued, it is hoped that this study is a part of the effort to achieve greater clarity.

Recommendations for Future Research

Recommendations for future research include:

1. Establishment of content validity of the characteristics listed on the SDDCT by review of a multidisciplinary panel of experts from the fields of religion, pastoral care, philosophy, sociology, psychology, etc.
2. Replication of the study with use of a "cue dictionary" so that the meaning of each characteristic would be common to all respondents.
3. Replication of the study using Delphi rounds in which the 31 validated cues of *spiritual distress* would be honed to a smaller cluster of most frequently identified cues.
4. Replication of the study with validation

of the presence and meaning of characteristics of *spiritual distress* through direct patient observation and interview.

Further study regarding the diagnosis of *spiritual distress* also needs to focus on validation of etiologies, goals, and nursing interventions for assisting patients to deal creatively with the state of *spiritual distress*.

Implications for Nursing

Although this particular study has focused on oncology patients, it is *not* inferred that *spiritual distress* is a problem only of those facing life-threatening illness; spiritual concerns are potentially a concern for any individual in a healthcare setting.

In light of the findings that spiritual needs are frequently expressed through nonspecific indicators of distress, nurse educators in basic and continuing nursing education programs need to include more emphasis on spiritual aspects of care. Basic and elective courses need to emphasize the manner in which inner spiritual turmoil may be expressed through emotional and physical dimensions of the person. In addition to focusing on cues that may indicate that a spiritual need exists, observations and questions that may be used to clarify whether the source of the distress is physical, psychosocial, or spiritual also need to be discussed.

Implications for direct care are based on the hope that the results of this study have helped to develop a clearer picture of the state of spiritual distress and of cues that point to the state. It is hoped that clarification of possible indicators of *spiritual distress* will assist nurses involved in direct patient care to have more confidence in assessing the state. This confidence will assist them to identify *spiritual distress* when it occurs so that appropriate interventions can be implemented to facilitate coping.

References

Brandt, B. (1987). The relationship between hopelessness and selected variables in women receiving chemotherapy for breast cancer. *Oncology Nursing Forum, 14*(2), 35–39.

Carey, R. G. (1974). Emotional adjustment in terminal patients: A quantitative approach. *Journal of Counseling Psychology, 21,* 433–439.

Carpenito, L. J. (1983). *Nursing diagnosis; Application to clinical practice.* Philadelphia: Lippincott.

Chadwick, R. (1973). Awareness and preparedness of nurses to meet spiritual needs. *The Nurse's Lamp, 22*(6), 2–3.

Clemence, M. (1966). Existentialism: A philosophy of commitment. *American Journal of Nursing, 66,* 500–505.

Colliton, M. (1981). The spiritual dimension of nursing. In I. Beland & J. Passos (Eds.), *Clinical nursing* (4th ed., pp. 492–501). New York: Macmillan.

Dickinson, C. (1975). The search for spiritual meaning. *American Journal of Nursing, 75,* 1789.

Dolan, J., Fitzpatrick, M., & Herrmann, E. (1983). *Nursing in society: An historical perspective.* Philadelphia: Saunders.

Ellis, D. (1980). Whatever happened to the spiritual dimension? *The Canadian Nurse, 80*(9), 42–43.

Fehring, R. (1986). Validating diagnostic labels; Standardized methodology. In M. Hurley (Ed.), *Classification of nursing diagnoses: Proceedings of the sixth national conference* (pp. 183–190). St. Louis, MO: Mosby.

Fish, J., & Shelly, J. (1983). *Spiritual care: The nurse's role.* Downer's Grove, IL: InterVarsity Press.

Frankl, V. (1963). *Man's search for meaning, an introduction to logotherapy.* New York: Washington Square Press.

Gibbs, H., & Acterberg-Lawlis, J. (1978). Spiritual values and death anxiety: Implications for counseling with terminal cancer patients. *Journal of Counseling Psychology, 25,* 563–569.

Gordon, M. (1985). *Manual of nursing diagnosis.* New York: McGraw-Hill.

Highfield, M., & Cason, C. (1983). Spiritual needs of patients: Are they recognized? *Cancer Nursing, 6*(3), 187–192.

Hubert, Sr. M. (1963). Spiritual care for every patient. *Journal of Nursing Education, 2*(2), 9–11.

Kalisch, P., & Kalisch, B. (1978). *The advance of American nursing.* Boston: Little, Brown.

Kim, M., McFarland, G., & McLane, A. (Eds.). (1984). *Classification of nursing diagnoses: Proceedings of the fifth national conference.* St. Louis, MO: Mosby.

Kim, M., & Moritz, D. (Eds.). (1982). *Classification of nursing diagnoses: Proceedings of the third and fourth national conferences.* New York: McGraw-Hill.

Miaskowski, C., & Garofallow, G. (1986). A study of nursing diagnoses in an oncologic patient population. In M. Hurley (Ed.), *Classification of nursing diagnoses: Proceedings of the sixth national conference* (pp. 465–468). St. Louis, MO: Mosby.

Miller, J. F. (1983). *Coping with chronic illness.* Philadelphia: Davis.

Nightingale, F. (1859/1969). *Notes on nursing.* New York: Dover.

Selye, H. (1976). *The stress of life* (2nd ed.). New York: McGraw-Hill.

Slaughter, T. (1979). *Identifying the spiritual needs of the oncology patient.* Unpublished master's thesis, University of Arizona, Tempe.

Sodestrom, K., & Martinson, I. (1987). Patients' spiritual coping strategies: A study of nurse and patient perspectives. *Oncology Nursing Forum, 14*(2), 41–51.

Stallwood, J., & Stoll, R. (1975). Spiritual dimensions of nursing practice. In I. Beland & J. Passos (Eds.), *Clinical nursing* (pp. 1086–1098). New York: Macmillan.

Vincent, K. (1986). The validation of a nursing diagnosis: A nurse consensus survey. In M. Hurley (Ed.), *Classification of nursing diagnoses: Proceedings of the sixth national conference* (pp. 207–214). St. Louis, MO: Mosby.

Weatherall, J., & Creason, N. (1987). Validation of the nursing diagnosis, spiritual distress. In A. M. McLane (Ed.), *Classification of nursing diagnoses: Proceedings of the seventh national conference* (pp. 182–185). St. Louis, MO: Mosby.

Validation of the Nursing Diagnosis *Sensory/Perceptual Alteration: Auditory*

Janice K. Janken, PhD, RN
Carol Lewis Cullinan, MSN, RN, C, FNP

The major defining characteristics for the nursing diagnosis *sensory/perceptual alteration: auditory* are disorientation in time, person, or place; altered abstraction; altered conceptualization; change in problem-solving abilities; reported or measured change in sensory acuity; change in behavior pattern; anxiety; apathy; change in usual response to stimuli; indication of body-image alteration; restlessness; irritability; and altered communication patterns (Carroll-Johnson, 1989). These defining characteristics theoretically are used by practicing nurses to make a diagnosis of *auditory sensory/perceptual alteration*, and suggest that a relationship exists between hearing impairment and changes in psychosocial functioning. However, the widely accepted assumption that hearing loss is associated with changes in psychosocial functioning has not been clearly demonstrated. Consequently, two purposes of this study were to (1) explore if psychosocial dysfunctioning is associated with hearing impairment and (2) evaluate the utility of using psychosocial changes as cues for making the nursing diagnosis *sensory/perceptual alteration: auditory.*

The current configuration of defining characteristics for *sensory/perceptual alteration* omits two variables that consistently appear in the literature as being related to hearing loss. They are increasing age (e.g., Kelly, 1985; Stone, 1987) and impacted cerumen (e.g., Bricco, 1985; Senturia, Goldstein, & Hersperger, 1983). Thus, a third aim of this study was to evaluate an alternative model of defining characteristics for predicting auditory impairment, one that incorporates age and impacted cerumen.

The specific research questions addressed were

1. What relationships exist between hearing ability and psychosocial functioning in acutely ill geriatric patients?
2. To what extent do changes in psycho-

The financial support for this project by Nurse Practitioner Associates for Continuing Education is gratefully acknowledged.

social functioning predict hearing impairment?

3. Do age and the presence of impacted cerumen significantly affect hearing ability?

Methods

Design

The design was a descriptive survey. The major defining characteristics for *sensory/perceptual alteration* were operationalized as seven variables: depression, cognitive function, social contact with children, social contact with relatives other than children, social contact with friends, self-reported hearing ability, and self-reported overall health status. Auditory sensory perception was operationalized as number of tones heard on the audiometric exam.

Sample

A random sample of 250 subjects was selected over a one-year period from English-speaking patients aged 65 years or older admitted to nonintensive care units of a large teaching hospital. Patients hospitalized more than once during the sampling period were eligible for selection only on their first admission. The computer in the hospital's admitting department was programmed to produce a daily list of admissions meeting the sample criteria. Every third day, the list was used in conjunction with a table of random numbers to select two or three subjects. Sampling every third day over a one-year period was done to ensure that admissions from all seven days of the week were represented, and to eliminate any seasonal bias.

Instruments

Mini-Mental Status Examination (MMSE)

The MMSE (Folstein, 1983) is an 11-question general-purpose screening examination that assesses several cognitive functions: consciousness, orientation, attention, thought content/form/processes, memory, language, general knowledge, and constructional ability (Foreman, 1987). This exam was used to determine the presence of the defining characteristics disorientation, altered abstraction, altered conceptualization, and change in problem-solving abilities.

Studies of test-retest reliability on this instrument have resulted in correlations of 0.56, 0.89, and 0.98, and studies of interrater reliability have produced coefficients of not less than 0.82 (Anthony, LeResche, Niaz, Van Korff, & Folstein, 1982; Folstein, 1983). Validity tests of the MMSE have achieved precision values ranging from 0.82 to 0.87 and specificity values ranging from 0.80 and 0.82 (Anthony et al., 1983; Foreman, 1987). Correlations between MMSE results and psychiatrists' clinical diagnoses yielded r values from 0.82 to 0.87 (Anthony et al., 1983). Together these results indicate that the instrument has acceptable reliability and validity in screening cognitive function. In this study the obtained reliability alpha coefficient was 0.84.

Geriatric Depression Scale (GDS) [short form]

The GDS (Yesavage, 1986) is a 15-item scale with yes/no questions that has been used as a screening device for depression in both physically well and physically ill elderly persons. Items ask about change in activity and feelings of boredom, fear, and lack of energy; thus, this scale was used to assess the defining characteristics of change in behavior pattern, anxiety, and apathy.

Reliability and validity studies of the GDS have been conducted (Yesavage & Brink, 1983). Cronbach's alpha was computed to assess internal consistency of the measure, yielding a coefficient of 0.94. Split-half reliability resulted in a coefficient of 0.94. When the scale was administered one week apart to 20 subjects, the test-retest reliability coefficient was 0.85. Validity was assessed by administering the scale to three groups of elderly persons: normal, mildly depressed, and severely depressed; the mean scores were ordered as predicted with normal subjects scoring the lowest and the severely depressed scoring the highest. In this study Cronbach's alpha was 0.87.

Hebrew Rehabilitation Center for Aged (HRCA) Social Contact Scale

The HRCA Social Contact Scale assesses the frequency of contacts that persons have with relatives and friends either face-to-face, via phone, or by letter, and their satisfaction with this amount of contact. Three of six components were used in this study: contact with children and grandchildren, contact with other relatives, and contact with friends. This instrument was used to assess the defining characteristic of altered communication patterns. Previously, reliabilities for internal consistency (Kuder-Richardson 20) had been computed for components of the scale using data from three samples; the values ranged between 0.63 and 0.95 (Sherwood, 1975). In this study, the internal consistency scores for the three scales used were social contact with friends 0.81, with other relatives 0.82, and with children 0.85.

Interview/medical record

An interview or the medical record were used to elicit data on age, sex, marital status, education, medical diagnosis, and living arrangements. In addition, subjects were asked to self-rate their hearing and their overall health as being either excellent, good, fair, poor, or bad. Self-rated hearing was used to assess the defining characteristic of reported change in sensory acuity, and self-rated health was used to operationalize indication of body-image alteration.

Otoscopic exam

An otoscopic exam of each ear canal was performed to determine the presence of im-pacted cerumen. Impacted cerumen was defined as an inability to visualize the tympanic membrane due to cerumen blocking the ear canal. Data were recorded as one ear canal occluded, both canals occluded, or neither ear canal occluded.

AudioScope

Finally, a geriatric version of the AudioScope was used to measure hearing. This instrument tests frequencies of 500, 1000, 2000, and 4000 Hertz (Hz) at an intensity of 40 decibels (dB), which are the standard criteria for screening of hearing loss in the elderly. The maximum score is to hear a total of eight tones or all four frequencies in both ears. Several studies (Bienvenue, Michael, Chaffinch, & Zeigler, 1985; Griffin, Bordenick, & Vernon, 1984; Hawke & Mansfield, 1984) have compared AudioScope results with those of conventional pure-tone air and bone conduction audiometric tests. Correlations between the two measures ranged from 0.9 to 1.0, indicating that the AudioScope is a valid instrument for detecting hearing impairment. Test-retest reliability coefficients from a sample of 182 subjects at the four test frequencies were all at least 0.98, indicating high reliability of the technique and repeatability of the results (Bienvenue et al., 1985).

Procedure

Potential subjects were approached on either the second or third day of hospital stay, informed of the study purpose, and asked to sign a consent form if they agreed to participate. After obtaining information on the demographic variables, self-reported hearing ability, and self-reported overall health status, the MMSE, GDS, and HRCA Social Contact Scale were administered, their order being randomized for each subject in order to avoid systematic bias. Following completion of these questionnaires, a hearing test was conducted with the AudioScope. Then the otoscopic exam was performed on each ear canal.

A companion study (Cullinan & Janken, 1990) evaluated the effect of removing impacted cerumen on restoring hearing ability. Thus, when impacted cerumen was observed, the nursing intervention of ear-canal irrigation was administered to clean the ear canal.

Results

Of the 250 subjects recruited for the study, 226 (90.4%) consented to participate. Forty-eight percent of the subjects were male (n = 109) and 52% female (n = 117). The ages of participants ranged from 65 to 99 years (M = 75.4, SD = 8.45). Years of education varied from 2 to 27 years, with a mean of 9.97 years (SD = 3.85). Only 7.1% (n = 16) of the sample were admitted to the hospital from a nursing home, while 33.6% (n = 76) lived at home independently and 59.3% (n = 134) lived at home with at least one other person.

Pearson product-moment correlations were computed to examine the relationships between depression; cognitive function; social contact with children, relatives, and friends; self-rated hearing; self-rated health; and hearing ability as assessed with the AudioScope. Significant, but at best moderate relationships (p < .0001) were found between hearing ability and self-rated hearing (r = 0.46), depression (r = −0.36), and cognitive functioning (r = −0.34). The negative sign before the depression and cognitive functioning values indicates an inverse relationship with hearing ability—in other words, subjects with depression and cognitive dysfunction tended to have poorer hearing. Significant weak correlations (p < .01) were found between hearing ability and social contact with friends (r = 0.72), self-rated health (r = 0.20), and social contact with relatives other than children and grandchildren (r = 0.20). The amount of contact with children and

grandchildren was not significantly related to hearing ability.

A multiple regression analysis was done to determine to what extent the changes in psychosocial functioning could predict hearing impairment. The seven variables representing the defining characteristics of *sensory/perception alteration* were used as potential predictors for the hearing score obtained on the AudioScope. Theoretically, these are the cues used in everyday nursing practice to make the diagnosis. Of the seven potential explanatory variables, only self-rated hearing and depression significantly added to the 29.5% explained variance in hearing ability. Table 1 shows the beta weights of the two variables, indicating their relative importance in explaining hearing ability. As can be seen, self-rated hearing was approximately two times stronger than depression as a predictor variable.

Potential predictor variables were expanded to include age and presence of impacted cerumen. As required for the computation of multiple regression, data on the three cerumen conditions of the ear canals were recoded into dichotomized or dummy variables: (1) cerumen occlusion of one or both ears versus clear ear canals, and (2) cerumen occlusion of one canal versus neither or both ears occluded. In this expanded model of 10 potential predictor variables, four significantly contributed to the 65.9% explained variance in hearing ability. As can be seen in Table 2, the contributing variables were age, impacted cerumen, and self-rated hearing with self-rated hearing being the only vari-

Table 1: Significant Beta Weights of Variables Representing Defining Characteristics Regressed on Hearing Score

Variable	Beta Weight
Self-rated hearing	0.416 (p < .00001)
Depression	0.227 (p < .01)

$r^2 = 0.295$

Table 2: Significant Beta Weights of Expanded Model Defining Characteristics Regressed on Hearing

Variable	Beta Weight
Wax versus no wax	0.673 ($p < .00001$)
Self-rated hearing	0.310 ($p < .00001$)
Wax, 1 ear versus the other	0.241 ($p < .00001$)
Age	0.171 ($p < .001$)

$r^2 = 0.659$

able currently serving as a defining characteristic.

Overall then, findings indicate that assessing psychosocial functions does not provide nurses with helpful cues for making the diagnosis *sensory/perceptual alteration: auditory.* Rather, results suggest that nurses can make a more accurate diagnosis merely by learning the patient's age and self-rating of hearing, and by checking ear canals for impacted cerumen.

Discussion

Although this study suggests that the currently accepted defining characteristics are invalid cues for making the *auditory sensory/perceptual alteration* diagnosis, it is far too premature to simply discard the diagnosis. A few points warrant consideration.

First, in contrast to some of the other nursing diagnoses, very little nursing research has focused on sensory impairment. This diagnosis is very broad with a singular list of defining characteristics provided for all five senses. Consequently, even though the currently accepted defining characteristics may not work well as predictors for auditory impairment, they may work better for the other four senses. Further study is recommended.

Second, this study focused on *chronic* hearing impairment. There may be a difference in how humans respond to *acute* hearing changes. Tracing the history behind the popular belief that sensory alterations are associated with psychosocial changes indicates that the notion stems from laboratory studies of acute sensory deprivation conducted on normal subjects during the 1950s and 1960s (Jackson & Ellis, 1971; Pollard, Uhr, & Jackson, 1963). Indeed, many of the symptoms exhibited by the normal subjects exposed to short-term sensory deprivation in the laboratory setting sound like the defining characteristics for *sensory/perceptual alteration.* However, laboratory results from normal subjects exposed to short-term sensory deprivation are not generalizable to patients in clinical settings who are experiencing the chronic progressive sensory losses associated with aging. In short, differences in defining characteristics for acute and chronic sensory alterations is another area that requires attention in future research.

Finally, even though these findings suggest that psychosocial changes do not serve well as defining characteristics or, in other words, as predictors for auditory impairment, there were significant associations between depression, cognitive dysfunction, social contact with friends and relatives other than children, and hearing impairment. These relationships should not be ignored. A look at the data relating depression and cognitive dysfunction to hearing ability illustrates the point.

On the GDS, scores greater than 5 indicate probable depression. Sixty-nine subjects (30.5% of the sample) had scores greater than 5. When their hearing was compared to those who were not depressed there was a significant difference; the depressed group heard an average of 3.47 out of the 8 possible tones in contrast to 5.06 tones for the nondepressed group. Similarly, on the MMSE, scores below 23 are indicative of cognitive impairment. Twenty-nine subjects (12.8%) had scores indicative of cognitive impairment. Their mean hearing score of 3.24 tones was significantly less than the mean number of tones (5.47) heard by the nonimpaired group.

These findings, along with the significant relationships between hearing ability and amount of social contact with friends and relatives other than children, suggest that once the diagnosis of impaired hearing is assigned, nurses should be alert to the possibility of these patients' increased risk for depression, cognitive impairment, and decreased social contact with friends and relatives other than children. Furthermore, rather than using alterations in psychosocial functioning as indicators for impaired hearing, as is currently done, these results suggest that perhaps impaired hearing should serve as a defining characteristic for the psychosocial diagnoses of *hopelessness, altered thought processes,* and *impaired social interaction.* This, too, is something that deserves exploration in future research.

References

Anthony, J. C., LeResche, I., Niaz, U., Van Korff, M. R., & Folstein, M. F. (1982). Limits of the "Mini-Mental State" as a screening test for dementia and delirium among hospital patients. *Psychological Medicine, 12,* 397–408.

Bienvenue, G., Michael, P., Chaffinch, J., & Zeigler, J. C. (1985). The AudioScope: A clinical tool for otoscopic and audiometric examination. *Ear and Hearing, 6,* 251–254.

Bricco, E. (1985). Impacted cerumen as a reason for failure in hearing conservation programs. *Journal of School Health, 55,* 240–241.

Carroll-Johnson, R. M. (Ed.). (1989). *Classification of nursing diagnoses: Proceedings of the eighth conference.* Philadelphia: Lippincott.

Cullinan, C. L., & Janken, J. K. (1990). Effect of cerumen removal on the hearing ability of geriatric patients. *Journal of Advanced Nursing, 15,* 594–600.

Folstein, M. F. (1983). The Mini-Mental State Examination. In T. Crook, S. Ferris, & R. Bartus (Eds.), *Assessment in geriatric psychopharmacology* (pp. 47–51). New Canaan, CT: Mark Powley Associates, Inc.

Foreman, M. D. (1987). Reliability and validity of mental status questionnaires in elderly hospitalized patients. *Nursing Research, 36,* 216–220.

Griffin, D. H., Bordenick, R. M., & Vernon, M. (1984). AudioScope in family practice: Field testing of a new instrument and a look at hearing loss in family practice. *Maryland State Medical Journal, 22,* 285–287.

Hawke, M., & Mansfield, D. (1984). Clinical evaluation of a screening audiometer and integral otoscope. *Modern Medicine of Canada, 39,* 200–203.

Jackson, C. W., & Ellis, R. (1971). Sensory deprivation as a field of study. *Nursing Research, 20,* 46–54.

Kelly, L. (1985, May). Hearing loss in the older person. *The Hearing Journal,* 24–27.

Pollard, J. C., Uhr, L., & Jackson, C. W. (1963). Studies in sensory deprivation. *Archives of General Psychiatry, 8,* 435–454.

Senturia, B., Goldstein, R., & Hersperger, W. (1983). Otorhinolaryngologic aspects of geriatric care. In F. U. Steinberg (Ed.), *Care of the geriatric patient* (pp. 482–492). St. Louis, MO: Mosby.

Sherwood, S. (1975). [Reliability data of HRCA Social Contact Scale.] Unpublished raw data, Hebrew Rehabilitation Center for Aged, Department of Social Gerontological Research, Boston.

Stone, J. T. (1987). Interventions for psychosocial problems associated with sensory disabilities in old age. In B. Heller, L. Flohr, & L. Zegans (Eds.), *Psychosocial interventions with sensorially disabled persons* (pp. 243–259). New York: Grune & Stratton.

Yesavage, J. A. (1986). The use of self-rating depression scales in the elderly. In *Handbook for clinical memory assessment of older adults* (pp. 213–217). Hyattsville, MD: American Psychological Association.

Yesavage, J. A., & Brink. T. L. (1983). Development and validation of a geriatric depression screening scale: A preliminary report. *Journal of Psychiatric Research, 17*(1), 37–49.

Impaired Skin Integrity: Clinical Validation of the Defining Characteristics

Janet Anderson, BAAN, RN
Aileen Thomson, BAAN, RN

Introduction

"In order to establish the independent professional status of nursing, a distinct knowledge base is required. This knowledge base can be credibly accomplished through scientific theory and research" (Hayes, 1987, p. 79). Integral to the development of a knowledge base, a language must be established to describe the clinical judgments upon which nursing care is based (Gordon, 1982). The term nursing diagnosis is used to describe the cluster of signs and symptoms (defining characteristics) derived from the nurse's assessment of the patient. Nursing diagnoses exclude problems that are treated by physician intervention.

Although nursing is in the process of establishing its independent professional status, the interdependent, collaborative functions are recognized. Gordon (1982) believed that nursing care consists of nursing diagnosis-related functions as well as delegated activities. These delegated activities include the implementation of disease treatment under medical orders or established protocols. According to Aydelott and Peterson (1987), practice is central to nursing and nursing diagnosis has been the primary instrument for refining the content upon which practice is based. Nursing diagnosis is supposed to be the "bridge over the knowledge–practice gap" (Bircher, 1986, p. 71).

Impaired skin integrity is one of the nursing diagnoses accepted for clinical testing by the North American Nursing Diagnosis Association (NANDA). The list of defining characteristics of the diagnosis has not been well developed, hence its validity has not been established. This study involved assessing patients with impairments of the skin in order to develop a list of defining characteristics that would contribute to these validation efforts.

Literature Review

The largest organ of the body, the skin, performs vital protective, insulative, and excre-

The authors would like to acknowledge the encouragement and support of Linda Cooper, MS, RN.

tory functions (Miller & Keane, 1983). Impairments in the skin, such as decubitus ulcers, pose a direct threat to the individual as they cause pain and discomfort, prolong illness, delay rehabilitation and discharge, and may even cause death (Davidson, 1987).

Concerns with the skin of individuals is high on the list of priorities in patient care as "any break in skin integrity interrupts the body's first line of defense again invasion of foreign matter" (Gosnell, 1987, p. 400). A study by Martin and York (1984) examined the incidence of nursing diagnoses and found that *impaired skin integrity* was high on the list. Care plans and nurses were randomly surveyed in an 800-bed hospital. From 160 care plans and 156 nurse interviews, a total of 411 nursing diagnoses were collected. *Impaired skin integrity* was among the top seven diagnoses. Metzger and Hiltunen (1987) included in their research a list of the 10 most frequently reported NANDA-accepted nursing diagnoses from 1980 to 1984. This list included *impairment of skin integrity*.

Caring for patients' skin is an important nursing activity. In the clinical setting, an assessment of a patient's skin may suggest the nursing diagnosis *impaired skin integrity*. Although many validation efforts have been made for various nursing diagnoses, research pertaining to *impaired skin integrity* is sparse. This review is not intended to be exhaustive but will highlight only relevant research material.

Impaired skin integrity from a nursing standpoint has been discussed mainly in terms of pressure sores or decubitus ulcers. A pressure sore has been defined as "an area of cellular necrosis usually over a bony prominence that has been subjected to pressure greater than capillary pressure for a period of time sufficient to cause cell death" (Davidson, 1987, p. 3).

Numerous publications discuss assessment and treatment of wounds and pressure sores (Cooper, Watt, & Alterescu, 1983; Gosnell, 1987; Horsely, 1981; Norton, McLaren,

& Exton-Smith, 1975; and Sklar, 1985). Cooper et al. (1983) estimated that between 5% and 30% of hospitalized patients develop pressure sores with another 20% at risk. The cost to the health care system for supplies, treatment, and staff is estimated at millions of dollars. Therefore research in the area of impaired skin has mainly focused on development, use, and testing of assessment tools for patients with or at risk for pressure-sore formation, treatment modalities, and incidence of pressure sores (Davidson, 1987; Horsley, 1981; and Sklar, 1985).

Norton et al. (1975) conducted an empiric study of factors involved in the production of pressure sores and their prevention. The researchers conducted three separate investigations. The first surveyed 250 patients who received a variety of local applications for routine prevention of pressure sores. The study revealed that use of local applications had no great effect on the incidence of pressure sores. The increased incidence of pressure sores was attributed to the patients' poor physical condition, old age, incontinence, diminished activity, and poor mental status. In the second project, a trial of four local applications on the skin of 218 patients revealed that local applications could not be relied on to prevent pressure sores. A third trial, carried out on 100 female patients, utilized frequent turning as a prophylactic measure for pressure-sore prevention. This measure showed marked reduction in incidence of pressure-sore formation.

Two articles specifically addressed *impaired skin integrity*. Fowler (1986) gave a brief account of expected outcomes and treatment modalities for patients with *actual impairment of skin integrity*. However, a focused view of impaired skin was taken as she addressed pressure sores only. Cattaneo and Lackey (1987) attempted to define *impaired skin integrity* operationally. They believed that operationalizing the nursing diagnosis would offer defining criteria that could be supported by empiric data. The authors compiled a list of defining characteristics identified by randomly selected enterostomal therapists throughout the United States. The list of characteristics identified contained a few phrases that required clarification. The use of the term bedsore or pressure sore requires a conclusion on the part of the assessor rather than observed characteristics of the particular wound being assessed. Perhaps the use of specific, descriptive terms would increase objectivity of the collected data (defining characteristics). According to NANDA (1987) "the more specific and discriminating the defining characteristics, the easier for the diagnostician to differentiate among diagnoses" (p. 119). An important recommendation by Cattaneo and Lackey was to survey staff nurses across the country in order to obtain their views of defining characteristics and to compare the results to those of the enterostomal therapists.

In order to minimize the occurrence of impaired skin, early recognition of signs and symptoms of damage is important. If nurses have a consistent cluster of defining characteristics for the diagnosis *impaired skin integrity*, they may promptly and accurately make the nursing diagnosis. This will then provide direction for the plan of care. Lackey (1986) suggested that "Practitioners of nursing care currently find most of the diagnostic categories very difficult to use in daily practice because they lack the concrete signs and symptoms necessary to make a diagnosis . . ." (p. 191).

Methods

Setting

Identified patients on 17 selected inpatient medical-surgical units at a large metropolitan teaching hospital were included in this study. The burn center, ICU, psychiatry, labor and delivery, and nursery units were excluded.

Sample

Nursing staff referred 109 patients with the previously identified nursing diagnosis *impaired skin integrity* to the researchers. Forty-eight of these patients were entered into the study. The nursing diagnosis *impaired skin integrity* was written on the nursing record on 19 of the 48 patients ($n = 50$). Six assessments were discarded, 3 test data and 3 because both researchers felt rushed. The remaining 61 referrals were not included in the study because either the areas had healed; the patient died, was discharged, or did not wish to participate; or the researchers were unable to obtain informed consent. The age range was 23 to 90 years, with a mean of 58 years.

Design

The design was a descriptive study using a quantitative analysis. It was based on Fehring's (1986) Clinical Diagnostic Validation (CDV) model. Nurses on the selected units notified the researchers when a nursing diagnosis of *impaired skin integrity* was identified, although the wording of the first part of the diagnosis varied somewhat; researchers accepted skin breakdown, alteration in skin integrity, impaired skin integrity, gangrene, infected site, and ulceration. The researchers visited the units on a weekly basis to obtain additional referrals.

Following subject identification, the researchers explained the purpose of the study to the patient and obtained an informed consent. Both researchers assessed each patient independently within one hour of each other. There was no treatment applied to any impaired area between assessments. Definitions of each item on the data-collection tool were utilized by each researcher during the assessments.

Data-Collection Tool

The data-collection tool consisted of a checklist of 41 characteristics of *impaired skin integrity*, completed after a thorough review of the literature. The tool was reviewed by four clinical nurse specialists, an enterostomal therapist, a plastic surgery nurse, and a nurse educator for input and revision. The tool was pretested and revisions were made. The final data-collection tool consisted of 38 items. Interrater reliability ratios on the test data were 80%, 83%, and 93%, respectively. Interrater reliability ratios on the 50 assessments ranged from 87% to 100% for an average of 94%.

Weighted interrater reliability ratios for each defining characteristic were calculated using Fehring's (1986) formula. A weighted interrater reliability ratio equal to or greater than 0.5 indicated a defining characteristic, and those equal to or greater than 0.8 indicated "critical" defining characteristics.

Results

Seven defining characteristics with a weighted interrater reliability ratio greater than 0.5 were identified: erythema (0.76), inflammation (0.75), subcutaneous tissue exposure (0.58), drainage (0.52), pain (0.52), and ulceration (0.52). No critical defining characteristics were identified. The total CDV score for the tool obtained by summing and averaging the ratio for each defining characteristic was 0.6. Figure 1 shows the CDV scores for the top 18 characteristics. The remaining 20 characteristics fell into one or more of the following categories: (a) never or rarely observed, (b) too many methodologic difficulties in ascertaining its presence, and (c) presence of the characteristic could not be determined without knowledge of the origin of the impairment.

Attempts to relate age to medical diagnoses, age to nursing diagnosis, medical diagnoses to nursing diagnosis, and activity levels to nursing diagnosis failed to show any significant relationships.

Discussion

The study was conducted on a small sample in one clinical setting, hence replication is required to render the results generalizable.

Different types of impairments (e.g., ulcers, surgical wounds, rashes) often had different characteristics. It may be beneficial, therefore, to study impaired skin according to type of impairment in order to capture the relevant defining characteristics. When all impairments were investigated together, the sample size of each is diminished and certain characteristics highly indicative of one type of impaired skin may be infrequently seen, and therefore appear insignificant. For example, bone/muscle/tendon exposure is indicative of impaired skin but was rarely seen and thus did not make the list of defining characteristics.

Fehring (1987) suggests that NANDA's defining characteristics be used in conjunction with the CDV model. The NANDA defining characteristics (disruption of skin surface, destruction of skin layers, invasion of body structures) account for visible characteristics only; any subjective characteristics are left out. The NANDA defining characteristics may be useful as headings for certain visible, descriptive, and specific characteristics, which could then be listed under the headings shown in Table 1.

When the nursing diagnosis *impaired skin integrity* is documented on the nursing care plan it would enhance communication among the health care team if type and location of the impairment were included. The diagnosis statement would then read *skin integrity impaired: actual (specify type and site)*.

The large number of referrals indicated that nurses were interested in caring for the skin of patients. The documentation pertaining to *impaired skin integrity*, however, was sparse. For many of the impairments assessed some form of medical treatment was in progress or a medical diagnosis indicating a skin

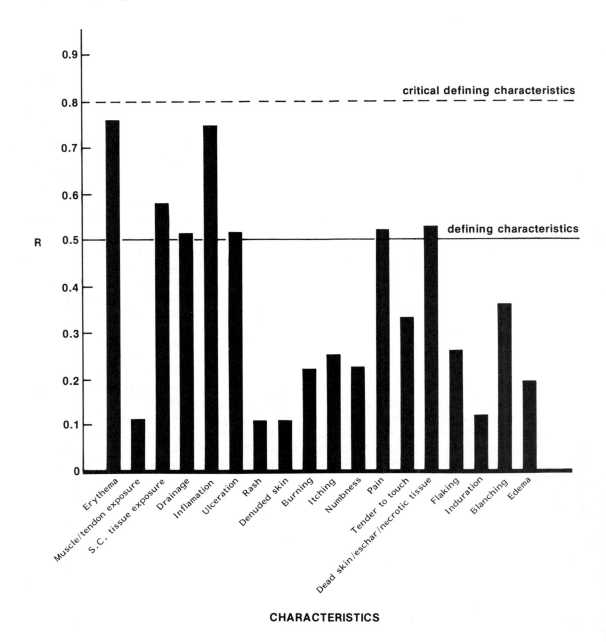

FIGURE 1 Defining characteristics recommended for further study.

impairment was documented on the patient record. Do nurses feel that if a medical treatment or diagnosis is documented there is no need for a nursing diagnosis as well?

Sklar (1985) discussed nursing diagnoses associated with *impaired skin integrity* such as *impaired physical mobility, altered tissue perfusion, altered nutritional status, altered elimination,* and *altered comfort.* As nursing is concerned with caring for the whole per-

Table 1: Specific Characteristics Categorized Under NANDA Defining Characteristics

Disruption of Skin Surface	Destruction of Skin Layers	Invasion of Body Structures
Denuded skin	Ulceration	Ulceration
Flaking	Dead skin/necrotic tissue/eschar	Muscle/bone/tendon exposure
Rash		
Edema	Induration	Dead skin/necrotic tissue/eschar
Induration	Drainage	
Inflammation	Inflammation	
	Subcutaneous tissue exposure	

son, it is important to examine associated nursing diagnoses. These associated diagnoses may influence the severity and duration of the skin impairment. In this study the documentation of diagnoses related to *impaired skin integrity* was not enough to draw any conclusions as to which may influence, or be influenced by, the specified nursing diagnosis.

Although ***actual*** impaired skin integrity is important as shown in the literature review, ***potential*** impaired skin integrity is equally important. Cooper et al. (1983) believed that while treatment of a pressure sore may end, prevention is ongoing. In addition, although a full-thickness impairment (i.e., extending into subcutaneous tissue) fills with scar tissue, it never achieves the same strength as normal skin. This has many important nursing implications, as preventive measures must be instituted to avoid the detrimental effects to individuals and high costs to the health care system.

The significance of the study lies in the questions that may form the basis of future study.

1. What does the staff nurse view as the defining characteristics of impaired skin integrity?

2. What factors contribute to the scanty documentation of nursing diagnoses?
3. At which level of skin destruction do specific subjective complaints occur?
4. Is the frequency of occurrence of the defining characteristics weighted too heavily in the formula?
5. What is the relationship between *impaired skin integrity* and the other related nursing diagnoses?
6. What are the defining characteristics of *potential impaired skin integrity?*

In order to answer these questions, nurses at the bedside must consistently be encouraged to document accurately all patient care activities and analyze critically the nursing diagnoses in existence. The clinical setting provides a rich source of information to assist in the generation, revision, and validation of nursing diagnosis.

References

Aydelotte, M. K., & Peterson, K. H. (1987). Keynote address: Nursing taxonomies—state of the art. In A. M. McLane (Ed.), *Classification of nursing diagnoses: Proceedings of the seventh national conference* (pp. 1–16). St. Louis, MO: Mosby.

Bircher, A. U. (1986). Nursing diagnosis: Where does the conceptual framework fit? In M. E. Hurley (Ed.), *Classification of nursing diagnoses: Proceedings of the sixth national conference* (pp. 66–97). St. Louis, MO: Mosby.

Cattaneo, C. J., & Lackey, N. R. (1987). Impaired skin integrity. In A. M. McLane (Ed.), *Classification of nursing diagnoses: Proceedings of the seventh national conference* (pp. 129–134). St. Louis, MO: Mosby.

Cooper, D. M., Watt, R. C., & Alterescu, V. (1983). *Guide to wound care.* Libertyville, IL: Hollister Inc.

Davidson, B. (1987). Preventing decubitus ulcers. *Wound Management, 1*(2), 1–4, 8.

Fehring, R. J. (1986). Validating diagnostic labels: Standardized methodology. In M. E. Hurley (Ed.), *Classification of nursing diagnoses: Proceedings of the sixth national conference* (pp. 183–190). St. Louis, MO: Mosby.

Fehring, R. J. (1987). Methods to validate nursing diagnoses. *Heart and Lung, 16,* 625–629.

Fowler, E. (1986). Nursing diagnoses: Actual impaired

skin integrity. *Journal of Gerontological Nursing,* *12*(10), 36–37.

Gordon, M. (1982). *Nursing diagnosis: Process and application.* New York: McGraw-Hill.

Gosnell, D. (1987). Assessment and evaluation of pressure sores. *Nursing Clinics of North America, 22,* 399–414.

Hayes, S. C. (1987). Strategies of research applicable to on-line clinical intervention. In A. M. McLane (Ed.), *Classification of nursing diagnoses: Proceedings of the seventh national conference* (pp. 79–95). St. Louis, MO: Mosby.

Horsley, J. (1981). *Preventing decubitus ulcers: CURN project.* New York: Grune & Stratton.

Lackey, N. R. (1986). Use of the Q methodology in validating defining characteristics of specified nursing diagnoses. In M. E. Hurley (Ed.), *Classification of nursing diagnoses: Proceedings of the sixth national conference* (pp. 192–195). St. Louis, MO: Mosby.

Martin, P. A., & York, K. A. (1984). Incidence of nursing diagnoses. In M. J. Kim, G. K. McFarland, & A. M. McLane (Eds.), *Classification of nursing diagnoses: Proceedings of the fifth national conference* (pp. 224–231). St. Louis, MO: Mosby.

Metzger, K. L., & Hiltunen, E. (1987). Diagnostic content validation of ten frequently reported nursing diagnoses. In A. M. McLane (Ed.), *Classification of nursing diagnoses: Proceedings of the seventh national conference* (pp. 144–153). St. Louis, MO: Mosby.

Miller, B. F., & Keane, C. B. (1983). *Encyclopedia and dictionary of medicine, nursing and allied health* (3rd ed.). Philadelphia: Saunders.

North American Nursing Diagnosis Association. (1987). *Taxonomy I revised.* St. Louis, MO: Author.

Norton, D., McLaren, R., & Exton-Smith, A. N. (1975). *An investigation of geriatric nursing problems in hospital* (pp. 193–238). Edinburgh: Churchill-Livingstone.

Sklar, C. G. (1985). Pressure ulcer management in the neurologically impaired patient. *Journal of Neurosurgical Nursing, 17*(1), 30–35.

Analyzing Expert Nursing Practice to Develop a New Nursing Diagnosis *Dysfunctional Ventilatory Weaning Response*

Jean Jenny, MSN, MEd, RN
Jo Logan, MEd, BScN, RN

The increased use of nursing diagnosis as a focus for nursing interventions has highlighted the pressing need for clinical practice theories to direct these interventions. Gordon (1989) has suggested that nursing diagnoses represent theoretical categories that identify specific practice areas for research, investigation, and theory generation. This paper describes how a new nursing diagnosis was derived during the development of a practice theory as part of a qualitative study to determine the knowledge, judgments, and actions used by expert nurses to wean patients from mechanical ventilation. The paper will address the methodology and the following findings: selected conceptual underpinnings that led to the perception of a new diagnosis, the rationale for the label and its definition, and the diagnostic attributes.

Background

A voluminous amount of literature on the subject of ventilatory weaning provided ample evidence that the process of weaning a patient from a mechanical ventilator is a source of confusion and frustration for many nurses (Norton, 1989). The findings that (1) as many as 20% of patients undergoing mechanical ventilation are unable to tolerate discontinuance (Tahvanainen, Salmenpera, & Nikki, 1983) and (2) that 19% of ventilated patients require up to one week to be weaned (Nett, Morganroth, & Petty, 1984) indicate that an undesirable response to weaning is not uncommon.

A survey of medical as well as nursing literature revealed no research on how nurses interpret and use information on weaning. The most common focus of medical literature has been predictors of ventilatory weaning success (Morganroth, Morganroth, Nett, & Petty, 1984) and, conversely, lists of problems perceived to inhibit success (Browne, 1984). Other prominent topics include the work of breathing (Lewis, Chawals, Benotti, Lakshman, O'Donnell, Blackburn, & Bistrian, 1988), muscle performance and respiratory muscle fatigue (Capps & Schade, 1988), and criteria for extubation (de Haven, Hurst, & Branson, 1986).

The nursing literature contains numerous prescriptive weaning articles but few are data based (Grossbach-Landis, 1980; Hagarty, 1984). Gosbee (1986) researched the relationship of physiologic weaning parameters and anxiety to length of time for patients with chronic obstructive lung disease (COLD) to wean from mechanical ventilation. A positive correlation was found among anxiety, knowledge of imminent weaning, and length of time to wean. There was no significant correlation between physiologic parameters and length of time to wean. Chambers, Anderson, York, and Drue (1987) reviewed charts of 20 patients who experienced difficulty in weaning and found low serum proteins, hemoglobin, and hematocrit as the factors most likely to be abnormal in patients unable to wean. No other studies were found that explored the nursing dimension in the weaning process.

Methods

The limited information available to explain how nurses interpret situational data and make clinical weaning decisions led to the selection of an inductive, qualitative method. Qualitative research methods have been suggested as particularly useful for concept generation if prior descriptive research has not been done in the area (Artinian, 1986). Melia (1982) advocates an inductive approach as essential to comprehend the world of nursing practice and pursue the questions that arise as one attempts to order the natural world through analysis. Chenitz and Swanson (1986) suggest that the elusive nature of the nursing process has inhibited research, and advocate the use of a qualitative research approach termed "surfacing nursing process" to capture the complex process dimension of nursing that is inherent and grounded in daily practice. Forsyth (1984) suggests a qual-

itative method is optimal to seek diagnostic causes or related factors, and that the final form emerging from the method is an integration of the conditions, contingencies, contexts, consequences, and strategies around a core variable, rich in conceptual detail and adequate to develop testable hypotheses.

The method selected for this study was consistent with the grounded-theory approach described by Strauss (1987). This method uses a detailed description of the study subject to generate theory that conceptualizes an underlying social process (Artinian, 1986). By this method theory is formulated through analysis of data systematically collected from the field, interviews, documentary or literary sources, or a combination of these sources (Simms, 1981). Grounded theory differs from other research methods in that it emphasizes observation or practice-based intuitive relationships among variables that can be tested empirically (Simms, 1981).

Study Design

In the belief that expert practice is an important original source of knowledge (Benner, 1984), nurses at the expert stage of skill acquisition, as described by Benner and based on the work of Dreyfus and Dreyfus (1980), were selected as study participants. Sixteen registered nurses in the intensive care unit (ICU) of a large university teaching hospital, who were identified as expert practitioners by their peers and supervisors, took part in the study. Their length of work experience in the unit ranged from 5 to 25 years, but many had previously worked in other ICUs. Written explanations of study participation and the ethical considerations were provided to volunteers.

Study informants provided a written description of a decisive incident from a recent weaning experience. Decisive incidents were defined as examples of either typical, unsuccessful, or demanding situations, or one in which the nurse's actions made a difference to outcome. The patients described in the incidents were male or female adults with a variety of indications for mechanical ventilation. The exemplars described both short- and long-term ventilation.

An interactive interview lasting approximately one hour was conducted in an ICU office at a time convenient for each participant. The written anecdote was used as the interview guide and directed the ensuing dialogue as the incident was probed for meaning. The interviews were tape recorded and the tapes were then transcribed verbatim for analysis. Participant observation may have strengthened the study but was not feasible in this setting.

The investigators conducted the interpretative analysis of data, which was facilitated by the use of a computer program called "The Ethnograph," designed by Seidel, Kjolseth, and Seymour (1988) for qualitative data analysis. Using the program simplified the mechanical tasks of data management, leaving more time for the conceptual work. Simultaneous data collection, coding, and analysis facilitated the emergent structure of the data categories and followed the constant comparative method of Strauss (1987) and Glaser and Strauss (1967). The following summarizes the procedure used.

Each datum incident identified in the transcripts was coded to create as many categories of analysis as possible. The unit of datum categorization was any segment of the narrative that reflected an observation, perception, judgment, decision, or action related to the weaning situation or to weaning in general. As data were coded and clustered into categories, the theoretic properties of each category were defined. When categories were saturated (i.e., no new coded data or properties were observed), the process was stopped.

Throughout the study the researchers selectively sampled the literature concerned with the specific themes or conceptual areas, e.g., perceived self-efficacy and respiratory muscle training. This helped to verify the theoretic constructions, provided the accepted terminology in that domain, and directed further data collection from the participants.

Reliability and Validity

Stern (1985) suggested that grounded theory has an inherent validity because it is derived from situation data, and that reliability is enhanced by the constant comparative method of data analysis that increases the internal consistency of the data sets from which the theoretic concepts were derived. By use of the member-check technique, study participants validated the theoretic data interpretations through repeated review of the findings. Other techniques to ensure reliability and validity followed the methods for trustworthiness outlined by Lincoln and Guba (1985) and have been described in detail elsewhere (Logan & Jenny, 1990).

Results

Conceptual Underpinnings of the New Diagnosis

The identification of a number of themes in the data provided the foundations for a grounded theory of the weaning process. These themes include knowing the patient, the work of weaning, the nurse-patient relationship, and the psychophysiologic patient power base.

1. *Knowing the patient* was the basis for expert nurses' judgments and decisions. It provided the authority for independent actions and consultative activities during the weaning process. This knowledge synthesized in the minds of nurses an ongoing assessment of the patient's current status, potential for work, presence of actual or impending problems, and probably situational responses.

... You know them like the back of your hand. You know how much he can do, and how much he can't. You know what upsets him and what doesn't ...

2. *The work of weaning* constituted the patient's role and was seen as both interactive and reciprocal with that of the nurse. This work included communicating, collaborating, and cooperating with the nurse to achieve progressive goals as well as the work of breathing.

> ... They have to be able to work hard and to really concentrate on their breathing and do all those routine things that we ask them to do ...

3. A *trusting relationship* was perceived as the necessary vehicle through which nurses effected weaning. When the relationship was weakened, patients were reluctant to work, manifested negative emotional responses, and were less successful in achieving weaning goals.

> ... A lot of it is getting the patient to trust you and work hard ... they have to know that you're going to be there and that you're not going to let them get into trouble ...

4. *The patient power base* representing those elements necessary to perform the work of weaning was constituted by two dimensions—physical energy and perceived self-control. As these functional constituents were eroded through patient's work or other adverse events, patients demonstrated progressively inadequate responses. A major nursing function was helping to reconstitute the patient's power base.

> ... It's sheer physical energy that has to go into their weaning work ... whether the weaning is done quickly or slowly, the patient must feel that he is in control.

5. *The situational factors* represented nurses' perceptions of elements necessary for a controlled, predictable environment and quality social support that would enhance patients' work efforts.

> ... I always think first of environment ... a calm environment, a feeling of security for the patient ... the feeling of rest and someone who is in control, someone who has a handle on things. The nurse's role is to create a positive environment ...

These conceptual elements provided the structure for theory development. They also represented that framework from which the problem aspects of weaning were perceived and explored.

Deriving the New Nursing Diagnosis

From the clinical vignettes volunteered by the nurses, it was apparent that not all weaning attempts were initially straightforward or successful. The category that first alerted us to the possibility of a new nursing diagnosis specific to weaning was that of "failure." This category was defined as the patients' failure to meet the current goals of weaning. The following describes a nurse's perception of failure:

> ... When you put the patient down to IMV 6, after about 3 minutes he was just tired out and it was a very rapid progression, and you can see it happen very quickly. The respiratory rate going up and the color getting dusky and heart rate going up ... it seems funny that the small increment would make such a big difference.

Once alerted to the concept of interference in the weaning progress, we identified a number of data categories that contributed a description of the weaning problem.

Selecting a Label

The patient's state or response to a health problem that occurs during the weaning process and that is problematic, unhealthy, potentially reversible, and can be diagnosed and treated by nurses was labeled *dysfunctional ventilatory weaning response (DVWR)*. The problem is defined as the temporary state in which a patient cannot adjust to lowered levels of ventilator support, which interrupts the weaning process.

The need for a weaning diagnosis had been perceived by the NANDA critical care nurses' interest group in previous years, and evoked discussion regarding the most appropriate label (Carroll-Johnson, 1988, p. 505). Some examples suggested were *failure to wean, inability to resume or sustain spontaneous ventilation*, and *ventilator dependency*. These labels were not acceptable for several reasons. They fail to differentiate a temporary situation from a permanent or terminal state. *Failure to wean* is nonspecific and could refer to a nursing problem rather than a patient state. *Inability to resume or sustain spontaneous ventilation* can suggest the need for intubation or continuing mechanical ventilation rather than weaning. *Ventilator dependency* is not clearly related to the weaning situation and is machine, not person, oriented. *Dysfunctional ventilatory weaning response* fulfills the requirements of a useful label. It describes a patient state or response to a health problem—ventilator dependency.

The qualifier "dysfunctional" was chosen deliberately as the prefix dys- signifies harmful or difficult. A weaning failure results in more than failure to reach goals (inadequate) or inability to maintain patient comfort (ineffective). It creates a new compound of dyspnea, anxiety, and increased muscle tension that increases metabolic energy expenditure and exacerbates respiratory muscle fatigue and patients' perceptions of loss of control. The problem definition, "the temporary state in which a patient cannot adjust to lowered levels of mechanical ventilator support, which interrupts the weaning process," indicates the nature of the subject (ventilated patient), the reason the state is dysfunctional

(interrupts the weaning process), the context of the problem (patient has begun weaning), and the possibility of reversal of the state (temporary). The term "dysfunctional response" is broad enough to encompass whatever specific behavior the patient has manifested that interrupts the weaning.

Defining Characteristics

Analysis of data indicated that the concept of comfort was the baseline state from which nurses judged patients' ability to continue with weaning. Comfort was defined as the absence of noxious stimuli and the presence of sufficient energy to meet the situational demands. Examples of noxious stimuli that reduce the comfort level include fatigue, pain, dyspnea, anxiety, and feelings of loss of control. Typical descriptions of patient comfort level were

. . . If they're feeling OK, then they're comfortable. To be comfortable, they're secure in their surroundings, they know their environment . . . they don't go flying off at every little sound . . . they don't pay attention to all that's going on around them, they can drift off to sleep. Heart rate, blood pressure, all down to normal, respiratory rate even, not gasping, ah, comfort . . . you can see comfort level in those things.

Some patients were weaned without ever feeling very uncomfortable because the nurses picked up subtle cues that the limits of the comfort zone were being reached and thus instituted a rest to reestablish energy levels in a controlled manner to prevent a setback. The ability to detect the defining characteristics of mild *DVWR* enabled the nurses to prevent progression.

The signs and symptoms described in the data have been tentatively clustered into three levels of *DVWR*—mild, moderate, and severe (see Table 1). These three levels were subsequently validated by the informants who thought the three levels would be useful in directing interventions. Although the

Table 1: Defining Characteristics of
Dysfunctional Ventilatory Weaning Response

Mild
- Expressed feelings of increased oxygen need, breathing discomfort, fatigue, warmth
- Queries about possible machine malfunction
- Restlessness
- Slight increased respiratory rate from baseline of less than 5 breaths/minute
- Increased concentration on breathing

Moderate
- Hypervigilance
- Decreasing cooperation
- Apprehension
- Diaphoresis
- Eye widening ("wide-eyed look")
- Decreased air entry on auscultation
- Color changes: pale, slight cyanosis
- Slight increase in blood pressure (<20 mm Hg)
- Slight increase in heart rate (<20 beats/minute)
- Baseline increase in respiratory rate (>5 breaths/minute)
- Slight respiratory accessory muscle use

Severe
- Agitation
- Profuse diaphoresis
- Deterioration in arterial blood gases from current baseline
- Increased blood pressure (>20 mm Hg)
- Increased heart rate (>20 beats/minute)
- Respiratory rate increased significantly from baseline
- Full respiratory accessory muscle use
- Shallow, gasping breaths
- Paradoxical abdominal breathing
- Discoordinated breathing with the ventilator
- Decreased level of consciousness
- Adventitious breath sounds, audible airway secretions
- Cyanosis

NOTE: From "Deriving a New Diagnosis Through Qualitative Research: Dysfunctional Ventilatory Weaning Response" by J. Logan and J. Jenny, 1990, *Nursing Diagnosis*, 1, pp. 37–44. Used by permission.

nurses agreed with the levels, they differed on the importance of some of the defining characteristics. These levels require further empiric testing.

Risk Factors

Risk factors increasing the possibility of patients' experiencing *DVWR* included patient characteristics or experiences that undermined the patient power base of physical energy or perceived control. Nurses readily identified types of patients who they judged might be difficult to wean.

. . . We talk about the anxiety, the length of time on the ventilator, their lung disease . . . often you can tell it'll be a difficult wean by these things. . . . With a noncooperative patient, you just have to hope for the best.
. . . The kind of patient who needs a slower wean is one who doesn't have many reserves. If you wear them out, you've wasted the physical stuff, plus psychologically you've lost a lot of ground.

Other risk factors identified in the data are included in Table 2.

Conclusion

The use of a qualitative research method, specifically the grounded-theory approach, was instrumental in facilitating the detection of a new nursing diagnosis from data collected to study how expert nurses weaned adult ventilated patients. Tanner (1988) has remarked, "There are no formal strategies of clinical judgment that can be described free of the context in which action occurs" (p. 430). A qualitative method is more successful in capturing the contextual nuances that color nursing actions, and brings a fresh perspective to a familiar situation. It also contributes a wealth of data about existing nursing diag-

Table 2: Risk Factors for *Dysfunctional Ventilatory Weaning Response*

- Extended history of ventilator dependence (more than 1 week)
- Weaning history of multiple unsuccessful trials
- Acute or chronic lung disease
- Multisystem disease
- Neuromuscular chronic disability
- Terminal illness
- Severe obesity
- High anxiety level or state anxiety
- Clinical depression or prolonged depressed state

noses, and provides material for the possible development of others.

The deliberate selection of a homogenous group of study subjects is a departure from the methods of traditional quantitative research, which seek a heterogenous, generalizable sample representing a normal curve of population distribution. Expertise is the distillation of knowledge and experience into the most efficient, effective practice. For new knowledge to be derived from practice it must come from the best examples of practice available and not a random sampling of what abounds. Benner (1984) has written, "Systematic documentation of expert clinical performance is a first step in clinical knowledge development" (p. 35) and this study has attempted to do just that.

Another benefit of using expert nursing practice for the field of study is the increased clinical utility of the theories derived. Concepts for guiding nursing practice must be "standardized, esteemed and fit for use" (Dickoff & James, 1989, p. 99). "It is self-evident that theory must be informed by real-world experience. . . . Nursing theory has not been adequately shaped by the practice of nurses. A theory is needed that describes, interprets and explains not an imagined idea of nursing, but actual expert nursing as it is practised day-to-day" (Benner & Wrubel, 1989, p. 5). The analysis and interpretation of nursing practice as performed by expert nurses that is offered in this study is intended to support the paradigm of the thinking–doer coined by Dickoff and James (1989) who write: "The big idea of the nursing diagnosis movement includes striving to keep doers of the most particularized nursing among those persons who participate strenuously in developing concepts for nursing" (p. 99).

References

Artinian, B. (1986). The research process in grounded theory. In C. Chenitz & J. M. Swanson (Eds.), *From practice to grounded theory: Qualitative research in nursing* (pp. 16–23). Menlo Park, CA: Addison-Wesley.

Benner, P. (1984). *From novice to expert: Excellence and power in clinical nursing practice.* Menlo Park, CA: Addison-Wesley.

Benner, P., & Wrubel, J. (1989). *The primacy of caring: Stress and coping in health and illness.* Menlo Park, CA: Addison-Wesley.

Browne, D. R. G. (1984). Weaning patients from mechanical ventilation. *Intensive Care Medicine, 10,* 55–58.

Capps, J. S., & Schade, K. (1988). Work of breathing: Clinical monitoring and considerations in the critical care setting. *Critical Care Nursing Quarterly, 11*(3), 1–11.

Carroll-Johnson, R. M. (Ed.). (1989). *Classification of nursing diagnoses: Proceedings of the eighth conference.* Philadelphia: Lippincott.

Chambers, P., Anderson, B., York, K., & Drue, S. (1987). Clinical validation of the nursing diagnosis of inability to wean from ventilators. In A. M. McLane (Ed.), *Classification of nursing diagnoses: Proceedings of the seventh national conference* (p. 278). St. Louis, MO: Mosby.

Chenitz, C., & Swanson, J. M. (Eds.). (1986). *From practice to grounded theory: Qualitative research in nursing.* Menlo Park, CA: Addison-Wesley.

de Haven, C. B., Hurst, J. M., & Branson, R. D. (1986). Evaluation of two different extubation criteria: Attributes contributing to success. *Critical Care Medicine, 14*(2), 92–94.

Dickoff, J., & James, P. (1989). Theoretical pluralism for nursing diagnosis. In R. M. Carroll-Johnson (Ed.), *Classification of nursing diagnoses: Proceedings of the eighth conference* (pp. 98–125). Philadelphia: Lippincott.

Dreyfus, S. E., & Dreyfus, H. L. (1980, February). *A five-stage model of the mental activities involved in directed skill acquisition.* Unpublished report supported by the Air Force Office of Scientific Research (AFSC), USAF. Berkeley, CA: University of California, Berkeley.

Forsyth, G. L. (1984). Etiology: In what sense and of what value? In M. J. Kim, G. K. McFarland, & A. M. McLane (Eds.), *Classification of nursing diagnoses: Proceedings of the fifth national conference* (pp. 62–72). St. Louis, MO: Mosby.

Glaser, B. G., & Strauss, A. L. (1967). *The discovery of grounded theory: Strategies for qualitative research.* Chicago: Aldine.

Gordon, M. (1989). Theoretical basis for nursing diagnosis. Paper presented at the University of Ottawa conference *Nursing theory, nursing diagnosis, nursing interventions: Putting it all together.* Ottawa, Canada.

Gosbee, R. A. (1986). Relationship of physiological weaning parameters and anxiety to length of time for patients with C.O.L.D. to wean from mechanical ventilation (Master's thesis, University of Toronto, 1985). *Masters Abstracts International, 24*(1), 57.

Grossbach-Landis, I. (1980). Weaning of ventilator-dependent patients. *Topics in Clinical Nursing, 2*(3), 45–65.

Hagarty, E. (1984). Weaning your COPD patient from the ventilator. *RN, 48,* 36–40.

Lewis, D. W., Chawals, W., Benotti, P. M., Lakshman, K. O'Donnell, C., Blackburn, G., & Bistrian, B. R. (1988). Bedside assessment of the work of breathing. *Critical Care Medicine, 16,* 117–122.

Lincoln, Y. S., & Guba, E. G. (1985). *Naturalistic inquiry.* Beverly Hills, CA: Sage.

Logan, J., & Jenny, J. (1990). Deriving a new diagnosis through qualitative research: Dysfunctional ventilatory weaning response. *Nursing Diagnosis, 1,* 37–44.

Melia, K. (1982). Tell it as it is—qualitative methodology and nursing research: Understanding the student nurse's word. *Journal of Advanced Nursing, 7,* 327–335.

Morganroth, M. L., Morganroth, J. L., Nett, M., & Petty, T. L. (1984). Criteria for weaning from prolonged mechanical ventilation. *Archives of Internal Medicine, 144,* 1012–1016.

Nett, L. M., Morganroth, M., & Petty, T. L. (1984). Weaning from mechanical ventilation: A perspective and review of techniques. In R. C. Bone (Ed.), *Critical care: A comprehensive approach* (pp. 171–182). Park Ridge, IL: American College of Chest Physicians.

Norton, L. C. (1989). Weaning the long-term ventilator-dependent patient: Common problems and management. *Critical Care Nurse, 9*(1), 42–52.

Seidel, J. V., Kjolseth, R., & Seymour, E. (1988). *The ethnograph.* Qualis Research Associates.

Simms, L. (1981). The grounded theory approach in nursing research. *Nursing Research, 30,* 356–359.

Stern, P. (1985). Using grounded theory method in nursing research. In M. Leininger (Ed.), *Qualitative research methods in nursing.* Orlando, FL: Grune & Stratton.

Strauss, A. L. (1987). *Qualitative analysis for social scientists.* New York: Cambridge University Press.

Tahvanainen, J., Salmenpera, M., & Nikki, P. (1983). Extubation criteria after weaning from intermittent mandatory ventilation and continuous positive airway pressure. *Critical Care Medicine, 11,* 702–770.

Tanner, C. (1988). Curriculum revolution: The practice mandate. *Nursing and Health Care, 8,* 427–430.

Interventions for the Nursing Diagnosis *Dysfunctional Ventilatory Weaning Response:* A Qualitative Study

Jo Logan, MEd, BScN, RN
Jean Jenny, MEd, MSN, RN

A qualitative study was conducted to explore the knowledge, judgments, and actions used by expert critical care nurses to wean adult patients from mechanical ventilation. Sixteen expert nurses from a tertiary care university-affiliated intensive care unit (ICU) provided written protocols and were subsequently interviewed about their impact on the weaning process. In the course of evaluating nursing's role in the weaning process, a new nursing diagnosis—*dysfunctional ventilatory weaning response (DVWR)*—became apparent (see page 133). *DVWR* was defined as the temporary state in which a patient cannot adjust to lowered levels of ventilator support, which interrupts the weaning process. The study methods and data analysis regarding the derivation of the diagnosis *DVWR* have been described elsewhere by Logan and Jenny (1990). Analysis of data provided a description of the actions used by the nurses to treat dysfunctional responses seen during the weaning process.

Findings

All the examplars quoted in this paper were provided by the expert nurse informants and are presented to indicate how the interpretations are grounded in the data.

Related Factors Directing Nursing Interventions

The related factors for *DVWR* were imbedded primarily in the category labeled "ready." Readiness was defined as a patient state in which the necessary physical and emotional resources to engage in the work of weaning were present.

. . . The patient was either psychologically or physically unprepared for the wean . . . I truly believe a large part of it is psychological.

The nurses repeatedly asserted that weaning was a psychophysiologic process. Determining that the patient was ready to start weaning was a judgment critical to the process because lack of readiness was seen to predispose the patient to a dysfunctional weaning response.

. . . You know, if moving gets him short of breath, you just know by those things if he's ready for it. If he can't tolerate anything more than an x-ray, there's no way you can have him go through a decrease in the amount of ventilation.

Readiness was a concept applied to the initiation of weaning and to the progression to the next step once the work of weaning had begun. The work of weaning was seen to occur in two phases. It included the preparatory as well as the active work, with nursing interventions occurring during one phase or the other with some degree of overlap.

Interventions used to treat *DVWR* were directed at the specific factors related to the problem. The interventions were interactive and a specific action would often affect more than one related factor. The interventions directly related to managing the diagnosis were imbedded in the following themes and categories: the work of weaning, ready, rest, failure, trust, and situation. The goals of the nursing interventions included optimizing the situational factors, restoring the lost energy resources, and regulating the energy demands during the two phases of the weaning process. Increasing the patient's sense of control was seen to be a crucial goal and is substantiated by the nursing literature (Boeing & Mongera, 1989).

Situational factors and interventions

The descriptions of incidents where patients failed to wean on the initial attempt, thus temporarily interrupting the weaning, indicated that the related factors and interventions included three dimensions—situational, physiologic, and psychologic. Situational factors were seen to contribute to the psychophysiologic readiness. These factors were frequently described as interrelated.

Situational-related factors included

- Insufficient trust in the nurse (e.g., extended nurse absence from bedside, unfamiliar nursing staff)
- Adverse environment (e.g., noisy, active)
- Negative events in the room (e.g., low nurse-patient ratio)
- Inappropriate or lack of social support
- Inappropriate pacing of diminished ventilator support
- Uncontrolled episodic energy demands or problems

The interventions for the situational-related factors were directed at reestablishing patient trust in the nurses, controlling social support, modifying the environment, and advocating for necessary changes in therapy or approach.

1. *Establishing patient trust.* Participants described the importance of gaining the patient's trust as a necessary factor in treating *DVWR*. The dysfunctional weaning response was associated not only with erosion of physical energy and negative emotional responses but also with patient distrust in the staff.

. . . When you're weaning, there are specific things to do, but a lot of it is getting the patient to trust you and to work.

Trust was defined as confidence in the nurse's willingness and ability to safeguard the patient's well-being. The initial trust felt by the patients was seen to diminish with each episode of failure to wean. Trust helped motivate the patient to engage in the work of weaning and reduced the negative psychophysiologic reactions resulting from a failure. Strategies to restore trust included a calm approach, demonstrating confidence in the patient's abilities and in positive outcomes, sharing information about oneself, demonstrating nursing competence by explaining and doing things with self-assurance, engaging the patient in collaborative activities such as care planning, proving one's honesty and reliability, providing individual attention, and taking the patient's feelings seriously. These attributes associated with the concept of trust were similar to those found in other studies (Meize-Grochowski, 1984). Strategies to reestablish and maintain a therapeutic relationship consisted of very deliberate actions used prior to and during the weaning process. With trust reestablished, nurses become part of the social support system for patients.

2. *Controlling and enhancing social support.* The nursing intervention of controlling and enhancing the social support system contributed to the treatment of *DVWR*. Restricting family access to patients during crucial working phases was seen to be necessary in certain situations.

. . . Sometimes families can have a very negative effect, whether they are just saying the wrong things or they don't understand, but the patient tends to get very worked up and they may not breathe as well on the machine. They might fight the ventilator, the blood pressure goes up, and they get restless and squirmy.

In contrast, when the support is seen as a positive factor, nurses actively incorporated this resource in the treatment.

. . . I allowed his fiancée to stay with him continuously, because I found her to be a great support. I brought her in because she really seemed to be his crutch.

Providing effective social support and opportunities for choice have been found to increase perceived control (Lindquist, 1986).

3. *Modifying the environment.* Nurses identified positive and negative weaning situations that suggested that modifying the weaning environment was an important adjunct to enhancing social support to treat *DVWR*. The following factors were mentioned repeatedly as conducive to successful weaning: personalized space; a quiet room; and confident, available staff. Similar suggestions were summarized by Dracup (1989) in her descriptions for tested interventions for reducing the potential harmful effects of the critical care environment.

4. *Advocacy.* Conflict arising over aspects of the weaning process led nurses to intervene in the form of advocacy. Advocacy involved ensuring that staff and others responded appropriately to the patient's needs or wishes. A source of conflict between medical and nursing staff was centered around the pacing of diminished ventilator support. The conflict reflected the nurses' unique knowledge of the patient's current state.

. . . Often it's the nurse who must decide if weaning is effective or whether another approach is necessary as the doctor often is not as familiar with the patient as the nurse. . . . Sometimes you really have to speak up and say "No, I don't think the patient is ready to be weaned," even though his gases may be fine. You're the patient's advocate. I don't care whose toes you're stepping on, this is for the patient's good.

Advocacy was an intervention used to secure necessary resources and agreement to pursue directions that were patient specific. Nurses directed their interventions to situational factors because they saw the situation as impacting directly on patients' physiologic and psychologic weaning responses.

Physiologic factors and interventions

Physiologic factors related to *DVWR* included

- Fatigue
- Sleep-pattern disturbance
- Inadequate nutrition
- Uncontrolled pain or discomfort
- Ineffective airway clearance.

Physiologic interventions were designed to restore patient energy reserves and to regulate the pattern of energy utilization.

1. *Ensuring availability of energy substrates.* Nursing measures to ensure the availability of energy substrates were directed at managing oxygen supply and nutrition. Strategies to protect an effective oxygen supply included adjusting oxygen therapy, suctioning, turning, and positioning. Managing feeding concerns ensured sufficient nutrients.

2. *Resting the patient.* Rest was defined as a period of ease or inactivity after working and included a reduction in activity level or an increase in ventilator support. It was a strategy designed to enhance the work performed by patients and was directed toward restoring energy levels to the point where the work of weaning could resume. Rest incorporated concern for discomfort from pain or psychologic distress. Methods to rest the patient were individualized.

. . . When we do the weaning, there's a period where you have a rest. Usually you make it once an hour—say you're making them work for 10 minutes and then they have the remainder of the hour to rest. Or you could do it over a period of a couple of hours and then rest, or you make them work in the daytime hours when people are more awake and there is more stimulation and then rest through the night.

Data suggested the intuitive nature of the assessments that expert nurses made to determine whether the patient was tolerating the lowered level of ventilator support or if the patient was becoming fatigued and required a rest. Resting the patient appropriately was described as preventing failure or setback in the process and also reflects current research. Ingersoll (1989) commented "The ideal approach may be one that allows alternate periods of training and resting, with careful monitoring of patients to determine when programs should be modified" (p. 14).

3. *Training techniques.* Training techniques included the strategies of pacing the tempo of weaning, push maneuver, and covert action. Slowing the tempo of the weaning plan was frequently mentioned for those who had failed previously or were identified as potentially difficult to wean. One nurse used the phrase "no-fail weaning" to describe a plan she negotiated with the doctor to reduce ventilator support in only one parameter by one unit a day, no matter "how good the patient looked on paper." This plan ensured each increment of success and minimized the possibility of failure, which, although deemed reversible in the nurse's eyes, would exact too great a toll on a patient who had few reserves.

Push is a therapeutic maneuver to increase the patient's respiratory muscle strength, endurance, and perceived self-efficacy, and is based on the judgment that the patient has further capabilities not yet demonstrated. Strategies include negotiating progressively further goals for reduced ventilator support, deliberately reducing ventilator support beyond the patient's comfort level, prolonging the duration of reduced ventilator support, and increasing the number of activities in the patient's daily routine. The following describe nurse and patient concerns during the push maneuver:

. . . You're providing a discipline that a patient can't provide for himself.
. . . Just to go a little bit farther . . . one better . . . it's like . . . a way to test themselves.

Negotiation is a very necessary part of the push technique because patients were willing to engage in this method only when they were sure of the nurse.

In contrast to the push technique (collaborative in nature) is a covert technique referred to as "sneak." Sneak was used to refer to a strategy that reduced ventilator support without the patient's knowledge in order to demonstrate the patient's capabilities. This technique was thought to be indicated when the patient was physiologically ready to progress but was extremely anxious and refusing any further ventilator reduction. The desired outcome was an increased sense of perceived efficacy and reduced anxiety, but sometimes it resulted in patient anger and distrust of staff. Turning down ventilator support against the patient's will often precipitated the negative emotional arousal states that led to physiologic responses that wasted limited energy. This interaction between the patient's emotional and physical responses resulted in further failures. The effect of these adverse psychologic responses on respiration have been described by Dudley and Pitts-Poarch (1980). The participants all noted the risk associated with this method and often felt guilty using it as its surreptitious nature appeared unethical. Ethical guidelines exist (Schmelzer & Anema, 1988) to substantiate the belief that when other measures had failed, there were situations when it was appropriate to adjust ventilatory support without telling the patient.

Psychologic factors and interventions

Psychologic factors contributing to a dysfunctional weaning response included

- Knowledge deficit of the weaning process
- Patient-perceived inefficacy about the ability to wean
- Decreased motivation
- Decreased self-esteem
- Moderate to severe anxiety
- Fear
- Hopelessness
- Powerlessness
- Diversional activity deficit.

Psychologic interventions were designed to enhance patient control in order to motivate the patient to try again and to try harder despite the onset of anxiety, fatigue, or other discomfort.

1. *Patient teaching.* Patient teaching was the major strategy employed to strengthen patients' sense of control by helping them to understand the importance of actively engaging in the work of weaning.

. . . Patients don't understand the weaning process—they don't realize what they have to go through to get the tube out.

One consequence of a setback was the patient's perception of failing.

. . . This patient definitely needed to go back physiologically, but psychologically we could see instantly that he perceived himself a massive failure.

Patient teaching involved reconceptualizing the previous failure and rationalizing the causes. Minimizing the setback was one approach. When the patient was disappointed in the progress, the nurses would minimize the setback by reframing the situation as a practice session. Nurses stressed the importance of setting achievable goals and explaining the process realistically, including the support that would be available to patients.

. . . We said "Here's the program. We follow you step-by-step and coach you along, but we go at your pace, whatever your pace is. We're going to try again, we're not going to just let you sit there."

2. *Normalizing.* Normalizing was a strategy used to treat *DVWR* related to impaired self-esteem and hopelessness. Normalizing included physical, emotional, and cognitive approaches. Attempts to improve the patient's appearance by grooming hair and nails, applying makeup, shaving beards, and using pajamas rather than hospital gowns were frequently cited. Getting the patients sitting up in a chair; diverting them with TV, music, reading; or taking the patient on trips outside the ICU were also employed. Conversation with the patients that included compliments or revealed personal activities of the nurse (e.g., Christmas or wedding plans) were efforts at sharing designed to convey a sense of ordinary life. Deliberate use of humor in good and bad times was another strategy. The nurses described examples of patient attempts to reward the nurse through some patient achievement. This effort was

greatly reinforced by the nurse, increasing the patients' control through reward power.

Providing predictability to the patient's day by collaborating to establish a care plan and then ensuring that everyone followed it appropriately was considered important. The normalizing activities provided the patient with individual attention, which conveyed a powerful message of caring intended to get the patient thinking positively.

3. *Improving perceived self-efficacy.* One effect of *DVWR* was the patient's loss of confidence in the ability to achieve the goal of extubation. Self-efficacy is a judgment of how well one can execute courses of action required to deal with prospective situations (Bandura, 1983). Bandura posits a theory of self-efficacy in which people's perceptions of their capabilities affect their behavior, level of motivation, thought patterns, and emotional reactions. The effects of perceived inefficacy include that potentially aversive events are viewed anxiously, that possible injurious consequences are imagined, and that avoidance behaviors increase. The nurses' observations of the effects of a patient's perceived inefficacy were congruent with the theory.

. . . I think in the end, the patient has to believe not just in the nurse, of course, that the nurse is right, but he has got to believe in himself, "I really can breathe. I really can go without the machine."

Intuitively the nurses were using strategies to enhance the precepts of self-efficacy similar to those discussed in the literature (Bandura, 1983). Providing mastery experiences was achieved by slowing the pace of weaning and thereby increasing chances of success. Nurses told the patient weaning-success stories in order to provide a vicariously successful situation. They used their extensive experience as a basis for the confidence they conveyed to patients regarding the patient's ability to achieve the goal. Finally, nurses encouraged feedback from patients regarding their state of comfort in order to teach them awareness of the early onset of fatigue. The strategies to enhance self-efficacy were centered around increasing the patient's exercise of control over the weaning process in order to reduce fear of trying again.

4. *Coaching.* Coaching involved getting patients to selectively attend to their breathing. Nurses achieved a balance between "psyching" the patient up and talking the patient down to an optimal level of attention and effort. Coaching patients through ineffective breathing patterns and anxiety was achieved by getting them to concentrate on their breathing. Essential coaching actions involved providing the patient with feedback, which kept the patient informed of what was happening, and supplying positive reinforcement and reward.

. . . As long as she knew every step of her improvement, she was agreeable to go on . . . encouragement and praise were lavishly given.

Continuous feedback was considered essential to keep the patient working, especially as the patient began to reach the limits of the comfort zone.

5. *Support.* When patients wasted energy through negative psychologic arousal, it worsened the depleted energy stores resulting from the work of weaning. Nurses described support strategies for dealing with the anxiety and fear associated with *DVWR*. Constant verbal reassurance to provide encouragement was a valuable strategy. A major strategy described to alleviate this effect was presencing—staying with the patient—which was often used in conjunction with touching and hand holding.

. . . You have to have a caring relationship and not to be afraid to sort of sit close to the patient and talk to them, and encourage them, and touch them on the hand and those kinds of things. I think that's the big part of it, as well as to acknowledge that you've got to get involved.

The constant demand for nurse presence and reassurance was considered essential, but was thought to be one of the most demanding tasks for nurses in the treatment of *DVWR*.

Interventions and the Levels of *DVWR*

The participants validated the levels of mild, moderate, and severe *DVWR* (see Table 1, page 138), and determined them useful for selecting interventions. For example, with mild *DVWR*, resting the patient by remaining at the same ventilator setting for a longer period and rewarding the patient were described as the needed interventions. For moderate *DVWR*, the resting would require a return to a higher setting for a predetermined period; in addition, more demanding emotional support and negotiating to attempt a push technique would be used. Following episodes of severe *DVWR*, the patient would be returned to the baseline of ventilator support for long rest periods. These episodes also required intense nurse presencing and reassurance with the possible use of the covert (sneak) action.

Conclusions

A major finding of this study is the nurses' emphasis on the psychologic aspects of the weaning process. That the work of weaning requires patients' physical energy resources is well documented. The importance of patients' perceptions of the situation is not. Nurses are very aware that they provide this missing perspective. Expert nurses perceive that readiness to wean involves physical and psychosocial resources that must be maintained during the process. Treating dysfunctional weaning responses is based on the nurse's knowledge of the interactive patterns of situational, physiologic, and psychologic events. The essence of the *DVWR* interventions is their continuous nature. That is only possible if the nurse can remain readily available to the patient's bedside.

Implications for further research include validating the defining characteristics of *dysfunctional ventilatory weaning response* and its three levels, determining the appropriateness of the interventions for each level, and refining and expanding the interventions.

References

Bandura, A. (1983). Self-efficacy determinants of anticipated fears and calamities. *Journal of Personality and Social Psychology, 45*(2), 464–469.

Boeing, M. H., & Mongera, C. O. (1989). Powerlessness in critical care patients. *Dimensions of Critical Care Nursing, 8*(5), 274–279.

Dracup, K. (1989). Are critical care units hazardous to health? *Applied Nursing Research, 1*(1), 14–21.

Dudley, D. L., & Pitts-Poarch, A. R. (1980). Psychophysiologic aspects of respiratory control. *Clinics in Chest Medicine, 1*(1), 131–142.

Ingersoll, G. L. (1989). Respiratory muscle fatigue research: Implications for clinical practice. *Applied Nursing Research, 2*(1), 6–15.

Lindquist, R. D. (1986). Providing patient opportunities to increase control. *Dimensions of Critical Care, 5*(5), 304–309.

Logan, J., & Jenny, J. (1990). Deriving a new nursing diagnosis through qualitative research: Dysfunctional ventilatory weaning response. *Nursing Diagnosis, 1*(1), 37–44.

Meize-Grochowski, R. (1984). An analysis of the concept of trust. *Journal of Advanced Nursing, 9*, 563–572.

Schmelzer, M., & Anema, M. G. (1988). Should nurses ever lie to patients? *Image, 20*(2), 110–112.

Health Patterns in Cancer Patients: Methods for Clinical Validation

M. Anne Woodtli, PhD, RN
Suzanne Van Ort, PhD, RN

Because of the increasing numbers of cancer patients, their earlier discharge from acute care settings, their increasing use of hospital outpatient services, and the continuing use of radiation therapy as a major part of a treatment regimen, cancer patients receiving outpatient radiation therapy are a population at risk. Even as early as 1982, it was estimated that over 50% of clients diagnosed with cancer received radiation therapy at some point in their treatment process.

Nurses play a valuable role in helping patients cope with the radiation therapy regimen and its potential consequences, and nursing diagnoses can be used to describe the phenomena of nursing related to the care of these patients. There is a need for consistent use of meaningful data that are tailored to the needs of cancer patients receiving external radiation. Currently these data are not available within a clinically validated nursing diagnosis framework and, therefore, valid patient outcomes and effective nursing interventions cannot be determined. There is little reported in the literature that is the result of research-based validation of either defining characteristics or nursing diagnoses in patients receiving external radiation therapy.

Literature Review

Radiation therapy is one of four major treatment modalities used to treat the cancer patient. In the current literature it is reported that at least half of all patients receive external radiation therapy as part of their treatment regimen (Eardley, 1986; Hanucharurnkul, 1989; Kubricht, 1984; Yasko, 1982). The American Cancer Society (1986) reported that 50% of patients treated with radiation therapy are treated to cure. Radiation therapy combined with other treatment modalities such as surgery or chemotherapy is frequently used in the treatment of patients with cancer of the head, neck, and digestive organs.

Cancers of the head and neck region represent 5.5% of all malignant disease (Strohl, 1987). In 1989, an estimated 31,000 new cases of oral cancers and 12,300 new cases of

The investigators wish to acknowledge funding for this project from the American Nurses Foundation and to thank them for their designation as American Journal of Nursing Scholars for 1988–1989.

laryngeal cancer were diagnosed (American Cancer Society, 1989). In addition, oral cancers caused an estimated 8,650 deaths, and approximately 3,700 deaths were attributed to cancer of the larynx in 1989 (American Cancer Society, 1989). Radiation therapy and surgery are the principal methods of treatment for cancers of the head and neck (Baker & Feldman, 1987). Cancers of the digestive organs represent 25% of all malignant disease, with an estimated 227,000 new cases of cancer of the digestive organs and 123,000 deaths reported in 1989 (American Cancer Society, 1989). Radiation therapy combined with other treatment modalities is commonly used to treat patients with cancer of the digestive organs.

Nursing diagnoses can be used to describe the phenomena of nursing related to the care of patients receiving radiation therapy for cancer (Gordon, 1987). Nursing diagnosis is one method that nurses can use to describe and document patients' functional pattern deficits and their nursing needs; the nursing diagnosis model provides a valid framework for examining nursing (Halloran & Kiley, 1984; Kritek, 1978). Each nursing diagnosis should be evaluated to determine its relevance and reflect the complexity of problems experienced by cancer patients (Herberth & Gosnell, 1989).

There is little in the nursing research literature related to nursing diagnoses for non-hospitalized cancer patients. Rains (1981) described patient problems related to functional health patterns of specific physiologic response, role function, and social relationships. Kubricht (1984) identified therapeutic self-care demands expressed by 30 subjects receiving outpatient radiation therapy. In a study of the expressed concerns of family members of adult cancer patients, Wright and Dyck (1984) found that family members were primarily concerned about symptom control. Grant (1986) described oral intake nursing interventions for cancer patients with actual or potential deficits in the Nutri-

tional–Metabolic functional health pattern. Most recently, Hanucharurnkul (1989) identified predictors of self-care in cancer patients in Thailand who were receiving radiotherapy.

Blank, Clark, Longman, and Atwood (1989) investigated the perceived home care needs of cancer patients who were receiving outpatient treatments. However, neither these nor other published researchers have specifically linked clinically identified signs and symptoms of patients receiving external radiation therapy to validated defining characteristics and their associated nursing diagnoses within specific functional health patterns.

Purpose

The long-range goals of this program of research are to describe nursing diagnoses, functional health patterns, expected patient outcomes, and nursing interventions for patients receiving external radiation therapy. The Woodtli Nursing Diagnosis Model Within the Nursing Process (Woodtli, 1988) has been used in three previous studies to describe the relationship among these components. The model served as the framework for the current study. The purposes of the current study were to describe patient symptoms, defining characteristics, nursing diagnoses, and functional health patterns, and to examine the relationships among these factors in patients with cancer of the head and neck and the digestive organs. To accomplish these purposes, it was first necessary to construct an instrument that would help identify patient symptoms and from those clinical data, determine the defining characteristics, nursing diagnoses, and associated functional health patterns. Instrument development is an extension of the assessment phase of the model. The focus of this manuscript is to describe research methods for developing a data-collection tool and an analysis protocol for identifying and validating health patterns in cancer patients receiving external radiation therapy in an outpatient setting.

Definitions

For the purpose of this study, the following terms were operationally defined:

- Symptom: Any consequence of radiation therapy that was reported by the patient
- Nursing diagnosis: Actual list of diagnoses approved for clinical testing in 1988
- Defining characteristic: Symptoms with a mean occurrence greater than or equal to 2.0 on the Radiation Symptom Scales (RSS)
- Functional health pattern: Structural framework for assessment composed of nine categories: Nutritional–Metabolic, Elimination, Activity–Exercise, Sleep–Rest, Cognitive–Perceptual, Self-perception–Self-concept, Role Relationship, Sex–Reproduction, and Coping–Stress (Gordon, 1987).

Methods

Development of the Instrument

An extensive review of the literature was conducted to identify signs and symptoms associated with external radiation therapy. Empiric data were obtained from clinical nursing specialists in oncology. These informational sources indicated that two sets of symptoms needed to be considered. Symptoms that were commonly found in all patients who received external radiation therapy were termed core symptoms; symptoms that were specific to the site of radiation, either head and neck or digestive organs, were termed site-specific symptoms.

Two parallel forms of the RSS were developed. Each form consisted of core symptoms common to both scales, and site-specific symptoms, targeted at either the head and neck or the digestive organs. Each item on both scales was keyed to one functional health pattern. For example, fatigue was keyed to the Activity–Exercise pattern, change in taste sensation was keyed to the Cognitive–Perceptual pattern, and interruption in sleep was keyed to the Sleep–Rest pattern.

Content validity

Although the scales had beginning content validity in that items were derived from the literature (Grant, 1986; Kubricht, 1984; Rains, 1981; and Yasko, 1982), they were further assessed by five expert judges according to the structured procedure described by Lynn (1986). One important element that was added to Lynn's procedure was the panel validation of each item within a specific functional health pattern. The final forms of the RSS consisted of 32 core items and 14 site-specific items in a 4-point Likert-type format and 1 open-ended item.

Both forms of the instrument were pilot tested. Subjects reported that the instruments were easy to understand and that they were able to complete them in approximately 10 to 15 minutes.

Reliability

The RSS was tested for reliability using Cronbach's coefficient alpha. Initial reliability estimates (coefficient alpha for total scale = 0.94, Form A = 0.91, Form B = 0.91) were within acceptable ranges. The instruments have now been revised to reflect the findings of this study.

Sample and Setting

The convenience sample was comprised of 30 adult patients who were currently receiving radiation treatments for either cancer of the head and neck or cancer of the digestive organs. Subjects were at least 18 years of age and had from 4 to 8 weeks of radiation treatments. Cancer sites of the head and neck and the digestive organs were selected because of the complexity of nursing care needs of patients with these diagnoses. The settings for the study were the radiation oncology clinic of a university medical center and a private facility providing radiation therapy.

Data Analysis

The overall data-analysis plan incorporated both primary and secondary data analysis. This report focuses on the initial data analysis; secondary data analysis is in progress. All data were analyzed for the total instrument, and data from each form of the RSS were analyzed separately. Responses to all items were analyzed using frequencies, percents, means, and standard deviations. Table 1 shows the analysis results for four sample items each from Form A and Form B. The items were then categorized within the specific functional health patterns with which they were associated.

Each symptom receiving a minimum mean

response of 2 (i.e., sometimes present) was considered as a defining characteristic within the one functional health pattern with which it was associated. Complete lists of functional health patterns with their defining characteristics were generated. Table 2 demonstrates the defining characteristics associated within the Nutritional–Metabolic pattern for patients receiving external radiation to the head and neck and to the digestive organs.

The lists of functional health patterns with their specific defining characteristics were submitted to a consensus panel of three expert nurses. The consensus panel members were considered expert because of their knowledge of and experience using nursing diagnoses, their clinical experience with patients receiving radiation, and finally their knowledge of oncology. None of these nurses was a member of the instrument content-validation panel. The consensus panel members clustered defining characteristics within each functional pattern and formulated nursing diagnoses. The interrater reliability measurements among the panel members were at a minimum 90% level of agreement. Final composite lists of functional health patterns, nursing diagnoses, and defining characteristics were generated.

Table 1: Sample Item Means from Radiation Symptom Scales, Forms A and B

Item	Mean[a]	Standard Deviation
Form A (head and neck)		
• Dry skin	2.93	1.34
• Loss of weight	2.4	1.24
• Feeling depressed	2.3	1.03
• Nausea	1.6	0.99
Form B (digestive organs)		
• Decreased energy: exercise	2.93	1.34
• Sleep interruption	2.4	1.24
• Loss of appetite	2.2	1.3
• Feeling angry	1.53	0.64

[a] 1 = never present
2 = sometimes present
3 = often present
4 = always present

Table 2: Defining Characteristics Associated with Nutritional–Metabolic Functional Health Pattern

Nausea
Loss of appetite
Loss of weight
Decreased food intake
Dry skin
Itching skin
Red skin
Swollen or puffy skin
Blisters and bubbles
Dry mouth
White/yellow patches in mouth
Cracks in lining of mouth
Difficulty swallowing
Weeping skin

Table 3: Nursing Diagnoses Associated with Nutritional–Metabolic Functional Health Pattern

Potential for infection
Nutrition: less than body requirements
Impaired swallowing
Altered mucous membrane
Impaired skin integrity
Impaired tissue integrity

Table 3 presents the nursing diagnoses associated with the Nutritional–Metabolic health pattern for patients receiving radiation to the head and neck and for patients receiving radiation to the digestive organs. The cluster of defining characteristics of *altered nutrition: less than body requirements* in patients receiving head and neck radiation or digestive organ radiation is shown in Table 4.

A composite list of functional health patterns and associated nursing diagnoses was then submitted to a validation panel of nurse experts for the content category validation. The validation panel members independently judged the validity of the placement of each nursing diagnosis with its associated defining characteristics within each functional health pattern. Only those patterns, diagnoses, and characteristics unanimously approved as relevant were included in the final database.

The second phase of the data-analysis pro-

Table 4: Defining Characteristics Associated with *Altered Nutrition: Less Than Body Requirements* as Identified by Consensus Panel

Loss of weight
Nausea
Loss of appetite
Decreased food intake
White/yellow patches in mouth
Cracks in lining of mouth
Difficulty swallowing

tocol incorporates a qualitative study in which subjects receiving external radiation to the head and neck and to the digestive organs will describe the symptoms that they experienced and identify as a consequence of radiation therapy. Data will be content analyzed. Defining characteristics, nursing diagnoses, and functional health patterns will then be derived.

The third phase of the protocol consists of a comparison of the findings from the quantitative and qualitative studies using multitrait–multimethod analysis. The final phase of data analysis is currently being refined and will incorporate a protocol including confirmatory factor analysis and latent variable modeling.

Significance

The significance of the process for instrument development and data analysis within a nursing diagnosis framework used in this study is related to five distinct areas:

1. Two parallel instruments that demonstrated initial reliability and validity were developed to provide clinically based data as a first step in assessing patient symptoms and identifying defining characteristics in a specific population.
2. A nursing diagnosis validation model within the nursing process used in previous studies was extended in scope and refined in practice.
3. Because defining characteristics, nursing diagnoses, and functional health patterns have been clinically derived and retrospectively validated for a population at risk, a beginning research database has been established that can be expanded, refined, or rejected through subsequent research efforts.
4. Nursing interventions and patient out-

comes related to research-based data can now be developed and tested.

5. Research data derived from quantitative methods have been established as a foundation for subsequent validation by qualitative methods. This combination of methods has the potential to provide real advancement in the development of nursing diagnosis theory and implementation of research-based practice.

References

American Cancer Society. (1986). *Cancer facts and figures—1986.* New York: Author.

American Cancer Society. (1989). *Cancer facts and figures—1989.* Atlanta, GA: Author.

Baker, K., & Feldman, J. (1987). Cancers of the head and neck. *Cancer Nursing, 10,* 293–299.

Blank, J. J., Clark, L., Longman, A. J., & Atwood, J. R. (1989). Perceived home care needs of cancer patients and their caregivers. *Cancer Nursing, 12,* 78–84.

Eardley, A. (1986). Radiotherapy: What do patients need to know? *Nursing Times, 82,* 16–22.

Gordon, M. (1987). *Nursing diagnosis: Process and application* (2nd ed.). New York: McGraw-Hill.

Grant, M. (1986). Nutritional interventions: Increasing oral intake. *Seminars in Oncology Nursing, 2*(2), 36–43.

Halloran, E., & Kiley, M. (1984). Case mix management. *Nursing Management, 15*(2), 39–45.

Hanucharurnkul, S. (1989). Predictors of self-care in cancer patients receiving radiotherapy. *Cancer Nursing, 12,* 21–27.

Herberth, L., & Gosnell, D. J. (1989). Nursing diagnoses for oncology nursing practice. *Cancer Nursing, 10,* 41–51.

Kritek, P. (1978). The generation and classification of nursing diagnoses: Toward a theory of nursing. *Image, 10*(2), 33–40.

Kubricht, D. (1984). Therapeutic self-care demands expressed by outpatients receiving external radiation therapy. *Cancer Nursing, 7,* 43–51.

Lynn, M. (1986). Determination and quantification of content validity. *Nursing Research, 35,* 382–385.

Rains, B. (1981). The non-hospitalized tube-fed patient. *Oncology Nursing Forum, 8*(2), 8–13.

Strohl, R. (1987). Head and neck implants. *Seminars in Oncology Nursing, 3*(1), 30–46.

Woodtli, A. (1988). Nursing diagnosis and defining characteristics: Two research models. *Research in Nursing & Health, 11,* 399–406.

Wright, K., & Dyck, S. (1984). Expressed concerns of adult cancer patients' family members. *Cancer Nursing, 7,* 371–374.

Yasko, J. (1982). *Care of the client receiving external radiation therapy.* Reston, VA: Reston.

NANDA versus the Johnson Behavioral Systems Model: Is There a Diagnostic Difference?

Brooke P. Randell, DNSc, RN

The University of California, Los Angeles (UCLA) Neuropsychiatric Hospital (NPH) currently utilizes the Johnson Behavioral Systems Model (JBSM) as a basis for the practice of psychiatric nursing. Nursing diagnoses are derived from this conceptual framework and represent statements reflecting behavioral-system imbalance. Prior to implementation of the JBSM, adult and geriatric psychiatry units utilized a modified set of NANDA diagnostic labels. This approach was discarded when the JBSM was implemented because of conceptual inconsistencies between NANDA and the model. This study was undertaken to determine the differences in diagnostic labels and kinds of problems identified when diagnostic reasoning emanated from a different conceptual schema.

Johnson Behavioral Systems Model

The nursing process as implemented at the UCLA NPH is based upon the JBSM as described by Auger (1976), Grubbs (1980), and Johnson (1980). Patients are assessed and behavioral data are classified by subsystem. In addition, the assessment examines the internal and external environment in relationship to behavioral efficiency. Nursing diagnoses are formulated that reflect the nature of the ineffective behavior and its relationship to the regulators in the environment. The environment is viewed as contextual to the behavioral difficulty, and critical environmental factors as well as behavioral inefficiency guide the nursing intervention. A JBSM diagnosis using NANDA syntax might read "*Insufficiency of the ingestive subsystem* related to delusion of poisoned food as evidenced by recent 20-lb weight loss and refusal to ingest any food." These labels are currently at the first level of a taxonomic structure; the taxa are represented by the subsystem labels and these diagnoses are at the broadest or most abstract level. It is believed that as clinical data are accumulated the second level of diagnostic labels can be derived. The language of these labels will be more generic and less specific to the JBSM.

Design

The study was descriptive based on retrospective chart review. It was designed to examine the most frequently occurring diagnoses generated using the NANDA categories and the JBSM labels. A sample of 34 patient records with NANDA nursing diagnoses was compared to 100 patient records with JBSM diagnostic labels. Defining characteristics and related factors from each set of diagnoses were compared to determine differences in problem identification using the two approaches.

Sample

The NANDA diagnoses were made on a group of 34 patients admitted to adult and geropsychiatry inpatient units. Twenty charts from adult psychiatry and 14 charts from geropsychiatry were reviewed. The patients ranged in age from 19 to 85 years with a mean age of 52 years. The sample was equally divided between males (18) and females (16). In the adult psychiatry population, the most frequently occurring psychiatric diagnosis was bipolar (45%), following by depression (25%). The geropsychiatry population was predominantly depressed (71%) (see Table 1).

The JBSM diagnoses were made on a group of 100 patients admitted to child, adolescent, adult, and geropsychiatric inpatient units. Seventy-one charts from adult and geropsychiatry and 29 charts from child and adolescent psychiatry were reviewed. The patients ranged in age from 4 to 105 years with a mean age of 44 years. The sample contained slightly more females (*n* = 57) than males (*n* = 43). In the adult and geropsychiatry populations the most frequently occurring psychiatric diagnosis was depression (Table 1). The diagnoses in the child/adolescent population were varied and included eating disorders, conduct disorders, psychotic disorders, de-

Table 1: Adult/Geropsychiatric Samples by Psychiatric Diagnosis

NANDA (*n* = 34)	Percent	JBSM (*n* = 71)	Percent
Adult Psychiatry			
• Bipolar	45	• Depression	31
• Eating disorders	20	• Psychotic	17
		• Bipolar	11
• Depression	25	• Schizo-affective	11
• Psychotic	10		
		• Eating disorders	6
		• Other	25
Geropsychiatry			
• Depression	71	• Depression	63
• Organic	14	• Dementia	9
• Other	14	• Bipolar	6

pression, autism, and mixed developmental disorders.

Methods

Each chart was reviewed recording the patient's age, sex, admitting psychiatric diagnosis, and all nursing diagnoses for each patient. In addition, the defining characteristics and related or etiologic factors identified were recorded. The three most frequently occurring NANDA diagnoses were identified and compared to the four most frequently occurring JBSM diagnoses in the Aggressive-Protective subsystem. Given the conceptual differences in the two schemas, a simple comparison of most frequently occurring diagnoses was not attempted. The Aggressive-Protective subsystem was the most frequently targeted. Four specific diagnostic labels were represented. These four diagnostic labels were then compared to the three most frequently occurring NANDA diagnoses by completing a detailed content analysis of the defining characteristics and related or etiologic factors.

Findings

A review of 34 patient records revealed a total of 97 NANDA nursing diagnoses were made, an average of 2.85 per patient. A review of 100 patient records revealed a total of 188 JBSM nursing diagnoses, an average of 1.88 per patient. The difference of approximately one less diagnosis per patient might in part be explained by the level of diagnostic label. The JBSM labels are broad and it is possible to diagnose problems across subsystems and to combine environmental factors in a manner that allows patient problems to be described using fewer diagnostic labels. As the labels move down the taxonomic hierarchy, this characteristic diminishes and there may be an increase in the level of diagnostic specificity and therefore in the number of JBSM diagnoses formulated.

The most frequently occurring NANDA diagnoses were *altered thought processes* (19%), *potential for injury* (18%), and *ineffective individual coping* (16%). Fifty-three percent of the diagnoses dealt with these three problems. The Aggressive-Protective subsystem was the most frequently targeted subsystem when the JBSM was used as a basis for diagnostic reasoning. Thirty-five percent of the nursing diagnoses dealt with insufficiency, discrepancy, dominance, or incompatibility problems in the Aggressive-Protective subsystem.

Discussion

The question remains of how to compare sensibly two different approaches to nursing diagnosis. One way is to compare the problems described by each set of diagnoses, identifying areas of agreement and disagreement. Obviously there is a relationship between *potential for injury* and the diagnoses in the Aggressive-Protective subsystem. Less obvious is the relationship between the *ineffective individual coping* diagnoses and the Aggressive-Protective diagnoses; however the definition of this subsystem, keeping self safe, is consistent with the idea of coping as psychologic safety. Problems in the Aggressive-Protective subsystem could be said to represent a narrow range of coping behaviors. Finally, the relationship between the *altered thought processes* diagnosis and the Aggressive-Protective diagnoses is seen in the fact that many of the latter identify thought disturbances as an etiologic factor.

Aggressive-Protective Subsystem

The Aggressive-Protective subsystem is concerned with protection, one means of which may be aggression. Protecting self from harm is the goal of the subsystem (Johnson, 1980). In developing the model, Johnson (1968, 1977) relied to a large extent on animal literature to substantiate the behavioral subsystems. Aggressive behavior in nonhumans is viewed as protective, hence the JBSM combines the words aggressive and protective to describe this subsystem. While some theories suggest that aggression is learned and is engaged in for the specific purpose of causing pain or injury to another, other theories suggest that aggression toward self or others is engaged in to protect self. For example, hitting another may serve to make one feel less vulnerable, but the effect in terms of safety tends to be short-lived and, in Johnson's view, ineffective or inefficient. From the perspective of the JBSM, then, behavioral assessment of this subsystem focuses on safety. Is the person able to keep him/herself safe? Are the behaviors effective and efficient?

Behavioral assessment examines individual behaviors to determine the level of effectiveness that has been achieved in relationship to the goal of personal safety. Given that 35% of the JBSM diagnoses in this sample dealt with this subsystem, it appears that psychiatric inpatients have difficulty protecting themselves.

A review of the defining characteristics associated with each diagnosis delineates the common problems associated with this subsystem. The defining characteristics suggest that the vast majority of these individuals have problems with suicidal ideation or gestures; physical aggression toward others; provocative, threatening verbal behaviors; and self-destructive behaviors (e.g., substance abuse, self-mutilation). Less frequently identified problems include poor judgment, risk-taking or impulsive behaviors, and property destruction. In addition, behaviors that reflected the person's inability to keep him/herself safe in the face of problems associated with their pathology or its treatment were included as Aggressive-Protective problems. The final group included patients at risk for falls secondary to drug-related side effects, patients at risk for falls or confusion secondary to electroconvulsive therapy (ECT), and patients at risk for a variety of unsafe situations secondary to discontrol of seizures.

Nurses using the JBSM in an acute psychiatric setting formulate four different types of Aggressive-Protective subsystem diagnoses focusing on different aspects of ineffective or inefficient approaches to protection/safety. They are (1) inability to feel safe, (2) unsafe behavior toward others, (3) unsafe behavior toward objects, and (4) inability to protect self from environmental hazard. How do these Aggressive-Protective problems compare with the problems diagnosed in a similar population using the NANDA labels?

Potential for Injury

Potential for injury is defined as "a state in which the individual is at risk of injury as a result of environmental conditions interacting with the individual's adaptive and defensive resources" (NANDA, 1989, p. 39). A small portion of the diagnoses identified risk factors that were consistent with this definition (e.g., physiologic deviations that impaired balance or gait, side effects of therapy that increased vulnerability). These prob-

lems were consistent with the JBSM labels associated with the problem of inability to protect self from environmental hazards.

The majority of the *potential for injury* diagnoses, however, were inconsistent with the definition; they focused on the individual's potential for self-injury as well as provocative or physically aggressive behavior toward others. This can be explained in part by the fact that the NANDA data in this study were collected prior to the approval and publication of the *potential for violence* diagnostic label. When given a forced choice, nurses used the *potential for injury* label to describe all unsafe behaviors despite the deviation from the definition and identified risk factors.

When the actual content of the diagnoses is identified, both groups of nurses (those using NANDA and those using JBSM) identified the same problems in this patient population. This comparison of divergent views suggests the universality of the *potential for injury* and *potential for violence* diagnoses. In addition, it suggests the divergent possibilities when behavior is viewed from the context of protection or safety. How is the problem of suicidality different when conceptualized as the inability to keep self safe as opposed to it being a potential for violence?

Environment

The JBSM views the person as a behavioral system and defines the environment as anything external to the behavioral system (Johnson, 1980). This is a unique way of conceptualizing the recipient of nursing care that has a significant impact on what counts as defining characteristics and what counts as etiologic factors. In developing the JBSM for clinical practice, the concept of environment was extended to include six regulators. Regulators represent specific units of the environment that simultaneously influence and are influenced by behavior. These regulators are both internal and external to the person. The internal environment is composed of the biophysical regulator, the psychologic regulator, and the developmental regulator. These are factors internal to the person that impact behavior. The external environment is composed of the sociocultural regulator, the family regulator, and the physical environmental regulator.

In formulating a nursing diagnosis using the JBSM, behaviors that appear to be ineffective in meeting the goal of a subsystem are listed as defining characteristics. Etiologic factors are drawn from the six regulators. The state of our knowledge is such that these factors are listed as contextual to the behavior, not causal. In the psychiatric population, the psychologic regulator is frequently identified as an etiologic factor in an Aggressive-Protective subsystem diagnosis. The assessment of the psychologic regulator involves an evaluation of mental status, self-esteem, and coping style. If the assessment of the psychologic regulator indicates that the patient has some sort of thought disorder or is hallucinating or delusional, this information is used as contextual or etiologic to the diagnostic label. A patient who expresses suicidal ideation or gestures in response to false beliefs about the environment would have neither an *altered thought processes* diagnosis nor a *sensory/perceptual alteration* diagnosis, according to NANDA. The diagnosis would focus on the patient's inability to keep him/herself safe, which is believed to be related to false beliefs about the environment.

When the JBSM data from this study were reviewed, 18% of the Aggressive-Protective subsystem diagnoses identified altered thought processes as a related factor. An additional 28% were related to other psychologic factors such as low self-esteem or limited coping abilities. Seventeen percent were related to family issues and 25% (predominantly in the geropsychiatric population) identified contributing biophysical problems. *Altered thought processes, low self-esteem*, and *ineffective coping* are never diag-

nosed as a problem using the JBSM, but are seen as factors contributing to behavioral problems expressed by the patient. Interventions then focus on the behavior in the context of related factors. Nursing care focuses on both the behavior and the identified etiologies. Aggressive behavior toward self or others is controlled and limited regardless of the etiology, but the manner in which that control is exercised is guided by the etiologic factors. The approach to the patient whose aggressive behavior reflects a thought disorder may be quite different from the approach to the patient who always employs an aggressive coping strategy.

Altered Thought Processes

Altered thought processes are defined as "a state in which the individual experiences a disruption in cognitive operations and activities" (NANDA, 1989, p. 95). Defining characteristics include inaccurate perception of the environment, cognitive dissonance, distractability, memory deficit problems, egocentricity, and hyper/hypovigilance. When the NANDA-based diagnostic labels and defining characteristics were reviewed there was minimal consistency as to what problems were actually being addressed.

Thirty-three percent of the diagnoses dealt with problems of orientation and appeared to represent an accurate interpretation of the label. The remaining diagnoses addressed a variety of problems such as concerns regarding living situations, the need for help with activities of daily living, uncooperative behavior, and depression. In each of these cases it appears that altered thought processes such as obsessive thoughts, paranoid ideas, and ruminative thoughts were viewed as etiologic factors that were related to the problems of living as experienced by these patients. One must conclude then that the diagnosis was frequently used incorrectly with nurses demonstrating that altered thought processes represent a context that guides their interventions for a variety of patient care problems.

The current NANDA taxonomic structure, unlike the JBSM, does not suggest what counts as etiology. Are altered thought processes per se the focus of attention of nursing intervention? Or does nursing intervention focus on the problems of living that the individual may experience in the context of these disrupted cognitive operations?

Ineffective Individual Coping

The NANDA diagnostic label of *ineffective individual coping* is defined as "the impairment of adaptive behaviors and problem-solving abilities of a person in meeting life's demands and roles" (NANDA, 1989, p. 60.) Destructive behavior towards self or others is just one of many defining characteristics associated with this label. As previously stated this diagnosis would not be made using the JBSM. Coping style or pattern is assessed as part of the psychologic regulator and is used as an etiologic factor for a variety of the behavioral problems manifested by psychiatric patients. Coping behavior is considered unique to the problem and the situation and therefore might manifest itself under a variety of labels (e.g., *potential for injury, potential for violence, altered nutrition,* or *social isolation*).

Thirty-one percent of the NANDA-based diagnoses in this sample appeared to deal with anxiety. The rest of the diagnoses covered a host of other problems including eating problems, provocative behaviors, helplessness, poor decision making, problems with activities of daily living, and relational problems. This particular diagnostic label appears to be so broad as to encompass all potential problems of the psychiatric patient. In the broadest sense one might say that all psychiatric hospitalizations are based on the patients' inability to cope effectively. In fact when the JBSM was introduced and the decision was made to abandon the NAN-

DA labels the nursing staff wanted to know what they were going to do without this particular label. It was noted that whenever nurses were in doubt as to the appropriate diagnosis, they could always use *ineffective individual coping* and not be wrong.

Because the process of formulating diagnostic labels is continually evolving, many of the labels lack the specificity to be truly definitive. However there is the potential to achieve such specificity; one wonders if such is the case with this label. Will it be possible to reach consensus on *ineffective individual coping* or does it represent such a broad category that other diagnostic labels, some already available and others yet to be developed, will prove to be more meaningful in defining human response?

Summary

This retrospective study compared diagnostic labels generated from the JBSM to those generated from an early NANDA list. The findings suggest the universality of the *potential for injury* and the *potential for violence* diagnoses. In addition it is suggested that the *potential for violence* diagnostic label does not represent the true nature of the problem presented by the suicidal patient. The conceptualization of the problem as an inability to keep oneself safe is offered as an alternative view. Comparing the two diagnostic approaches also raises the etiologic issue. The JBSM helps distinguish what counts as a problem and what counts as etiology, calling into question existing labels such as *altered thought processes* and *ineffective individual coping*.

Our science is still young and none of our conceptual frameworks nor the NANDA taxonomy represent finished works. Approaching the diagnostic dilemmas from a variety of perspectives will help us identify areas of agreement and areas where our thoughts are divergent. Multiple approaches to the diagnostic process add richness to our data and force us to examine the assumptions that underlie our decisions to label a human response in a particular way.

References

Auger, J. R. (1976). *Behavioral systems and nursing.* Englewood Cliffs, NJ: Prentice-Hall.

Grubbs, J. (1980). An interpretation of the Johnson Behavioral System Model for nursing practice. In J. Riehl & C. Roy (Eds.), *Conceptual models for nursing practice* (2nd ed.). New York: Appleton-Century-Crofts.

Johnson, D. E. (1968, April). *One conceptual model of nursing.* Paper presented at Vanderbilt University, Nashville, TN.

Johnson, D. E. (1977). *The behavioral system model for nursing.* Paper presented at the Unviersity of Delaware, Newark, DE.

Johnson, D. E. (1980). The behavioral systems model of nursing. In J. Riehl & C. Roy (Eds.), *Conceptual models for nursing practice* (2nd ed.). New York: Appleton-Century-Crofts.

North American Nursing Diagnosis Association. (1989). *Taxonomy I revised.* St. Louis, MO: Author.

A Proposed Model for Assessing Compliance within the Unitary Man/Human Framework Based on an Analysis of the Concept of Compliance

Mary Kontz, MSN, RN

The purpose of this analysis was to provide clearer understanding of the concept of compliance and to develop propositional statements indicating the effect of variables on client compliance. The following questions were answered:

1. What are the definitions of compliance?
2. What are the critical attributes of compliance?
3. What variables influence client health-related behaviors?

Methods

A modification of Wilson's (1963) strategy for concept analysis was used; the steps included

1. Isolate the question of the concept (i.e., noncompliance) from other questions.
2. Locate and roughly map the area occupied by the concept, including defining the concept.
3. Review the literature to extract explicit or implicit meanings of the concept.
4. Extract provisional criteria that may be used in naming the occurrence of the phenomenon.
5. Examine such factors of social context, underlying anxieties, and application of varying means in different social situations (Wilson, 1963).

Literature perceived to be relevant to adult health nursing was reviewed. The initial concept analysis was conducted in 1984 (Kontz, 1984) and updated with current findings in the theoretical literature.

Definitions of Compliance

A complete analysis of the theoretical and operational definitions has been previously published (Kontz, 1989). To summarize:

Theoretical definitions, when stated by researchers, are similar to the definition of compliance provided by Haynes (1979) as "the extent to which a person's behavior, such as taking medications, following diets, or executing lifestyle changes, coincides with medical or health advice" (p. 3). Researchers' definitions of compliance reflected the entire health care regimen and encompassed any preventive, therapeutic, or maintenance care.

The theoretical definitions of compliance were congruent in the desired outcome of following the recommended therapeutic regimen. The theoretical definitions were not congruent with respect to the level of participation and responsibility the client should have in achieving the desired outcome.

From the analysis of the theoretical definitions of compliance, the following definition was proposed: "Compliance is a complex phenomenon in which an individual exhibits behaviors consistent with his or her definition of health and health-related activities. In cases where the individual has received health-related advice from health care professionals, the individual assumes responsibility for incorporating perceived relevant advice into his or her daily activities. In the areas in which the individual does not perceive the advice to be relevant, the health care professional assumes responsibility to intervene appropriately. This intervention should be goal oriented, consistent and realistic to the individual's case. The individual should make informed decisions as to the health-related advice he or she wishes to follow, and the health care provider should accept these decisions and assist the individual to maintain health within these restrictions" (Kontz, 1989, p. 58).

This definition explicates the role of the health care provider and that of the client. Furthermore, the responsibilities of the health care provider and client are delineated. The proposed definition suggests a much broader perspective on the compliance issue.

Operational definitions varied from simple (e.g., keeping appointments) to complex (indirect and direct measurements of compliance). Many operational definitions could not be replicated, such as those implied by the methods used to score the measurement instrument. This finding was supported in the literature (Caron, 1985; Sackett & Snow, 1979). In addition, each direct and indirect measurement of compliance had inadequacies so that a combined approach to measurement was necessary to draw conclusions (Gordis, 1979). Because of the various ways in which compliance was operationalized, each study had to be evaluated on its own merits and comparisons of findings was problematic.

Unitary Man/Human Framework

The Unitary Man/Human Framework was selected as the organizing framework for the vast amount of literature reviewed in this analysis. Research was initially conducted prior to the endorsement of this framework by NANDA as Taxonomy I. The framework, definitions of the nine interactional patterns, and assumptions were used as set forth in the proceedings from the third, fourth, and fifth national conferences on nursing diagnoses (Kritek, 1984; Roy, 1978, 1982a, 1982b).

The framework had several identifying components not included in Taxonomy I. However, they remain important to the concept analysis presented here. First, the nine interactional patterns were grouped under three major constructs of moving, interaction, and action. These constructs were not defined in the NANDA proceedings, nor was it clear in more recent publications when and why these concepts were removed from the framework. For this concept analysis, these constructs were used to group the interactional patterns and to illustrate the propositional statements. Second, the nine patterns were called "interactional" patterns. Interaction is defined in the Random House Dictionary of the English Language (1987) as "to act one upon another." In 1986, these interactional patterns became known as human response patterns.

Critical Attributes of Compliance

The critical attributes of compliance were isolated using the criteria of (1) frequent citations in the literature and (2) limited incongruence in the empirical research findings. For each critical attribute inconsistencies were found in the empirical research reviewed; however, some support was found for the following:

1. *Perceiving*
   a. Client verbalization of
      1) perceived susceptibility to health condition
      2) perceived severity of consequences of illness
      3) perceived benefits of therapy
2. *Knowing*
   a. Client verbalization of need for health-related information
3. *Feeling*
   a. Client verbalization of increased self-esteem or low anxiety levels
4. *Exchanging* No critical attributes found
5. *Communicating*
   a. Client verbalization of confusion over explanations given by different health care providers requiring clarification
6. *Relating*
   a. Client verbalization of
      1) supportive family or friends during times of illness or crisis
      2) willingness of family and friends to assist client or past assistance with therapeutic regimen
      3) a positive relationship with health care provider
      4) effective communication with health care provider
   b. Objectively, the client demonstrated

accurate performance of therapeutic regimen.
7. *Choosing*
   a. Client verbalization of enough information to make an informed decision
   b. Objectively, client
      1) exhibits effective coping strategies.
      2) exhibits a realistic approach to the treatment regimen.
      3) seeks needed information to make a health-related decision.
      4) participates in the decision-making process.

The majority of the critical attributes identified were subjective, suggesting that health care professionals must rely on the client's accurate verbalizations with regard to compliance.

Variables Influencing Compliance

Concepts Classified under the Construct *Moving*

Perceiving

The Perceiving pattern was defined as the "reception of information" (Roy, 1984, p. 29). The theoretical and empirical literature reviewed included the Health Belief Model (HBM) (Rosenstock, 1974) and Neisser's (1978) model of the perceptual cycle.

The HBM differed from the perceptual schema described by Neisser (1978). Neisser suggested perception was developed or modified through reception of information, while the HBM focuses on current perception, not past experience or behavior. Perhaps this limitation of the HBM explains the inability of the health care provider to effectively predict compliance over time. The Neisser model has not been used specifically in the research literature on compliance.

Empirical literature of the HBM was reviewed by Mikhail (1981) and included 31 research studies. The purpose of Mikhail's review was to determine (1) empirical adequacy of the HBM, (2) the contribution of the study to understanding of the HBM, and (3) the usefulness of the HBM in predicting compliance. Her findings regarding empirical adequacy included

1. The variable of perceived susceptibility was more supported than any other variable in the model
2. Perceived susceptibility was positively related to preventive health actions and adherence to the therapeutic regimen
3. Perceived severity of the health condition was positively correlated to adherence behaviors in preventive and chronic illness
4. Perceived benefits were associated with higher compliance rates when the recommended health action reduced the threat to the person
5. Perceived costs were found to be negatively associated with compliance behaviors, and
6. Health motivation was positively correlated with preventive health behavior.

The HBM provides some understanding of why people behave as they do in certain situations and of the variables that affect their decision-making process. Mikhail (1981) noted that operationalization of the constructs in the model is confusing in the empirical literature and that it is unclear how much influence independent variables have on health-related behavior. Mikhail found minimal empirical support that health beliefs are potentially modifiable. Variables within the HBM can be manipulated to produce desired changes in health behavior, however it is unclear whether the manipulated variable actually produces either a change in health beliefs or a sustained change in health behavior.

Several other critiques of the HBM identified some of the same findings as Mikhail (Haynes, Taylor, & Sackett, 1979; Redeker, 1988; and Wallston & Wallston, 1984). Haynes et al. (1979) addressed the interaction that Mikhail stated was difficult to support, suggesting that the combined effects of perceived susceptibility, severity, and benefits of therapy were more likely to be positively correlated with compliance behaviors. On the other hand, Wallston and Wallston (1984) suggested that the HBM was basically a catalog of variables rather than a well-articulated model that specified the relationship among its variables. They agreed with Mikhail that there were inconsistencies across empirical studies in the operationalization and measurement of the variables making it virtually impossible to compare findings across multiple investigations. The recommendations were that further refinement of the model was needed and that instrumentation was critical for future research endeavors.

Champion (1984) reviewed the instruments used to collect HBM data and summarized the instruments' inadequacies as follows: (1) tools were largely untested for validity or reliability, (2) operational definitions had wide variance from one study to another, (3) studies used only one or two items for measuring a concept, and (4) concepts were operationalized at a nominal level so that only descriptive statistics could be used. Champion's critique of the limitations of the HBM instruments to predict compliance was supported by the empirical literature reviewed for this analysis.

Most of the literature supported positive relationships between compliance and perceived susceptibility of illness, severity of illness, and benefits of therapy. However, inconsistent findings cited (Haynes et al., 1979; Mikhail, 1981; and Rutledge, 1987) suggested that perception cannot be studied in isolation from other intervening variables.

For example, Tirrell and Hart (1980) found that a person's perceived susceptibility to the illness was negatively associated with compliance and influenced by personal problems. Thus patient priorities and coping behaviors influence compliance. Furthermore, fear or anxiety levels stimulated by perceptions may affect coping behaviors. When clients were viewed individually, specific determinations about anxiety, fear, and compliance behaviors can be assessed.

Perceived barriers consistently decreased compliance. Based on this finding it was inferred that perceived barriers may have a more powerful effect on compliance than other constructs in the HBM. Many barriers influence compliance: personal problems (Tirrell & Hart, 1980); financial cost, transportation available and accessibility, side effects of medications (Watts, 1982); and incorporation of drug schedules into daily routines (Hershey, Morton, Davis, & Reichgott, 1980). Medication compliance was related to frequency and timing of dosing rather than to number of medications; as dosage schedules were streamlined, medication compliance increased (Fujii & Seki, 1985).

Findings varied with regard to the ability of the HBM to predict compliance over time for chronically ill clients. Except for perceived barriers, which decreased compliance and was more consistently supported than other variables, inconsistencies were found within each perceptual category of the HBM.

Propositional statements consistent with the findings in the literature were formulated for the variable of Perceiving as

1. Perceived susceptibility to illness, severity of illness, and benefits of treatment increases compliance.
2. Perceived barriers to the treatment regimen decrease compliance with the regimen.

Knowing

The Knowing pattern was defined as "meaning associated with information" (Roy, 1984,

p. 29). Findings in the empirical literature did not support specific educational strategies that enhance compliance; however, client teaching was found to increase client knowledge regardless of the method used (Haynes, 1976; Mills, Barnes, Rodell, & Terry, 1985; and Spelman, 1984). There was some evidence that combining client education with other strategies such as counseling increased compliance (Green, 1979, p. 165; and Haynes, 1979), that tailoring the educational strategy to the individual increased knowledge and compliance (Marshall, Penckofer, & Llewellyn, 1986; and Wyka, Levesque, Ryan, & Mattea, 1980), and that implementation of structured teaching programs increased compliance (Marshall et al., 1986).

Knowledge alone was not linked to positive effects on compliance. Educating the patient resulted in increased knowledge, but knowledge was not consistently associated with improved outcome behaviors (Bille, 1977; Brown, Wright, & Christensen, 1987; Haynes et al., 1979; and Kerr, 1985). Clients who asked for information were just as successful in learning as those given the information without asking (Bille, 1977). This implied that information sought and information gained passively may be assigned the same meaning. Also, because group education was found effective and enhanced compliance in a group of voluntary subjects (Wyka et al., 1980), relationships or bonds established with other clients and health care providers may be the intervening variable.

The propositional statement that summarized the materials reviewed on Knowing was

1. Combined strategies for teaching and counseling clients increases compliance.

Feeling

The Feeling pattern was defined as "subjective awareness of information (Roy, 1984, p.

29). Limited empirical research was found concerning feeling and compliance. Some feeling states, such as fear and anxiety, have been studied as they related to communication.

In a study by Lum, Chase, Cole, Johnson, Johnson, and Link (1978), a questionnaire was administered to 57 oncology subjects to determine the effect of self-esteem on compliance. Enhanced self-esteem was linked to reduced anxiety and compliance, suggesting that lower anxiety levels could enhance compliance. Linkages were also found between enhanced self-esteem and compliance.

While there was evidence in the literature that dealt with anxiety as a stimulus and motivator to conduct information searches, no studies were found to link anxiety and compliance. Barnlund (1976) suggested anxiety that accompanies illness may affect the learning process and disrupt effectiveness of communication. Therefore, several linkages to compliance could be proposed. For example, anxiety may be produced if an individual perceives the illness to be severe. Anxiety may cause the individual to engage in an information search including seeking health care. Anxiety produced by illness may result in ineffective learning and communication with health care providers. Altered feeling states (e.g., anxiety) may produce decreased compliance indirectly associated with the client's perception, knowledge, and communication. Support for these linkages was not found however.

The propositional statements that summarized the literature reviewed on Feeling were

1. Increased self-esteem increases compliance.
2. When decreased anxiety levels are associated with increased self-esteem, compliance increases.

Concepts Classified under the Construct *Interaction*

Exchanging

The Exchanging pattern was defined as "mutual giving and receiving" (Roy, 1984, p. 29). Exchanging was previously defined as the "interchange of matter and energy between man and environment" (Roy, 1982, p. 244). Assessment factors for Exchanging include eating, drinking, eliminating, breathing, and giving/receiving approval and advice. The Exchanging pattern is primarily made up of physiologic responses and targets the disease process. An underlying assumption of this concept analysis was that compliance is not disease dependent (Haynes, 1979; Kontz, 1989; and McCord, 1986). While there was some evidence to support that symptomatology may affect behavior, there are no direct linkages that the disease process affects and sustains behavior. No propositional statements could be made in the Exchanging pattern.

Communicating

The Communicating pattern was defined as "sending messages" (Roy, 1984, p. 29). None of the patterns of Unitary Man/Human Framework can be completely analyzed without communication. The hidden meanings and content of communication were not well documented in the literature; neither were studies determining the effectiveness of the communication process. Nevertheless, it is postulated that content and effectiveness of the communication process influence understanding of the information and, thus, influence compliance.

Influencing variables on communication and compliance were identified in four areas—role modeling, effectiveness of written drug information, effectiveness of communication, and fear communications. In a study to determine nurses' knowledge of insulin administration (Villeneuve, 1982), findings demonstrated that nurses in the hospital did not perform insulin administration in the same way patients were taught. Nurses were providing conflicting messages to clients through their nonverbal role modeling, thus increasing clients' confusion about what was taught and subsequently decreasing compliance with the appropriate administration of insulin. While further research is needed to determine the relationships among teaching, role modeling, and their influence on compliance, this study provided insight into the health care providers' influence on compliance.

The influencing variables identified on effectiveness of written drug information and compliance were

1. Use of written drug information enhances compliance with short-term therapy, but does not affect compliance behavior in long-term therapy (Morris & Halperin, 1979).
2. Written drug information increases the client's knowledge about drug information (Morris & Halperin, 1979).
3. Combining written drug information and counseling over time enhances compliance (McKenny, Slinig, Henderson, Devins, & Barr, 1973; Morris & Halperin, 1979). The act of counseling suggests a relationship or rapport between the client and the provider. Whenever more time is spent with a client, the effects of rapport cannot be ignored or confused with communication.

Effectiveness of communication was addressed in three studies. The type of communication used (written, verbal, or nonverbal) may influence the effectiveness of the communication process and compliance (Brown et al., 1987; Hulka, 1979; and Kasch & Knutson, 1987).

Fear communication has been studied for its motivation on the client's health behavior. Findings in the literature were inconsistent; fear communications were found to influence compliance both positively and negatively. There was evidence that the intensity of fear communication was an influencing variable of compliance; however the intensity of the fear communication that motivates clients to change behavior has not been established (Best & Block, 1979; Blackwell, 1976; Esler, 1978; and Mikhail, 1981).

In summary, communication and counseling used in combination effectively improved compliance according to the research reviewed (Green, 1979; Haynes, 1979; and Morris & Halperin, 1979). Combined strategies were more effective in producing positive effects on compliance. This last finding also suggested that continuity of care, client-provider relationships, and benefits derived from counseling were important influencing variables improving compliance.

The propositional statements summarizing the literature reviewed on Communicating were

1. Conflicting messages between verbal and nonverbal communication from the health care professional lead to confusion over expected compliance behaviors and therefore decrease compliance.
2. Written and verbal communication used in combination improves learning and will improve compliance over time.
3. Use of written drug information (a) increases compliance with short-term therapy and (b) does not increase compliance behavior in long-term therapy.

Relating

The Relating pattern was defined as "establishing bonds with other persons or objects" (Roy, 1984, p. 29). The empirical literature reviewed on Relating included social support and client-provider relationships.

Social support. While social support was found to positively affect compliance, two intervening variables affect social support—locus of control and the effect of time on relationships. Locus of control influences the type and amount of social support needed by the client and the effectiveness of that support (Gerzewski, 1983). Norbeck (1981) suggested that the health care provider and the client may have different perceptions of who is the supportive significant other. This finding was supported in a study by Hilbert (1985) in which spouse support following myocardial infarction was not found to be significantly related to compliance. Two other studies found that subjects' adherence was significantly related to their beliefs about what others thought they should do (McMahon et al., 1986; Miller et al., 1988). Norbeck (1981) also suggested that the characteristics of the person can influence the amount and type of social support needed, thus locus of control may influence social support, as reported by Gerszewski (1983).

Another variable, the strength of the relationship over time (Norbeck, 1981), was supported by O'Brien (1982). The relationships gained stability over time, but the importance of the relationship changed. Norbeck's (1982) explanation for the change in relationships over time was that the intensity of social support needed changes over time based on the duration of support required. For example, chronically ill persons have low intensity of support needed on a continuous basis. This can deplete social support networks and could explain the increased intensity of the relationship between the client and provider (O'Brien, 1980). The provider continues to offer the client support to cope with stressors of illness.

The propositional statement summarizing the effect of social support on compliance was

1. Social support perceived as helpful by the individual increases compliance.

The client–provider relationship. Many variables were found in the client–provider relationship. First, communication that enhanced the relationship improved compliance. Specific communications influencing the relationship were (1) lack of explanation, which negatively influenced the relationship and decreased compliance; (2) a combination of written and verbal communication, which positively affected the relationship and improved compliance (Stickney, Hall, & Gardner, 1980); and (3) communication of client expectations by the health care provider, which improved compliance (Hulka, 1979).

Client verbalization that the client-provider relationship was satisfactory enhanced compliance (Haynes et al., 1979); however, factors contributing to a satisfactory relationship were not enumerated consistently. The suggested factors defining a satisfactory relationship were the amount of instruction given, justification of drug usage, receptivity of provider to client, responsiveness of provider to client complaints and admission of noncompliance, inclusion of the family in the treatment regimen, and professional competence. Support was found in the literature that a satisfactory relationship coupled with explicit communication enhanced compliance (Hulka, 1979). Thus it was inferred that a positive client-provider relationship enhances the effectiveness of communication.

Hulka (1979) defined the effectiveness of communication as the difference between information given and information retained. However information retained does not mean the information was understood and applied. This was supported by Hulka's findings that information retained did not result in reduced drug error rates. The implication of this finding was that effectiveness of communication must be determined by performance of a desired behavior.

The propositional statements that could be derived from the literature with respect to the effects of client–provider relationships were

1. Communication between the client and the health care provider that is perceived effective by the client improves the relationship and increases compliance.
2. Communication by the health care provider that provides the client with instructions and expectations increases compliance if used over time.
3. When the health care provider is receptive to the client's admissions of noncompliance and illness complaints, the client–provider relationship improves and compliance increases.

Concepts Classified under the Construct *Action*

Valuing

The Valuing pattern was defined as "the assigning of worth" (Roy, 1982, p. 244). Valuing includes the client's philosophic beliefs regarding health, the meaning of life and health, religious practices and beliefs, and health goals and priorities. Roy (1982) described locus of control as an empirical indicator of the Valuing pattern.

Locus of control. The concept of locus of control distinguishes differences between internally and externally controlled behaviors; however the research using the concept of locus of control offered little evidence that it was a predictor of compliance (Arakelian, 1980; and Haynes et al., 1979). There was some evidence to support that characteristics of and strategies employed by internally and externally controlled people change over time (Lowery & Ducette, 1976). In addition, Wallston & Wallston (1978) found that an understanding of internally and externally controlled individuals contributes to the health

professional's interventions and enhances client compliance.

In a study by D'Altroy, Blissenbach, & Lutz (1978) support was found for tailoring treatment regimens to the client's locus of control. Similarly, the Wallston & Wallston (1978) study demonstrated client weight loss was achieved through structured programs tailored to client's locus of control.

Some contradictory findings were noted by comparing results in the literature on self-esteem and locus of control. Increased self-esteem has been shown to enhance compliance (Lum et al., 1978). The literature on locus of control suggested that externally controlled persons had less self-esteem but were more compliant (Schroeder & Miller, 1983). These conflicting results suggest other intervening variables, untested in the studies, may have interfered with compliance.

The propositional statement that summarizes the literature reviewed on locus of control was

1. Effectiveness of treatment regimens depends on tailoring the regimen to an individual's locus of control tendency.

Moving

The Moving pattern was defined as "activity within the environment" (Roy, 1982, p. 244). Assessment factors included degrees of mobility, and empirical indicators are locomotion characteristics, control of intentional movement, joint flexibility, goal-directed movement, and activity tolerance. Factors in the compliance literature that interfere with goal-directed movement include actual barriers to health care such as cost of care, environmental conditions, transportation, physical barriers, and long waiting periods in clinics and physician offices. In this analysis, a distinction was made between perceived barriers (Perceiving) and actual barriers (Moving).

There was limited empirical evidence regarding actual barriers to compliance. Studies did not include the effects of physical barriers on compliance, such as deficits in vision, hearing, and mobility/flexibility (e.g., difficulty removing pill container tops).

Haynes et al. (1979) summarized the reasons clients gave for noncompliance. These included transportation (eight studies) and weather (three studies). Tirrell and Hart (1980) supported weather as a cause for clients not following the recommended exercise regimen during winter months.

A study conducted by Stickney et al. (1980) found that scheduling follow-up appointments improved compliance rates, suggesting that psychiatric clients were less likely to take responsibility for follow-up. Problems with keeping appointments (e.g., clinic error, confusion over appointment, loss of appointment slip, and waiting time at the clinic) were also identified as interfering with compliance (Haynes et al., 1979). The classic research on the relationship between waiting time and compliance was performed by Rockhart and Hofmann (1969), whose findings showed that reducing waiting times decreased the rates of no show.

Employment was identified as a major cause of noncompliance in six studies (Haynes et al., 1979), which found that a regimen that interfered with work or that required clients to take time off from work to keep appointments resulted in decreased compliance.

The propositional statement that summarizes the literature on Moving was

1. Actual barriers in the health care system, such as lack of continuity of care, inaccessibility to transportation, and long waiting periods, decrease compliance.

Choosing

The Choosing pattern was defined as "the selection of alternatives" (Roy, 1984, p. 29). The theoretical and empirical literature reviewed on Choosing included the decision-making process (Simon, 1976) and the Health Decision Model (Eracker, Korscht, & Becker, 1984). These theorists emphasized the need for clients to participate actively in their regimen, a position gaining increasing legal support. This position relates to the health care provider's unrealistic expectations of client compliance behavior. Based on knowledge and experience, the health professional often sets goals of optimum control of the client's disease state, knowing possible ramifications, and complications of high-risk states. Thus the health professional's goals involve total care to reduce risk factors.

Research on client's decision making as it related to compliance was sparse. The studies reviewed did not control for other intervening variables that may affect compliance, such as ethical considerations or rapport established with the client.

The literature reviewed on decision making suggested that contracting was a useful tool in enhancing compliance (Kosnar, 1987; Steckel, 1974, 1976; and Steckel & Swain, 1977). Contracting may be a successful intervention because (1) realistic goals are established for clients because of their active participation in decision making, (2) client control over the situation is increased, (3) the treatment regimen is reduced to more manageable portions instead of trying to accomplish many behaviors at one time, and (4) the client-provider relationship offers guidance and support for effective coping strategies.

Active participation was a variable tested in a study on 268 elderly women by Chang, Uman, Linn, Ware, and Kane (1985). Holding individual differences constant, they found active participation was not significantly related to intent to adhere to the therapeutic regimen. The other variables have not been tested in the empirical literature on contracting.

Several variables found to influence a mother's decision to accept or reject amniocentesis in a study by Cox, Sullivan, and Roghmann (1984) were insurance coverage for the procedure, experience with birth defects, physician support or nonsupport for the procedure, and social group attitudes toward the procedure. Also, education level influenced the number of sources available for consultation and influenced the final decision. Ethical aspects were not addressed in this study.

It appears from the literature reviewed on decision making that researchers are looking for effective interventions before establishing exact criteria to measure compliant behavior.

The propositional statements summarizing the literature reviewed on decision making were

1. Active participation by the client in the health care decision-making process enhances perceived control over the situation and increases compliance.
2. The individual's active participation in health-related decisions enhances realistic and achievable goal-setting, which increases compliance.
3. Active participation by the client in the health care decision-making process enhances perceived control over the situation and increases compliance.

Demographic Variables

The literature reviewed demonstrated inconsistencies in the demographic variables that affected compliance. The two findings with most support in the literature were that

1. Older individuals were more likely to follow recommended regimens (Haynes et al., 1979; Marston, 1970).
2. Ethnicity affects compliance when individual priorities are perceived more important than following physician orders (O'Brien, 1982).

Sex, marital status, occupation, and religion were not found to increase or decrease compliance with any consistency.

Conclusions

The propositional statements were diagrammed in the three dimensions—moving, interaction, and action—indicating the direction and effect of the variables on compliance. The propositional statements were then used to construct a model for assessing compliance. Figure 1 illustrates the interrelationships of the nine interactional patterns of the Unitary Man/Human Framework and their direction and effect on compliance. The changing patterns of unitary man (Roy, 1984) were supported by the findings of this analysis. Change in any pattern influences the other patterns and can alter its direction and effect on compliance. The Perceiving pattern can influence all others as demonstrated in the figure.

It is postulated that the nurse, using the model to assess compliance, can diagram variables that influence compliance for each client. While the HBM was limited to assessing four perceptions, this model represents a more comprehensive assessment of client perceptions and patterns. Compliance is not a simple act, but a complex, dynamic concept influenced by many intervening variables.

Recommendations

Major recommendations for further study based on this analysis include

1. Further refinement of the theoretical and operational definitions of compliance to reflect the complexity of the concept and the roles and responsibilities of the client as currently reflected in the literature.
2. Development of a measurement instru-

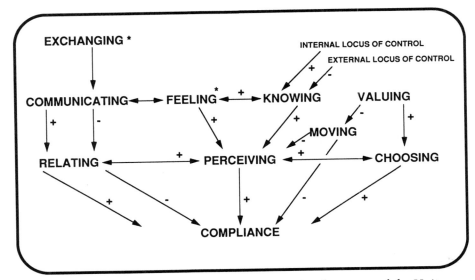

FIGURE 1 Interrelationships of the nine interactional patterns of the Unitary Man/Human Framework illustrating the direction and effect of the variables of compliance. Refer to original research study which included 30 propositional statements (Kontz, 1984). + = positive relationship; − = negative relationship; * = insufficient evidence to support any statements between variables.

ment to assess factors contributing to compliance from the proposed model for assessing compliance.

3. Development of tools to study the effects of several variables (e.g., the effect of fear communications) on compliance.

4. Further use of the Unitary Man/Human Framework to clarify the definitions of the major constructs and interactional patterns.

5. Review of the nursing diagnosis *noncompliance* for accuracy of definition and representativeness of the defining characteristics.

6. Determination of a comprehensive set of nursing diagnoses that more accurately describes the complexity of the concept of compliance.

References

Arakelian, M. (1980). An assessment and nursing application of the concept of locus of control. *Advances in Nursing Science, 3*(1), 25–42.

Barnlund, D. C. (1976). The mystification of meaning: Doctor-patient encounters. *Journal of Medical Education, 51,* 716–725.

Best, J. A., & Block, M. (1979). Compliance in the control of cigarette smoking. In R. B. Haynes, D. W. Taylor, & D. L. Sackett (Eds.), *Compliance in health care* (pp. 202–222). Baltimore: Johns Hopkins University Press.

Bille, D.A. (1977). A study of patients' knowledge in relation to teaching format and compliance. *Supervisor Nurse, 8*(12), 55–62.

Blackwell, B. (1976). Treatment adherence. *British Journal of Psychiatry, 129,* 515–531.

Brown, C. S., Wright, R. G., & Christensen, D. B. (1987). Association between type of medication instruction and patients' knowledge. *Hospital Community Psychiatry, 38*(1), 55–60.

Caron, H. S. (1985). Compliance: The case of objective

management. *The Journal of Hypertension, 3,* 811–822.

Champion, V. L. (1984). Instrument development for the health belief model constructs. *Advances in Nursing Science, 6*(3), 73–85.

Chang, B. L., Uman, G. C., Linn, L. S., Ware, K. E., & Kane, R. L. (1985). Adherence to health care regimes among elderly women. *Nursing Research, 34,* 27–31.

Cox, C. L., Sullivan, J. A., & Roghmann, K. J. (1984). A conceptual explanation of risk-reduction behavior and intervention development. *Nursing Research, 33,* 168–173.

D'Altroy, L. H., Blissenbach, H. F., & Lutz, D. (1978). Patient drug self-administration improves regimen compliance. *Hospitals, 52,* 131–136.

Eracker, S. A., Kirscht, J. P., & Becker, M. H. (1984). Understanding and improving patient compliance. *Annals of Internal Medicine, 100,* 258–268.

Esler, A. (1978). Attitude changes in an industrial hearing conservation program: Comparative effects of directives, educational presentations and individual explanations as persuasive communications. *Occupational Health Nursing, 26,* 15–20.

Fujii, J., & Seki, A. (1985). Compliance and compliance improving strategies in hypertension: The Japanese. *The Journal of Hypertension, 3,* 819–822.

Gerszewski, S. A. (1983). The relationship of weight loss, locus of control, and social support. *Nursing Research, 32,* 43–47.

Gordis, L. (1979). Conceptual and methodological problems in measuring patient compliance. In R. B. Haynes, D. W. Taylor, & D. L. Sackett (Eds.), *Compliance in health care* (pp. 23–45). Baltimore: Johns Hopkins University Press.

Green, L. W. (1979). Educational strategies to improve compliance with therapeutic and preventive regimens: The recent evidence. In R. B. Haynes, D. W. Taylor, & D. L. Sackett (Eds.), *Compliance in health care* (pp. 157–173). Baltimore: Johns Hopkins University Press.

Haynes, R. B. (1976). Strategies for improving compliance: A methodological analysis and review. In D. L. Sackett & R. B. Haynes (Eds.), *Compliance with the therapeutic regimens* (pp. 69–82). Baltimore: Johns Hopkins University Press.

Haynes, R. B. (1979). Determinants of compliance: The disease and the mechanics of treatment. In R. B. Haynes, D. W. Taylor, & D. L. Sackett (Eds.), *Compliance in health care* (pp. 49–62). Baltimore: Johns Hopkins University Press.

Haynes, R. B., Taylor, D. W., & Sackett, D. L. (Eds.). (1979). *Compliance in health care.* Baltimore: Johns Hopkins University Press.

Hershey, J. C., Morton, B. G., Davis, J. B., & Reichgott, M. J. (1980). Patient compliance with antihypertensive medication. *American Journal of Public Health, 70,* 1081–1088.

Hilbert, G. A. (1985). Spouse support and myocardial infarction. *Nursing Research, 34,* 217–220.

Hulka, B. S. (1979). Patient-clinician interactions and compliance. In R. B. Haynes, D. W. Taylor, & D. L. Sackett (Eds.), *Compliance in health care* (pp. 63–77). Baltimore: Johns Hopkins University Press.

Kasch, C. R., & Knutson, K. (1987). A descriptive analysis of caregivers' compliance gaining strategies, parts I and II. *Dialysis and Transplantation, 16,* 89–91, 129–131.

Kerr, J. A. (1985). Adherence and self-care. *Heart & Lung, 14,* 24–30.

Kontz, M. (1984). *A proposed model for assessing compliance within the unitary man/human framework based on an analysis of the concept of compliance.* Unpublished master's thesis. University of Miami, FL.

Kontz, M. (1989). Compliance redefined and implications for home care. *Holistic Nursing Practice, 3*(2), 54–64.

Kosnar, A., (1987). Contracting for care. *AAOHN Journal, 35,* 493–495.

Kritek, P. B. (1984). Report of group work on taxonomies. In M. J. Kim, G. K. McFarland, & A. M. McLane (Eds.), *Classification of nursing diagnoses: Proceedings of the fifth national conference* (pp. 46–58). St. Louis, MO: Mosby.

Lowery, B. J., & Ducette, J. P. (1976). Disease-related learning and disease control in diabetics as a function of locus of control. *Nursing Research, 25,* 358–362.

Lum, J. L., Chase, M., Cole, S. M., Johnson, A., Johnson, J.A., & Link, M. R. (1978). Nursing care on oncology patients receiving chemotherapy. *Nursing Research, 27,* 340–345.

Marshall, J., Penckofer, S., & Llewellyn, J. (1986). Structured postoperative teaching and knowledge and compliance of patients who had coronary artery bypass surgery. *Heart & Lung, 15,* 76–82.

Marston, M.-V. (1970). Compliance with medical regimens: A review of the literature. *Nursing Research, 19,* 312–323.

McCord, M. A. (1986). Compliance: Self care or compromise? *Topics in Clinical Nursing, 7*(4), 1–8.

McKenny, J. M., Slinig, J. M., Henderson, H. R., Devins, D., & Barr, M. (1973). The effect of clinical pharmacy services on patients with essential hypertension. *Circulation, 48,* 1104–1111.

McMahon, M., Miller, P., Wikoff, R., Garrett, M. J., & Ringel, K. (1986). Life situations, health beliefs, and medical regimen adherence of patients with myocardial infarction. *Heart & Lung, 15,* 82–86.

Mikhail, B. (1981). The health belief model: A review and critical evaluation of the model, research, and practice. *Advances in Nursing Science, 4*(1), 65–82.

Miller, P., Wikoff, R., McMahon, M., Garrett, M. J., &

Ringel, K. (1988). Influence of a nursing intervention on regimen adherence and societal adjustments postmyocardial infarction. *Nursing Research, 37,* 297–302.

Mills, G., Barnes, R., Rodell, D., & Terry, L. (1985). An evaluation of an inpatient cardiac patient/family education program. *Heart & Lung, 14,* 400–406.

Morris, L. A., & Halperin, J. (1979). Effects of written drug information on patient knowledge and compliance: A literature review. *American Journal of Public Health, 69,* 47–52.

Neisser, U. (1978). Perceiving, anticipating, imagining. In C. W. Savage (Ed.), *Perception and cognition: Issues in the foundations of psychology, Minnesota studies in the philosophy of science* (vol. 9). Minneapolis: University of Minnesota Press.

Norbeck, J. S. (1981). Social support: A model for clinical research and application. *Advances in Nursing Science, 3*(4), 43–58.

Norbeck, J. S. (1982). The use of social support in clinical practice. *Journal of Psychiatric Nursing and Mental Health Services, 20*(12), 22–28.

O'Brien, M. E. (1980). Hemodialysis regimen compliance and social environment: A panel analysis. *Nursing Research, 29,* 250–255.

O'Brien, M. E. (1982). Pragmatic survivalism: Behavior patterns affecting low-level wellness among minority group members. *Advances in Nursing Science, 4*(3), 13–26.

Random House Dictionary of the English Language (2nd ed.). (1987). New York: Random House.

Redeker, N. S. (1988). Health beliefs and adherence in chronic illness. *Image: Journal of Nursing Scholarship, 20*(1), 31–35.

Rockhart, J. F., & Hofmann, P. B. (1969). Physician and patient behavior under different scheduling systems in a hospital outpatient department. *Medical Care, 7,* 463–470.

Rosenstock, I. M. (1974). Historical origins of the health belief model. In M. H. Becker (Ed.), *The health belief model and personal health behavior.* Thorofare, NJ: Charles B. Slack.

Roy, C. (1982a). Theoretical framework for classification of nursing diagnosis. In M. J. Kim & D. A. Moritz (Eds.), *Classification of nursing diagnoses: Proceedings of the third and fourth national conferences* (pp. 215–220). New York: McGraw-Hill.

Roy, C. (1982b). Historical perspective of the theoretical framework for the classification of nursing diagnosis. In D. A. Moritz (Ed.), *Classification of nursing diagnoses: Proceedings of the third and fourth national conferences* (pp. 235–245). New York: McGraw-Hill.

Roy, C. (1984). Framework for classification systems development: Progress and Issues. In M. J. Kim, G. K. McFarland, & A. M. McLane (Eds.), *Classification of nursing diagnoses: Proceedings of the fifth national conference* (pp. 26–40). St. Louis, MO: Mosby.

Rutledge, D. N. (1987). Factors related to women's practice of breast self-examination. *Nursing Research, 36,* 117–121.

Sackett, D. L., Haynes, R. B., Gibson, E. S., et al. (1975). Randomized clinical trial of strategies for improving compliance in primary hypertension. *Lancet, 1,* 1205–1207.

Schroeder, P., & Miller, J. F. (1983). Qualitative study of locus of control in patients with peripheral vascular disease. In J. F. Miller (Ed.), *Coping with chronic illness: Overcoming powerlessness* (pp. 149–162). Philadelphia: F. A. Davis.

Simon, H. A. (1976). *Administrative behavior* (3rd ed.). New York: Free Press.

Spelman, M. R. (1984). Back pain: How health education affects patient compliance with treatment. *Occupational Health Nursing,* 649–651.

Steckel, S. B. (1974). The use of positive reinforcement in order to increase patient compliance. *Journal of American Association of Nephrology Nurses and Technicians, 1,* 39–41.

Steckel, S. B. (1976). *Influences of knowledge and of contingency contracting on adherence to hypertensive treatment regimens.* Doctoral dissertation, University Microfilms, University of Michigan.

Steckel, S. B., & Swain, M. A. (1977). Contracting with patients to improve compliance. *Hospitals, 51,* 51–54.

Stickney, S. K., Hall, R. C., & Gardner, E. R. (1980). The effect of referral procedures on aftercare compliance. *Hospitals and Community Psychiatry, 31,* 567–569.

Tirrell, B. E., & Hart, L. K. (1980). The relationship of health beliefs and knowledge to exercise compliance in patients after coronary bypass. *Heart & Lung, 9,* 487–493.

Villeneuve, M. E. (1982). The patient compliance puzzle. *Nursing Management, 13,* 54–56.

Wallston, B., & Wallston, K. (1978). Locus of control and health: A review of the literature. *Health Education Monographs, 6,* 107.

Wallston, B. S., & Wallston, K. A. (1984). Social psychological models of health behavior: An examination and integration. In A. Baum, S. Taylor, & J. E. Singer (Eds.), *Handbook of psychology and health, vol. IV: Social psychological aspects of psychology.* Hillsdale, NJ: Erlbaum.

Watts, R. J. (1982). Sexual functioning, health beliefs, and compliance with high blood pressure medications. *Nursing Research, 31,* 278–282.

Wilson, J. (1963). *Thinking with concepts.* London: Cambridge University Press.

Wyka, C. A., Levesque, P. G., Ryan, S. L., & Mattea, E. G. (1980). Group education for the hypertensive. *Cardiovascular Nursing, 16*(1), 1–5.

Utility of the Nursing Minimum Data Set in Validation of Computerized Nursing Diagnoses

Connie W. Delaney, PhD, RN
Peg Mehmert, MSN, RN, C

The quality of nursing practice depends on the ability of professional nurses to diagnose a client's actual and potential health deficits, establish effective and efficient nursing interventions, and continuously reassess movement toward optimal health. The diagnostic process rests on the validity of the diagnostic labels. Models of validation of nursing diagnoses depend on access to comparable nursing data at local, regional, national, and international levels. McCloskey (1988) and others have repeatedly emphasized the use of information technology and clinical databases to support validation studies. Through enhanced taxonomy development, nursing information systems will augment the efficiency and effectiveness of technology to serve nursing practice.

The Nursing Minimum Data Set (NMDS) work of Devine and Werley (1988), Werley and Lang (1988), Werley and Zorn (1988), and others has focused attention on identifying the minimum set of data items necessary to meet information demands of such a nursing practice. These efforts are responsive to the recommendations of the Secretary's Commission on Nursing (1988) to enhance efficient and effective use of nursing resources through the use of computerized systems, as well as the National Center for Nursing Research's research agenda emphasizing refinement of nursing information systems. It has been proposed that coupling the use of the NMDS with computerized information systems may offer the most efficient, cost-effective approach for meeting the access and comparability needs essential for validating diagnostic labels.

Purpose

This research was initiated to ascertain the utility of the NMDS in addressing numerous clinical practice questions. Phase 1 of this work is reported here. The purpose of Phase 1 was to assess the utility of the NMDS for validating the defining characteristics of the nursing diagnostic labels associated with *alterations in fluid balance*. Specific questions were

1. Is there a significant relationship between each diagnostic label and demographic characteristics of age, sex, race, length of stay, and place of discharge?
2. What are the major and minor defining characteristics of each of the diagnoses associated with *alterations in fluid balance*?
3. What is the documented incidence of risk factors associated with the label *potential fluid volume deficit*?

Methods

This descriptive pilot study was conducted in a 265-bed midwestern community hospital. The site was selected based on its long-term use of the NANDA taxonomy, having a computerized nursing information system in place since 1984, and commitment to ongoing quality assurance and staff development activities demonstrating effective use of nursing diagnosis and computers. The computerized care planning system is available for use on a Spectra 2000 Medical Information System. The pathway contains the NANDA-approved diagnostic labels, definitions, defining characteristics, and related factors. In addition, expected outcomes and nursing order sets explicit for each label have been developed and are continually updated.

The NMDS instrument (version for inpatient acute care) as described in *Nursing Minimum Data Set: Data Collection Manual* (Werley, Devine, & Zorn, 1988) was used to guide data collection. Negotiations were begun to establish an electronic transfer of the NMDS elements. In the meantime, a systematic random sample (n = 191) was selected from the 400 computerized patient discharge care plan summaries for the previous calendar year from patients diagnosed as having one or more of the nursing diagnoses related to *alterations in fluid balance*. Extraction of the NMDS elements, defining characteristics, and related factors was completed.

These data elements were stored in a research relational database. Interrater reliability was established. A report generator, *R & R Relational Report Writer*, was used to extract data subsets for analysis. Subsets were uploaded to an IBM mainframe system where Statistical Analysis System was used for data analysis.

Sensitivity measures were the statistical method selected to determine validation of the defining characteristics. Sensitivity was defined as the proportion of subjects that exhibit certain defining characteristics of a given diagnosis to the total number of subjects with the respective diagnoses. In addition, because the interest was in identifying the *minimum* data set, focus was also placed on identifying the defining characteristics with very low or no sensitivity. Sensitivity levels of individual characteristics were evaluated consistent with the definition of major and minor characteristics according to NANDA guidelines. The sensitivity of combinations of groups of characteristics was also determined. Attention was focused on identifying those groups of characteristics having zero sensitivity. To summarize, the sensitivity of individual defining characteristics and groups of characteristics determined validation.

Results

The sample consisted of 191 subjects (see Table 1). Ages ranged from newborn to 94 years, with a mean age of 45.4 years. Approximately 50% of the subjects were female, and 95% were white. The average length of hospital stay was 8.3 days with more than one half having stays of 5 days or less. Ninety-two percent of the subjects were discharged to their homes. The distribution of diagnostic labels was *fluid volume deficit related to active loss*, 41.1% (n = 78); *fluid volume deficit related to failure of regulatory mechanisms*, 14.6% (n = 28); *fluid volume excess*, 14.6%

Table 1: Demographic Factors by Nursing Diagnosis

	Fluid Volume Deficit Related to Regulatory Mechanism	Fluid Volume Deficit Related to Active Loss	Fluid Volume Excess	Potential Fluid Volume Deficit	Total
N	28	78	28	57	191
Sex M	12 (44%)	39 (52%)	10 (37%)	19 (36%)	80 (44%)
F	15 (56%)	36 (48%)	17 (63%)	34 (63%)	102 (56%)
Age in years ($\bar{X}$)	54.7	40.7	68.3	35.4	45.2
Race White	25 (89%)	73 (97%)	28 (100%)	53 (91%)	178 (95%)
Non-White	3 (11%)	2 (3%)	0	5 (9%)	10 (5%)
Place discharged to					
Home	25 (89%)	73 (94%)	23 (82%)	54 (95%)	175 (92%)
Other	3 (11%)	5 (6%)	5 (18%)	3 (5%)	16 (8%)
Length of stay in days ($\bar{X}$)	6.2	6.5	16.3	7.7	8.3

($n = 28$); *potential fluid volume deficit,* 29.7% ($n = 57$). No significant differences were noted between the diagnostic categories and sex, race, and discharge deposition. However, those who exhibited *fluid volume excess* were significantly older and had longer lengths of hospital stay ($p < 0.05$). Subjects from newborn to 14 years of age had more *fluid volume deficit related to active loss* than other fluid volume diagnoses. *Fluid volume deficit related to active loss* was most prevalent for subjects aged between 15 and 65 years; in this age group *fluid volume excess* was least prevalent.

Validation of the defining characteristics of *fluid volume deficit related to failure of regulatory mechanisms* demonstrated that no characteristics qualified as major; only two characteristics met the criterion for a minor characteristic. Based on sensitivity of individual and group characteristics, the defining characteristics for this label could be reduced from 14 to 6 specific characteristics (see Table 2).

Validation of the defining characteristics of *fluid volume deficit related to active loss* revealed that no characteristics met criteria for major or minor characteristics. The 25 defining characteristics of the label could be re-

duced to 10 or less according to individual and group sensitivity (see Table 2).

Validation of the characteristics of *fluid volume excess* concluded that no items qualified as major; two characteristics met criteria for a minor characteristic. Individual

Table 2: Sensitivity of Five Highest Ratings of Individual Defining Characteristics for Each Diagnosis

Fluid volume deficit related to failure of regulatory mechanisms ($n = 28$)
• Dry skin, mucous membranes	57%
• Weakness	57%
• Increased skin turgor	39%
• Increased body temperatures	32%
• Thirst	21%

Fluid volume deficit related to active loss ($n = 78$)
• Decreased skin turgor	42%
• Decreased urine output	39%
• Concentrated urine	23%
• Altered body temperature	22%
• Output greater than intake	10%

Fluid volume excess ($n = 28$)
• Dependent edema	68%
• Dyspnea	61%
• Fatigue	36%
• Rales	21%
• Change in mental status	18%

and group sensitivity revealed that the list of 25 characteristics could be substantially reduced.

Sensitivity of the risk factors of *potential fluid volume deficit* could be reduced from four to three items.

Conclusions

Validation of the nursing diagnoses related to *alterations in fluid balance* was accomplished using the computerized NMDS with a modified definition of the nursing diagnosis component and the use of the NMDS-enhanced comparison of patient demographics within and among diagnostic categories. The use of sensitivity in conjunction with NANDA guidelines was effective in isolating numerous redundant, nondifferentiating defining characteristics for each diagnostic label for this sample. Several issues, however, emerged related to NMDS definition, system design, data retrieval, and data storage and processing.

The definition of the nursing diagnosis element of the NMDS should be expanded to include defining characteristics. In addition, adding etiologies as well as dates of diagnosis resolution will facilitate the use of the NMDS for addressing numerous other practice questions, including cost analysis.

Design of the nursing information system impacts the type of analysis possible. For example, when defining characteristics are linked to a specific diagnosis, frequency measures and sensitivity estimates can be determined. On the other hand, specificity, in the strict statistical sense, is not possible. That is, determining the ratio of the number of subjects with a specific diagnosis among those with a specific defining characteristic to the total number of subjects with the respective defining characteristic is restricted. System design that incorporates free text entry may minimize this concern. However, staff nurses' use of this option may be negligible in the reality of nursing practice.

Data retrieval technique is crucial. Sampling by nursing diagnosis again precluded the determination of specificity measures. Random sampling, however, if completed in a system without linkage of defining characteristics to specific diagnosis, will allow both sensitivity and specificity analysis. The efficiency of such a system, however, would possibly be compromised in actual practice. Manual retrieval of the NMDS from computer output is time consuming. Electronic retrieval is essential for efficient data collection. To date, electronic retrieval of subsequent data sets has been accomplished in this project. Three downloads of the NMDS including additional nursing diagnoses have effectively occurred. Data analysis is currently underway.

This study has demonstrated the effectiveness and efficiency of establishing a research database from a computerized clinical information system. A database separate from the hospital information system improves efficiency of statistical analysis and optimal use of resources in both the practice and academic settings.

Continued collaboration between practice and academia and the use of this methodology can facilitate the development of an increasingly efficient clinical system. This has the potential for a significant impact on the quality of the delivery of nursing care.

Recommendations

Recommendations include replication of the study to a larger and geographically more diverse sample. In addition, the next phase of this study involves validating all defining characteristics of all NANDA-approved diagnoses using this system. Moreover, analysis of this pilot study data continues by addressing research questions associated with related factors, relationship of diagnoses to diagnosis related group (DRG) category, nursing order sets, hours of care and associated nursing care costs, and outcomes actualized.

References

Devine, E., & Werley, H. (1988). Test of the nursing minimum data set: Availability of data and reliability. *Nursing Research, 11,* 97–104.

McCloskey, J. (1988). The nursing minimum data set: Benefits and implications for nurse educators. *Perspectives on Nursing 1987–89* (pub. no. 41-2199). New York: National League for Nursing.

Secretary's Commission on Nursing (vols. 1 & II). (1988). Washington, DC: Department of Health and Human Services.

Werley, H., Devine, E., & Zorn, C. (1988). *Nursing minimum data set: Data collection manual.* Milwaukee, WI: University of Wisconsin–Milwaukee.

Werley, H., & Lang, H. (Eds.). (1988). *Identification of the nursing minimum data set.* New York: Springer.

Werley, H., & Zorn, C. (1988). Integrating the nursing minimum data set with computerization of nursing and health care information systems. In N. Daly & K. Hannah (Eds.), *Proceedings of the third international symposium on nursing use of computers and information systems science* (pp. 378–386). St. Louis, MO: Mosby.

Validation of *Hopelessness:* Perceptions of the Critically Ill (Author's Abstract)

Anne LeGresley, MS, RN

A person who has been burned suffers one of the most severe traumas that human beings can survive. The injury itself is frightening and during the prolonged hospitalization the victim must face pain, helplessness, hopelessness, dependency, and the possibilities of disfigurement, deformity, and death. It is truly remarkable that under the most difficult circumstances, notwithstanding almost overwhelming evidence to the contrary, most people can maintain (if only covertly) the spark of hope that somehow, someday the situation will take a turn for the better. Without hope, humans lose the capacity to achieve, grow, and develop. The only wish of the hopeless person is to give up.

The purpose of this study was to describe the nature of the phenomena of hopelessness and hope from the perspective of individuals and family members who had experienced a critical burn injury. The study sought to answer the question: What are the constituents of the lived experiences of hope and hopelessness? A qualitative research method was employed, with emphasis on the phenomenologic approach. The sample consisted of nine individuals who had sustained major burn injuries and their significant others. Data were gathered through the use of an open-ended, semistructured interview. Three major themes emerged from the data: hope, hopelessness, and the distinct phase of physical and psychologic recovery. The data supported the assumption that hope and hopelessness are not mutually exclusive, and that hope is not the complete absence of hopelessness.

Based on the findings of the study, the diagnosis of hopelessness will be reviewed. The definition, defining characteristics, and etiologic factors will be examined and implications for nursing practice, education, and research will be discussed. It is the author's premise that qualitative research is critical to provide validation for many of the nursing diagnoses currently accepted by NANDA. It is only through rigorous examination of complex phenomena, such as hopelessness, that we will come to understand and articulate the multifaceted nature of the art and science of nursing.

IV

Panel Presentations

Methodologies for
Nursing Diagnosis Research

Qualitative Methods for Nursing Diagnosis Research

Elizabeth A. McFarlane, DNSc, RN

Over the past decade there has been an explosion of interest in qualitative methods. While the utility of qualitative methods had been acknowledged during the 60s and 70s, their use as an accepted method of scientific inquiry was continually debated. Sociologists, psychologists, anthropologists, and nurse scientists fertilized the research fields of their disciplines in the 60s with their qualitative studies. Yet the issues of empiric- versus theory-based research and deductive versus inductive approaches continued to be raised.

While the debate related to research methods will continue, its focus for nurse scientists has changed from one of whether qualitative methods are appropriate to one of determining when to use qualitative methods. Moccia (1988) addresses the issue of when to use qualitative or quantitative methods or a combination of both by determining whether the aims of the nurse scientist are directed toward the control of human phenomena or the explanation and understanding of human phenomena.

The focus of the "new" debate on research methods has implications for nursing diagnosis research. The need to identify and validate nursing diagnoses has been a priority for nurses supporting the development of a taxonomy since the meeting of the First National Conference on the Classification of Nursing Diagnoses in 1973 (Gebbie & Lavin, 1975). Although almost two decades have elapsed, research supporting the development and refinement of nursing diagnoses has been limited. Kim (1989), in her review of nursing diagnosis research, noted an increase in research published in referred journals, but pointed out that the majority of nursing diagnosis research continues to be presented at the biennial national conferences on classification of nursing diagnoses and is published in the conferences' proceedings. While some qualitative, quantitative, and integrated methods have been used for the development and validation of nursing diagnoses, the need to analyze the application of these methods and to generate new approaches has been evident. In response to this need, the idea of an invitational conference on research methods for validating diagnoses was conceived. The idea became a reality in April 1989.

This paper will summarize the three papers presented at the conference that addressed specific qualitative methods (Dreher, 1990; Knafl, 1990; Strauss & Corbin, 1990), the responses that presented ways in which a specific method could be applied to nursing diagnosis research (Gordon, 1990; Miller, 1990; Thomas, 1990), and a synthesis of the conference's qualitative session (Kerr & Fitzpatrick, 1990). The qualitative methods addressed at this session of the conference included grounded theory, concept development, ethnography, and phenomenology.

Grounded Theory

Anselm Strauss's (1990) stimulating paper on "Grounded Theory's Applicability to Nursing Diagnosis Research" addressed general and specific features of grounded theory and presented it as an appropriate and useful method for nursing diagnosis research. The inductive nature of grounded theory, as well as the nature of the data collection (through interview, observation, analysis of documents), provide a means to explore and generate descriptive data. The exploratory approach in grounded theory has a specific purpose: the generation and development of theories. Data collection and analysis are interrelated, and concepts and hypotheses come from the data and are continually "worked" in relation to the data being collected. Concepts and hypotheses must be considered provisional and must earn their way into the evolving theory. "This grounding in the data is what gives grounded theory its theory-observation congruence" (p. 8).

Strauss specified nine features that should be present in studies being done in the grounded theory tradition:

1. **Concepts are the basic unit of analysis.** The researcher works with conceptualizations of data rather than with the actual data.
2. **Categories must be developed and related.** Certain concepts become categories, i.e., higher level, more abstract, and more thoroughly developed concepts.
3. **Sampling proceeds on theoretical grounds.** Sampling is done in terms of concepts and their dimensions after preliminary selective sampling and analysis of the first data.
4. **Analysis makes use of constant comparisons.** An incident is noted and compared against other incidents, resulting concepts are labeled and, in time, compared and grouped.
5. **Patterns and variations must be accounted for.** Data are examined for regularity; patterns and variations in a particular phenomenon are identified.
6. **Basic underlying processes must be identified.** Process(es) can signify a phenomenon that can be described in phases or steps or a purposeful action that does not necessarily have a linear progression.
7. **Writing theoretical memos is an integral part of doing grounded theory.** Theoretical memos provide a system for tracking categories, properties, conceptual relationships, and hypotheses evolving from the analytical process.
8. **Hypotheses about relationships among categories are developed and verified as much as possible through the research process.** The hypotheses, once formulated, are taken back to the field and "tested"; constant revision occurs until the hypotheses hold true for the phenomena under study. While grounding theory in data requires an inductive approach, the verification process requires the researcher to engage in deduction.
9. **Broader structural conditions must be brought into the analysis, however microscopically focused it is.** The analysis must be expanded beyond conditions seeming to have an immediate bearing on the phenomenon to include conditions that could have an indirect impact on the phenomenon.

The procedures used in a grounded theory approach require that action be studied as it takes place within contexts. Upon review of the nursing diagnosis literature, Strauss found the diagnostic concepts to be too abstract, too simple, and likely to ignore or underplay context. He recommends grounded theory be used to assist in specifying relevant contexts and, more specifically, to identify contextual patterns that hinder or support effective diagnosing. Contextual influences that impact on the identification and interpretation of defining characteristics and risk factors also must be recognized if diagnoses are to be made with any certainty.

Mary Durand Thomas's (1990) response to Strauss's paper reviewed four nursing studies not focusing on diagnosis but using grounded theory. Examination of the studies revealed two characteristics—process and context—that could have an impact on nursing diagnosis studies. Diagnosis research must focus on process rather than a particular response at a specific time in order to develop a frame of reference for seemingly diverse responses occurring over time. The consideration of context will have an impact on process in that different conditions or structure can alter or expand the process.

Two operations within grounded theory methodology were identified by Thomas as being useful in differentiating closely related diagnoses or in identifying more specific diagnoses from a diagnostic category. The use of *constant comparisons* implies that indicators of a concept (nursing diagnosis) are compared for similarities and differences in meaning, resulting in a "sharpening" of the concept. *Dimensionalizing* involves making distinctions, resulting in dimensions and subdimensions as products.

The attention given to process and context provides a more holistic approach in assessing a patient, making a nursing diagnosis, and determining the focus for nursing intervention. Use of certain grounded theory procedures, such as constant comparisons and dimensionalizing, allows for more individualized and specific diagnosing.

Concept Development

Acknowledging the need for refinement of existing diagnostic concepts, Knafl (1990) explored the applicability of qualitative research strategies to such efforts. Specifically, she addressed the intersection of concept analysis and qualitative research in terms of a hybrid approach to concept development as described by Schwartz-Barcott and Kim (1986) and as adapted to Knafl's research on family management styles.

Discussion of the nature of concept analysis provided a foundation for the paper and incorporated a comparison of proposed approaches to concept analysis. Analytic purposes, the focus and extent of the literature review, and the place of case development were found to vary among the approaches. Knafl advises that "given the availability of alternate approaches and the differences among the approaches, it is important to match one's overriding purpose with that of the approach to concept analysis" (p. 42).

Examination of the nature of qualitative research results in the identification of commonalities and differences among specific methods. Common themes included viewing inquiry as an interactive process between the researcher and participants, immersing self in the everyday life of the study setting, and valuing perspectives of participants. Differences were related to the aim, focus of the research question, conceptual framework, sampling techniques, data collection and analysis activities, and final product. As in choosing an approach to concept analysis, Knafl recommends that selection of a specific qualitative method should be based on "fitting one's research question and purpose to the strengths and intent of the approach" (p. 45).

Schwartz-Barcott and Kim's (1986) hybrid model of concept development is described by Knafl as promising and as one that offers a framework for combining concept analysis and qualitative research. The model interfaces theoretical analysis with empirical observation, and consists of three sequential phases: theoretical, fieldwork, and final analytical. As an example in using the hybrid model for concept development, Knafl presented an informative overview of her efforts to develop the concept of family management style. Her work supports her supposition that once concepts (nursing diagnoses) are named and validated, they must be nurtured and refined. A hybrid model for concept development can be useful in elaborating existing diagnostic concepts and contributing to the development of the classification for nursing diagnoses.

In her response, Gordon (1990) supported Knafl's assertion that concepts/nursing diagnoses must be nurtured and refined if they are to be meaningful. Application of a hybrid model for the purpose of refinement and validation of diagnostic category components was supported by Gordon. Using this qualitative approach, four outcomes should be sought: (1) a useful level of generality of diagnostic concepts, (2) distinctiveness of diagnostic concepts, (3) validity or clinical representativeness of diagnostic concepts, and (4) concept–concept relations.

Gordon provided relevant examples that emphasized the need to pursue achievement of the four identified outcomes. She pointed out that some nursing diagnoses are actually taxonomic categories and, therefore, too inclusive to be useful in determining interventions. Validation of the sets of empirical referents/defining characteristics of diagnostic concepts is also needed in order to assure accurate description of one concept as opposed to another. Diagnostic concepts often lack clarity and must therefore be explored in terms of (1) naming a concept (Is the name representative of the concept?) and (2) determining the validity of subjective cues for a particular concept (Are certain feelings and perceptions identified by patients?). And finally, in the interest of taxonomic develop-

ment, relationships must be specified among diagnostic concepts in terms of inclusivity and developmental and causal relationships.

Ethnographic Methods as Diffentiated from Phenomenology

Melanie Dreher (1990) approached the task of differentiating ethnographic and phenomenologic methods by first exploring unsettled issues surrounding the concept of nursing diagnosis—issues that could be addressed through qualitative methods. Distinguishing medical and nursing diagnoses was identified as the first issue. Dreher described the concepts of disease and illness as being used to distinguish most medical and nursing diagnoses—medical diagnoses being described as focusing on disease as defined within the parameters of scientific medicine, while nursing diagnoses tend to focus on responses to illness as experienced and defined by the patient and family. Using this means of comparison, the common ground is *sickness*—"sickness interpreted by medicine and sickness interpreted by nursing" (p. 8).

A second issue relates to nursing's progress in generating a classification system for diagnostic concepts. To that end, nurses must continue to search for patterns and regularities in health and illness behavior. According to Dreher, "whether nursing grows to maturity as a science will depend upon the progress it makes in describing and classifying human behavior in health and illness" (p. 81).

The limited nature of the definition of nursing diagnosis, that is, its focus being more on what the nurse can do than on what the patient is experiencing, was presented as a third issue. Due to contextual variations, the patient conditions that are amenable to nursing interventions are simply an artifact of place and time.

To address these issues, Dreher proposed

that nursing research take at least two directions: (1) "continue to observe, classify, and label patterns of behavior surrounding health and illness" (p. 84) and (2) "focus on nursing technology—specifically, a description of what nurses do and on the nature of the nurse-patient relationship in clinical decision making" (p. 85). To achieve these ends research methods must support the comprehensive and holistic nature of practice and embrace the total human experience. Ethnography and phenomenology are inductive methods that can be employed as one attempt to understand the meaning of human behavior.

These two methods share similarities, although derived from different philosophic perspectives and serving different purposes. Both methods are interested in the actor's or informant's perspective, which enlightens the investigator; both approach human behavior without preconceived expectations, variables, or categories; and both are based upon the assumption of holism.

Differences and merits of each approach were noted by Dreher in considering application to nursing diagnosis research. Phenomenology attempts to take into account the meaning that events have for the actors. Sickness, health, and caregiving would be explored from the perspective of the informant who could be a patient or a nurse, and the context in which events occur would be relevant only from this perspective.

In contrast, ethnography moves beyond informants' perceptions of experiences, and attempts to understand phenomena from the actor's perspective while describing and explaining deviations in actual behavior. In relation to context, observed patterns of behavior are explained through lengthy, continuous firsthand involvement of the investigator in the setting. Of the two strategies for conceptualization used in ethnographic description, the "emic" approach (derived from the term phonemic) is more closely related to phenomenology, using in-depth interviewing as a primary data-gathering technique. The "etic" approach (derived from the term phonetics) is based on intense, direct observations of behavior as opposed to in-depth interviewing. Dreher emphasized that "reliance on one approach to the exclusion of the other would not do justice to the complexities of human behavior and most ethnographers embrace both emic and etic strategies in their attempt to describe and explain behavior" (p. 91).

Dreher supported ethnography as providing opportunities to develop a more comprehensive database and consequently a more comprehensive understanding of behavior in contextual terms. Judith Fitzgerald Miller (1990), in her response to Dreher's paper, described the utility of both phenomonologic and ethnographic research methods and stressed their value in identifying diagnostic concepts and indicators and in validating diagnoses. The flexible, open-ended research technique used in phenomenology and the immersion of the researcher through the participative-observer techniques employed in ethnography offer separate yet supporting approaches. Miller's distinction of the conceptual origins and purposes of the two approaches offers guidance in determining the approach most suitable for achieving the specific aims of research to be done.

Miller noted that the opportunities to engage in qualitative research are available in everyday clinical practice. She suggested that master's prepared practitioners should incorporate qualitative approaches in the gathering of data in their routine practices. Ongoing documentation of the nature of patient experiences and "unique interpretations" of experiences and resulting nursing diagnoses and indicators would provide rich data. The ethnographic and phenomenologic methods "focus increased attention on collecting data and validation with persons experiencing the diagnosis and/or content analysis of patient records" (p. 109).

Synthesis of the Qualitative Session

Mary Kerr provided a concise yet comprehensive synthesis of the wealth of information provided by the presenters and respondents participating in the qualitative session of the invitational conference (Kerr & Fitzpatrick, 1990). Kerr stressed that findings generated from qualitative research provide "the ground work for the identification of further research questions" (p. 114) leading to the further development of nursing knowledge.

The qualitative approaches to nursing research support nursing's holistic perspective of the person. In choosing a specific qualitative approach, the nurse researcher must expand considerations beyond the holistic perspective and examine a considered approach in terms of its underlying philosophy, its aims or purposes, and suitability of data collection and analysis techniques. These must be considered in relation to the proposed research's purpose and the question to be answered.

Kerr and Fitzpatrick (1990) identified four domains in which qualitative methods can be used to enhance the knowledge of nursing: clinical judgment, contextual issues, clinical application, and philosophic inquiry. Related to clinical judgment, factors influencing nurses' abilities to make a diagnosis can be identified. Contextual issues, specifically the influence of context on nursing diagnosis, can be thoroughly examined through use of a qualitative research approach. The ease with which qualitative methods can be applied in clinical settings makes them useful in research seeking to identify new diagnoses and to clarify existing diagnoses. Qualitative methods can be particularly helpful in addressing the issue of the level of abstraction of current and future diagnosis. Philosophic critiques of nursing knowledge, past and present, can assist in examining the assumptions and methods of the discipline of nursing as well as the evolution of context. Qualitative methods can provide the vehicle for such examination, which will, in turn, enhance the generation of future knowledge.

Summary

The papers presented at the conference on qualitative methods expanded the possibilities of generating new diagnoses, validating current diagnoses, and developing a diagnostic classification scheme. To make the possibilities become realities, a variety of research methods must be applied to the research problems identified by nurses. Use of qualitative approaches in the examination of these problems will assist in describing diagnostic processes and identifying diagnostic concepts in terms of process. The context and structure impacting on the "diagnostic experience," whether from the "perspective" of the diagnostician or the person being diagnosed, would also be explored. Ultimately, understanding of diagnostic concepts would be expanded and diagnosis labels, definitions, indicators, and classification would be refined and further developed.

References

Dreher, M. (1990). Ethnographic methods as differentiated from phenomenology. In *Monograph of the invitational conference on research methods for validating nursing diagnoses* (pp. 78–97). St. Louis, MO: North America Nursing Diagnosis Association.

Gebbie, K. M., & Lavin, M. A. (1975). (Eds.). *Classification of nursing diagnoses: Proceedings of the first national conference*. St. Louis, MO: Mosby.

Gordon, M. (1990). Concept development: Reaction paper. In *Monograph of the invitational conference on research methods for validating nursing diagnoses* (pp. 64–77). St. Louis, MO: North American Nursing Diagnosis Association.

Kerr, M. E., & Fitzpatrick, J. J. (1990). Qualitative research methodologies: Synthesis and recommendations. In *Monograph of the invitational conference on research methods for validating nursing diagnoses* (pp. 114–120). St. Louis, MO: North American Nursing Diagnosis Association.

Kim, M. J. (1989). Nursing diagnosis. In J. J. Fitzpatrick, R. L. Taunton, & J. Q. Benoliel (Eds.), *Annual review of nursing research* (Vol. 7). New York: Springer.

Knafl, K. A. (1990). Concept development. In *Monograph of the invitational conference on research methods for validating nursing diagnoses* (pp. 37–63). St. Louis, MO: North American Nursing Diagnosis Association.

Miller, J. F. (1990). Differentiating phenomenologic and ethnographic research approaches: Reaction paper. In *Monograph of the invitational conference on research methods for validating nursing diagnoses* (pp. 98–113). St. Louis, MO: North American Nursing Diagnosis Association.

Moccia, P. (1988) A critique of compromise: Beyond the methods debate. *Advances in Nursing Science 10* (4), 1–9.

Schwartz-Barcott, D., & Kim, H. (1986). A hybrid model for concept development. In P. Chinn (Ed.), *Nursing research methodology: Issues and implementation.* Rockville, MD: Aspen.

Strauss, A., & Corbin, J. M. (1990). Grounded theory's applicability to nursing diagnostic research. In *Monograph of the invitational conference on research methods for validating nursing diagnoses* (pp. 4–24). St. Louis, MO: North American Nursing Diagnosis Association.

Thomas, M. D. (1990). Grounded theory and nursing diagnosis: Reaction paper. In *Monograph of the invitational conference on research methods for validating nursing diagnoses* (pp. 25–36). St. Louis, MO: North American Nursing Diagnosis Association.

Quantitative Methods for Nursing Diagnosis Research

Mary Ann Schroeder, PhD, RN

This paper presents a synthesis of quantitative methods presented at the Conference on Research Methods for Validating Nursing Diagnoses, held in Palm Springs, California in April 1989. Major topics addressed reliability and validity issues related to nursing diagnoses, the potential for the use of epidemiologic research designs to validate nursing diagnoses, and the need for more sophisticated statistics for validation research.

The complexity and scope of research endeavors required for further validation of nursing diagnoses and consequential nursing interventions to achieve desired patient outcomes are significant. The intent of this paper is not to overwhelm, but to challenge readers to create a vision of the great potential of these methods when applied to the validation of nursing diagnoses.

Nursing is at an exciting stage of development in terms of the possibilities and potential for the use of quantitative methods for the clinical validation of nursing diagnoses. The descriptive and correlational methods used to date have provided the foundation for NANDA Taxonomy I as well as an awareness of problems inherent in these methods. This information can also be used to raise our consciousness of the potential use of the more sophisticated multivariate quantitative methods for validating nursing diagnoses by more accurately representing the complexity of the phenomenon under investigation.

In essence this paper will (1) describe and assess the adequacy of appropriate quantitative methods used for the clinical validation of nursing diagnoses, (2) address the issues associated with the use of quantitative methods for nursing diagnosis research, and (3) identify directions for future research. Before beginning, however, it is necessary to state that the use of quantitative research methods is appropriate only after qualitative methods have adequately identified and described defining characteristics associated with a nursing diagnosis, and that these characteristics have then been used to develop a clinical definition for a specific nursing diagnosis. Nursing should not support the quantitative-versus-qualitative argument but use both qualitative and quantitative methods, as the research question warrants, to validate nursing diagnoses more adequately.

Quantitative methods appropriate for nursing diagnosis research can be described as a trajectory of quantitative methods that can be used for the clinical validation of nursing diagnoses. This trajectory (see Figure 1) represents three stages of developmental research. Stage I represents quantitative methods used to identify, describe, and initiate definition of nursing diagnoses and their associated defining characteristics using descriptive statistics and correlation coefficients associated with content validity and interrater reliability. Stage II represents multivariate quantitative statistical methods that further establish the predictive criterion and construct validity of actual nursing diagnoses. Stage III is much the same as stage II but suggests quantitative methods using prevalence rates to predict potential nursing diagnoses and Bayesian statistics to provide data from which decisions such as nursing interventions can be made and implemented. These stages occur within a developmental progression achieving interrater reliability and content validity prior to predictive and construct validity.

Stage I
- Descriptive Methods
  Frequencies
- Content Validity
  Diagnostic Content Validity
  Clinical Diagnostic Validity
- Interrater Reliability Correlation Coefficients

Stage II
- Predictive Validity
  Discriminant Analysis
  Logistic Regression
- Construct Validity
  Correlation Coefficients
  Factor Analysis
  Cluster Analysis

Stage III
- Predictive Validity
  Same as Stage II
  Epidemiologic Methods (Prevalency Rates)
  Bayesian Statistics (Potential Nursing Diagnoses)
- Construct Validity
  Same as Stage II

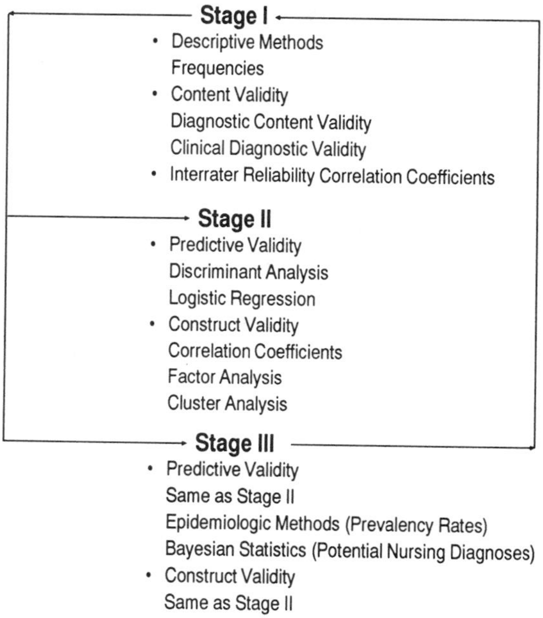

FIGURE 1 Quantitative trajectory nursing diagnosis research.

Quantitative Trajectory for Nursing Diagnosis Research

Stage I

Quantitative methods associated with stage I include descriptive statistics and correlation coefficients to establish content validity and reliability.

Descriptive methods

The bulk of validation measures for various nursing diagnoses has been in the form of descriptive research that identifies defining characteristics associated with various nursing diagnoses. The predominant mechanism used by many clinicians has been to record the frequencies of the incidence of defining characteristics related to a nursing diagnosis (Dalton, 1985; Hurley, 1986). From these defining characteristics, nursing diagnoses have been defined and submitted to NANDA for inclusion in Taxonomy I. Research to validate nursing diagnoses within and across settings has been progressing very slowly. McLane and Fehring (1984) expressed concern over the paucity of published articles relating to research and validation of nursing diagnoses. In response, an entire session of NANDA's Seventh National Conference in 1986 was devoted to research and methodologic issues related to nursing diagnoses.

Content validity

Methods of content validation have been used extensively in nursing research to define the domain of content by content experts who come to consensus on the inclusion or exclusion of, for example, defining characteristics believed to be associated with a specific diagnosis. One of the major problems with the estimation of content validity, however, is that it is subjective in nature and, according to Bohrnstead (1983) "there are no rigorous ways to access it except by using methods of construct validation" (p. 100).

Methods of content validation require scientific rigor and include judgment, establishing a criterion for content validity, and most important, use of decision rules to define the domain of content related to a specific nursing diagnosis. Lack of attention to scientific rigor jeopardizes decisions in terms of the inclusion or exclusion of defining characteristics within a nursing diagnosis (Fitzmaurice, 1990). Scientific rigor is evidenced by the selection of expert judges who will provide a valid judgment in a specific content area. Although content validity is subjective in nature, its objectivity can be increased by the significant positive correlations between nurses and nurse and patient perceptions of the meaning attributed to a specific phenomenon. Further research should be performed to correlate patients' and nurses' perceptions of the same phenomenon. This should be extended over various settings to increase the external validity of the findings.

The work of Gordon and Sweeney (1979) and Fehring (1986, 1987) has provided promising models in estimating content validity of nursing diagnoses. Some clinicians (Metzger & Hiltunen, 1987) have used Fehring's Diagnostic Content Validation (DCV) model to identify *and rate* defining characteristics pertinent to a nursing diagnosis. Thus, the models developed by Fehring, based on the work of Gordon and Sweeney, provide a more precise method for validation, because a quantitative method has been developed that provides a tentative and arbitrary value below which defining diagnosis characteristics will be deleted. Thus a procedure is described that attributes clinical significance to identified defining characteristics.

These models represent a stage in the development of quantitative methods to validate nursing diagnoses and, as such, have assisted practitioners in the clinical decision-making process of identifying those defining characteristics most representative of a specific nursing diagnosis. The result, however, is not only the rather simplistic dichotimization of complex phenomena, but also the lack of validity of this dichotimization across clinical settings. The complex interaction of defining characteristics within and across diagnoses suggests the use of linear, nonlinear, and additive multivariate quantitative models to capture the essence of the interaction of multiple variables.

Reliability

Reliability, in general, refers to the concept of repeatability. Reliability associated with nursing diagnosis refers to the degree to which defining characteristics of a diagnostic category can be used to *consistently* arrive at the same nursing diagnosis (Gordon, 1987). The three most common types of reliability are interrater reliability, test-retest reliability, and internal consistency reliability. Interrater reliability is the most frequent form of reliability reported in nursing diagnosis research. Interrater reliability is most used in studies using either Fehring's DCV model or Content Diagnostic Validity (CDV) model.

The CDV model, used by expert clinicians, generates a weighted interrater reliability ratio for each defining characteristic. The DCV model generates a content validity index, a measure of the experts' ratings of the relative importance of defining characteristics associated with a nursing diagnosis. Some clinicians (Metzger & Hiltunen, 1987) have used the DCV model to identify and rate defining characteristics pertinent to a nursing diagnosis. Each diagnosis is rated on a scale from 1 to 5 where 1 indicates not at all characteristic of the diagnosis being tested and 5 equals very characteristic. These ratings are then converted to a scale ranging from 0 to 1 with $1 = 0$, $2 = 0.25$, $3 = 0.5$, $4 = 0.75$, and $5 = 1$. These ratios are then converted to major and minor characteristics. Major characteristics are indicated by a score of 0.8 or greater; minor characteristics are those between 0.5 and 0.79. A total DCV score can be computed by summing the individual ratio scores greater than 0.5 and dividing by the total number of defining characteristics. It is suggested that nursing diagnoses that have DCV and CDV total scores below 0.6 be further refined or removed from the NANDA taxonomy. Test-retest reliability should be incorporated in diagnostic research studies to determine the stability of the CDV and DCV models over time.

Internal consistency reliability refers to the homogeneity of items that measure a concept. Internal consistency reliability is encountered primarily in terms of the construction of instruments to measure clinical phenomena. The items should be moderately correlated among themselves, but the responses to the items should vary across respondents. One mechanism for increasing internal consistency is to increase the structure of observation guides (Padilla, 1990). Another, which has already been addressed, is the rigorous methods used to include or exclude defining characteristics from a nursing diagnosis. The use of inclusion or exclusion criteria would tend to increase the homogeneity of the items within a nursing diagnosis and therefore increase the internal consistency of the observation guide.

Stage II

Quantitative measures associated with stage II include those statistical procedures that provide estimates of predictive and construct validity.

Predictive validity

Content validity is a logical prerequisite for criterion-related predictive validity. Criterion-related validity refers to the correlation between a measure and some criterion of interest that exists in the present or may be predicted in the future. The presence of apparent predictive criterion-related validity is evidenced by 13 of the categories in Taxonomy I that refer to potential nursing diag-

noses, which are accompanied by risk factors (Fitzmaurice, 1990). A potential state is a predicted rather than an actual state and intervention is directed at reducing risk factors. A large number of studies have been reported in the nursing diagnosis literature describing risk factors associated with potential problems; however, there is a great need to develop and implement systematic studies to achieve the predictive criterion validity associated with these potential diagnoses. This is especially evidenced by the lack of description of an actual diagnosis for eight of the potential diagnostic categories. It would appear, therefore, that there is a great deal of research that needs to be done not only to identify risk factors associated with potential diagnoses and to validate each potential diagnosis across multiple samples, but also to define the actual diagnosis associated with each potential diagnosis. This research would provide the framework for epidemiologic studies to determine the prevalence rates for defined nursing diagnoses.

The use of Fehring's (1986) Etiological Correlation Rating (ECR) model generates an index of predictive validity that has not been extensively used in practice and, thus, illustrates the need and future direction for further research. The validity index computed with this model represents the strength of the association between a specific nursing diagnosis and a proposed etiology for the diagnosis. The basis for this type of validation is the absence of a direct cause-and-effect relationship of the etiologies with most nursing diagnoses (Fehring, 1986). The importance of the etiologic correlation coefficient is that it is a reflection of the strength of the etiology's ability to predict the existence of a diagnosis.

Construct validity

Construct validity refers to the degree to which an instrument measures a construct of interest. A construct is an abstract representation of reality and can be thought of as a dimension inferred from a network of interrelationships (Rossi et al., 1983). Construct validity is the most difficult form of validity to achieve, but it is the most essential in validating nursing diagnoses. This is true because each diagnosis is composed of a number of defining characteristics. Therefore, each diagnosis could be considered as a concept that is unique and different from others. In the real world, however, this is not the case. An example is in the overlap between the two nursing diagnoses *anxiety* and *fear*. Some physiologic characteristics of both human experiences have been reported to be exhibited in both diagnoses (Yocom, 1984).

Construct validation is determined by two types of relationships. The first is the relationship between the defining characteristics and the underlying, latent, unobserved concept referred to as *within*-concept validity. The second is the relationship among the defining characteristics referred to as *between*-concept validity. The notion of a concept implies that the defining characteristics within the domain of content correlate together because they reflect the same underlying construct. Furthermore, if the defining characteristics within one domain correlate with defining characteristics from another domain it is because the constructs themselves are related. An example of the application of the two relationships associated with construct validity may clarify this point.

For purposes of this example, consider the two nursing diagnoses *powerlessness* and *self-esteem disturbance*. Each of these two diagnoses has empirically derived defining characteristics. The first hypothesis would confirm that there is an interrelationship among the defining characteristics within each diagnosis. This could be determined by a matrix of bivariate correlations, and the relationship of each characteristic with the underlying, unobservable concept of powerlessness could be estimated by confirmatory factor analysis. The factor loading for each defining characteristic provides an estimate of the correlation of that defining characteristic with the nursing diagnosis. The second hypothesis would postulate that there is an inverse relationship between powerlessness and self-esteem: that is, the greater the perception of powerlessness, the less the perception of self-esteem.

The construct validity within and external to each nursing diagnosis should be further developed. Factor and cluster analyses are methods of estimating construct validity within a concept while discriminant analysis estimates construct validity external to a concept. The statistical techniques applicable to the construct validation of nursing diagnoses are discriminant analysis, factor analysis, and cluster analysis.

Discriminant analysis. Stepwise discriminant analysis and logistical regression are two special cases of multiple regression in which the dependent variable is either nominal or ordinal. The defining characteristics for each nursing diagnosis would serve as independent variables to predict membership to that specific diagnosis. Stepwise discriminant analysis serves as a technique to predict membership into a group (nursing diagnosis) according to specific variables (defining characteristics). The predicted group membership is then compared to the a priori group membership. Logistical regression does much the same thing but is interpreted as calculating the risk of belonging to one of two groups. Both models serve as mechanisms for construct validation for nursing diagnosis because the actual and predicted group membership should be consistent. Construct validity would be achieved if defining characteristics associated with different nursing diagnoses were used to classify patients to the appropriate nursing diagnosis group based on knowledge of the a priori group membership.

Factor analysis. Factor analysis and cluster analysis are statistical techniques used to reduce a large number of variables to a smaller number of presumed underlying variables.

Factor analytical techniques are performed to extract a smaller number of factors from a large number of variables. Names are applied to the extracted factors based on the content of the items.

Cluster analysis. Cluster analysis is often referred to as the poor man's factor analysis because the computations are simpler than factor analysis and it does not require as large a sample as does factor analysis. Cluster analysis differs from discriminant analysis in that the number and characteristics of the groups are derived from the data with no prior knowledge of group membership. Thus, cluster analysis could be very useful in nursing diagnosis to identify diagnostic categories associated with a specific nursing diagnosis. The defining characteristics would be used as the classification variables and patients would be assigned to nursing diagnoses based on their symptoms. One of the intuitively appealing characteristics of cluster analysis compared with factor analysis is that each variable (defining characteristic) is assigned to only one cluster. In factor analysis, variables are assigned to more than one factor and thus variability for each variable is shared across factors.

Stage III

The techniques outlined for predictive and construct validity in stage II would be generalized to stage III. In addition, epidemiologic methods could be selected to predict the probability of experiencing a potential nursing diagnosis based on actual risk factors. Bayesian statistics could be used as a decision-making process in determining nursing interventions using previous knowledge related to the association between etiologies, defining characteristics, and potential nursing diagnoses. Descriptive epidemiologic studies have been reported in the NANDA proceedings, but these are descriptive rather than epidemiologic studies because prevalence rates are not reported and small, convenience samples are used (Alexander, 1990; Norris, 1990). Bayesian statistics are an alternative to the classical inferential statistics used to draw conclusions from data in samples of populations for which no data exist. Bayesian inference, however, is tailored to the research process starting with the initial uncertainty about the variables and upgrading this uncertainty in the face of information obtained from data derived from repeated studies. The advantage of Bayesian over classical statistical inference is that the data are derived from prior research and it is not necessary to start from the very beginning for each research study. Both epidemiologic studies and Bayesian statistics assume that previous qualitative and quantitative methods have been used to provide the data.

Issues Associated with the Clinical Validation of Nursing Diagnoses

The issues associated with the use of quantitative methods include the interface among the conceptual, substantive, and methodologic domains of research. The conceptual aspect reflects some content that is of interest. The identification and development of the operational definition for each nursing diagnosis are the conceptual domain. Each diagnosis accepted by NANDA is a concept that must be operationalized and validated. The substantive or empirical aspect is the observed defining characteristics or cues exhibited by patients classified for each nursing diagnosis. The methodologic domain is represented by the techniques or procedures by which the validity of measurement instruments developed to tap specific nursing diagnoses can be estimated. Validation of nursing diagnoses must be addressed not as a unitary concept but as a component of the conceptual framework that guides the practice of nursing.

One of the persistent problems in the identification of defining characteristics associated with nursing diagnoses is the uniqueness of these characteristics to a specific nursing diagnosis. There is a great need to identify the uniqueness of diagnostic cues so that there is no overlap between or among diagnoses. Cluster analysis would be one quantitative statistical mechanism to achieve this, but in the real world this is not possible and overlap remains a persistent problem. This overlap also represents a pesky statistical problem. Examples of overlap include the defining characteristics associated with *anxiety* and *fear* and another between the proposed nursing diagnoses of *apathy* and *depression.* It is particularly difficult when one nursing diagnosis may be a precursor of another. For example, is *apathy* a precursor of *depression,* or is *apathy* a personality characteristic separate from *depression*? These questions refer to the validity of the diagnoses. If one is to consider *depression* as a consequence of *apathy*, the estimation of predictive criterion validity through multiple regression techniques would be appropriate. If, on the other hand, *apathy* is conceptualized as a personality trait, it may be differentiated from and not causally associated with *depression.*

These examples illustrate some of the conceptual problems that show the need for further research—particularly the estimation of extensive external validity or generalizability to obtain further measures to validate the conceptual meaning of defining characteristics that share variability across various nursing diagnoses. Evidence is beginning to emerge that may demonstrate the complexity of validating nursing diagnoses. It would appear that there are differences in the number and intensity of defining characteristics associated with various nursing diagnoses *across clinical settings* such as acute care settings and community health care agencies. Thus, there must be a delicate balance among the conceptual, empirical (clinical), and methodologic (statistical) domains used to validate nursing diagnoses.

Another issue is the need to increase confidence in the content validity of a nursing diagnosis by comparing patient and nurse perceptions of cues nurses identify as defining characteristics for a specific nursing diagnosis. Although content validity is subjective in nature, its objectivity can be increased by the significant positive correlations between nurse and patient perceptions of the meaning attributed to a specific phenomenon. Further research should be performed to correlate patients' and nurses' perceptions of the same phenomenon across various settings.

Directions for Future Research

There can be no dispute about the need for research to clarify further the issues related to (1) the predictive, criterion, and construct validity of the defining characteristics and etiologies associated with nursing diagnoses, (2) the relationship between nursing diagnoses and planned nursing interventions, and (3) the further development testing of these diagnoses within theoretical models. The clinical validation of nursing diagnoses is a complex process involving the careful use of both qualitative and quantitative methods to assure the interface among the empirical, substantive, conceptual, and methodologic domains. The suggested steps for validating nursing diagnoses include:

1. Development of standardized instruments to enhance comparability of defining characteristics across settings
2. Continued efforts to estimate content validity of nursing diagnoses within and across clinical settings
3. Estimation of construct validity within and across diagnostic categories
4. Epidemiologic studies to determine the incidence and prevalence of various nursing diagnoses
5. Use of multivariate statistical models to predict diagnoses

6. Studies to correlate patients' and nurses' perceptions of diagnostic-related cues
7. Efforts to correlate nursing diagnoses and their associated etiologies
8. Studies to determine the effectiveness of diagnosis-specific nursing interventions.

The development of standardized instruments will not only maximize the internal consistency of measures but will enhance comparability of defining characteristics across settings. Concept analysis should be used to arrive at the operational definition of the diagnosis. Are the defining characteristics internal or external to the domain? Are these characteristics validated within and across settings? Epidemiologic studies may be useful in providing group data to identify those patients at risk for a potential nursing diagnosis based on risk factors. Risk factors may vary with different groups based on what diagnoses are being applied. Discriminant analysis or logistical regression could then be used to discriminate defining characteristics among groups. Multivariate statistics, such as discriminant analysis or logistical regression, and factor or cluster analysis would be appropriate to provide a more realistic representation of the complex interactions of defining characteristics within and across diagnoses and settings.

Finally, Bayesian statistics could be used in decision making in planning nursing interventions based on prior data. Decision making involves combining previous knowledge with other information to choose among actions (Pollard, 1986). This method represents the ultimate quantitative method in the validation of nursing diagnoses but assumes prior clinical validation achieved through rigorous scientific clinical research.

Clinical researchers have provided the groundwork for more sophisticated quantitative methods to achieve the clinical validation of nursing diagnoses. There is much work to be done; carefully planned strategies will involve using both qualitative and quantitative methods. There is a need for research and a multitude of available quantitative research designs and statistical analyses to achieve the goals. Nurses must welcome the challenge to refine and further define the taxonomy of nursing diagnoses using a variety of qualitative and quantitative methods appropriate to the research question and design.

References

Alexander, C. (1990). Epidemiologic approaches to validation of nursing diagnosis. In *Monograph of the invitational conference on research methods for validating nursing diagnoses* (pp. 121–136). St. Louis, MO: North American Nursing Diagnosis Association.

Afifi, A., & Clark, V. (1984). *Computer-aided multivariate analysis.* Belmont, CA: Lifetime Learning Publications.

Bohrnstead, G. (1983). Measurement. In P. H. Rossi, J. D. Wright, & A. G. Anderson (Eds.), *Handbook of survey research.* New York: Academic Press.

Dalton, J. (1985). A descriptive study: Defining characteristics of the nursing diagnosis cardiac output, alterations in: Decreased. *Image: The Journal of Nursing Scholarship, 17*(4), 113–116.

Fehring, R. J. (1986). Validating diagnostic labels: Standardized methodology. In M. E. Hurley (Ed.), *Classification of nursing diagnoses: Proceedings of the sixth national conference* (pp. 183–189). St. Louis, MO: Mosby.

Fehring, R. J. (1987). Methods to validate nursing diagnoses. *Heart & Lung, 6,* 625–629.

Fitzmaurice, J. (1990). Tool development: Validity related to nursing diagnosis: Response to Schroeder. In *Monograph of the invitational conference on research methods for validating nursing diagnoses* (pp. 121–136). St. Louis, MO: North American Nursing Diagnosis Association.

Gordon, M. (1987). *Nursing diagnosis: Process and application* (2nd ed.). New York: McGraw-Hill.

Gordon, M., & Sweeney, M. A. (1979). Methodological problems and issues in identifying and standardizing nursing diagnoses. *Advances in Nursing Science, 2*(1), 1–15.

Hurley, M. E. (Ed.). (1986). *Classification of nursing diagnoses: Proceedings of the sixth national conference.* St. Louis, MO: Mosby.

McLane, A., & Fehring, R. J. (1984). Nursing diagnosis: A review of the literature. In In M. J. Kim, G. K. McFarland, & A. M. McLane (Eds.), *Classification of nursing diagnoses: Proceedings of the fifth national conference* (pp. 525–540). St. Louis, MO: Mosby.

Metzger, K. L., & Hiltunen, E. R. (1987). Diagnostic content validation of ten frequently reported nursing diagnoses. In A. M. McLane (Ed.), *Classification of nursing diagnoses: Proceedings of the seventh national conference* (pp. 144–153). St. Louis, MO: Mosby.

Norris, J. (1990). Epidemiologic approaches to validation of nursing diagnosis: Response to Alexander. In *Monograph of the invitational conference on research methods for validating nursing diagnoses* (pp. 137–146). St. Louis, MO: North American Nursing Diagnosis Association.

Padilla, G. (1990). Tool development: Reliability and related statistics. In *Monograph of the invitational conference on research methods for validating nursing diagnoses* (pp. 121–136). St. Louis, MO: North American Nursing Diagnosis Association.

Pollard, W. E. (1986). *Bayesian statistics for evaluation research: An introduction.* Newbury Park, CA: Sage.

Yocom, C. J. (1984). The differentiation of fear and anxiety. In M. J. Kim, G. K. McFarland, & A. M. McLane (Eds.), *Classification of nursing diagnoses: Proceedings of the fifth national conference* (pp. 352–355). St. Louis, MO: Mosby.

Integrated Methods for Nursing Diagnosis Research

Mi Ja Kim, PhD, RN, FAAN

The topic of an integrated approach to nursing diagnosis validation research suggests an integration of qualitative and quantitative methods. To a large extent, this is true. Because both methods should be used for validation studies to the extent possible, separation of qualitative methods from quantitative methods for nursing diagnosis validation studies is quite arbitrary. A pluralistic approach to research methodology for validation of nursing diagnoses would do more to enlighten us about the universe of nursing than any single approach (Allen, Benner, & Diekelmann, 1986).

Munhall (1986) expresses concern for nursing's emphasis on what she terms "structural truth." The potential problem of giving attention to structural truth rather than to the search for a dynamic meaning of nursing is aptly captured in the following excerpts that have implications for nursing diagnosis research:

Are we measuring our lives in coffee spoons? (p. 1)

There are more things in heaven and earth than are dreamt of in our hypothesis, and our observations should be open to them. (p. 2)

Take the knotted, anomalous, confounded world and make it orderly and sometimes predictable but report occasionally on an *n* of 1. (p. 2)

Let us not make methodological issues another issue for the submissive aggressive syndrome. (p. 4)

Two points to be gleaned from these quotations are that our attempts to validate/standardize the description of patient problems are difficult at best, and yet we cannot dwell on the debate over methodologic issues.

For any nursing diagnosis validation study, there are three basic elements that must be present, which are

1. There must be an operational definition of the nursing diagnosis and its defining characteristics. Without a definition to set the theoretical basis for a given concept (in this case the nursing diagnosis and its accompanying defining characteristics), the validity of the study result can be questioned.
2. It is essential that measurement criteria for each defining characteristic be established before proceeding with validation of the nursing diagnosis. Because

defining characteristics are vital components that characterize the parameters of a given nursing diagnosis, it is imperative that these be operationally defined with measurement criteria, using norms if possible.

3. A conceptual framework must be developed or selected to guide the development of the nursing diagnosis. A conceptual framework will help nurse researchers define the universe of nursing's clinical phenomena and guide boundary setting for our clinical concerns.

As corollaries to the above three basic elements are the specificity and sensitivity of individual nursing diagnoses. Because nursing diagnoses are inferred from patient problems that require nursing therapy, acceptable levels of specificity and sensitivity along with validity and reliability of these diagnoses are prerequisite for appropriate nursing therapy/interventions.

Because nursing diagnoses are concepts, techniques used for concept development also are relevant for nursing diagnosis. The development of concepts is achieved by systematic literature review (Rodgers, 1988), case development and concept analysis (Chinn & Jacobs, 1987; Walker & Avant, 1988). The major foci of systematic literature reviews are sample design, disciplinary boundaries, and historical development (Rodgers, 1988). Whereas the systematic literature review is usually used for refinement of existing concepts (diagnoses), the case development method is usually used for new concepts that have not been studied extensively (Knafl, 1990).

Concept analysis can be done by either a theoretical or an empirical process. The theoretical approach entails the use of the research literature (and at times empirical referents to augment the analysis). This approach has been used primarily to evaluate or refine existing concepts. On the other hand, empirical processes such as phenomenology, grounded theory, and ethnography can be used to discover new concepts as well as to refine existing ones (Knafl, 1990).

An integrated approach, using both qualitative and quantitative methods, is an ideal way to conduct nursing diagnosis validation research. A brief description of the theoretical distinctions between qualitative and quantitative approaches will address potential variations in integrated approaches.

Qualitative Methods

Common themes across qualitative approaches are: Each entails immersion in the everyday life of the setting chosen for study, values participants' perspectives on their worlds and seeks to discover those perspectives, views inquiry as an interactive process between the researcher and the participants, and is primarily descriptive and relies on people's words as the primary data (Marshall & Rossman, 1989, p. 11).

Qualitative research methods in nursing include ethnography, phenomenology, and grounded theory. Dreher (1990) states that the ethnographic approach is a research method associated with the discipline of anthropology. The goal is to describe and explain both patterns and deviations in social behavior, often relying on cultural comparison. The ethnographer observes human behavior and responses with no preconceived expectations, variables, or categories; there is no attempt to validate a designated theoretical framework. Ethnography is a naturalistic, qualitative, inductive, comparative method aimed at studying human behavior and attitudes through observations made in natural settings (Dreher, 1990).

Phenomenology and grounded theory are other frequently used qualitative approaches. Although both often use similar data, there are important differences between these two approaches. Knafl (1990) compares them (see Table 1).

Table 1: Comparison of Study Designs Using Phenomenology and Grounded Theory

	Phenomenology	Grounded Theory
Aim/Purpose	Describe lived human experience	Develop data-based theory
Research question	Focus on lived experience and essential structure	Focus on social-psychologic problems and processes to resolve them
Conceptual framework	Bracketing, silence	Symbolic interactionism
Sample	Purposive	Theoretic
Data-collection activities	Activities aimed at intuiting phenomena (e.g., observing, reading, imagining, listening)	Activities aimed at developing theory (e.g., observing, interviewing, document review)
Data-analysis activities	Extracting significant statements, formulating meanings, clustering themes, describing	Open coding, category identification, conceptual refinement
Final product	Description of general essence of phenomenon	Conceptual presentation in terms of social process
Key terms, buzz words	Lived experience, bracketing, intuiting, essential structure	Constant comparison, theoretical sample, core category, BSP

NOTE: From "Concept development" by K. Knafl, 1990, in *Monograph of the invitational conference on research methods for validating nursing diagnoses*, pp. 37–63. Copyright © NANDA, 1990. Used with permission.

Quantitative Methods

The quantitative approach to nursing diagnosis validation research is governed by the empirical–analytical paradigm, which distinguishes itself from the qualitative approach by "the emphasis on theory, the centrality of observation and measurement and the ideal of experimental designs" (Allen et al., 1986, p. 24). Two assumptions are made when using quantitative approaches: (1) that the world is structured by lawlike regularities, which can be identified and manipulated, and (2) that the world is ordered and can be broken down into a system of independent variables. In the quantitative approach under the empirical–analytical paradigm, knowledge is generated when hypotheses can be tested and reproducible findings are used to make improvements in concept development such as nursing diagnosis. Variables of theory/concept must be operationalized into precise and distinct definitions (Allen et al., 1986).

Epidemiologic/survey research methods that can be used in nursing diagnosis research include cohort design, cross-sectional design, and case-control design. These methods are not necessary for the validation of individual nursing diagnoses per se, but are useful methods to survey more general use of nursing diagnoses.

A cohort design is also called a prospective or longitudinal design in which the factors of interest (e.g., nursing diagnoses) are collected for all subjects at the beginning of the time period. Investigators follow the subjects over a specified period in which those who develop a change in a given health status (i.e., nursing diagnosis) are identified (Alexander, 1990).

In a cross-sectional design, on the other hand, information on a health problem (i.e., a nursing diagnosis) and exposure to risk factors are collected concurrently at a given time in order to describe characteristics of a target population. This design uses retrospective information to determine a relationship between the health problem and exposure to risk factors (Alexander, 1990).

Case-control design matches cases (subjects with health problems) to noncases (subjects without health problems) on a set of potentially confounding variables, which improves statistical precision in estimating relationships between health problems and exposure. This design is less costly than cohort or cross-sectional designs because of the sampling process and study period (Alexander, 1990).

Content validity and construct validity are two statistical concepts/methods that can be used for validation studies. Concept validity is defined as the degree to which the domain of content has been sampled (Schroeder, 1990). Content validity has been used most commonly by researchers for nursing diagnosis validation research to date. However, content validity has fundamental limitations for the measurement of theoretical concepts (Fitzmaurice, 1990).

Construct validity, on the other hand, is defined as the degree to which the construct of the nursing diagnosis of interest is measured (Schroeder, 1990). Factor analysis, cluster analysis, discriminant analysis, and multiple regression are statistical methods that can be used for development of construct validity of a nursing diagnosis. Clearly, more research focusing on the construct validity of nursing diagnoses is needed. However, this requires a more comprehensive and systematic approach with larger sample size.

Reliability refers to a property of a tool that ensures consistency when measuring a given value of a phenomenon. That is, there is evidence to support the reproducibility of a number assigned to a given value of the phenomenon (Padilla, 1990). Statistical concepts/methods that address the reliability aspect of a given nursing diagnosis are (1) interrater and intrarater reliability, (2) stability, (3) equivalence, and (4) internal consistency. Interrater reliability refers to the consistency with which two or more raters yield data using a given instrument. Intrarater reliability refers to the consistency with which a single rater yields measures on multiple administration of an instrument. A

Pearson product moment correlation coefficient can be used to determine reliability for norm-referenced measures when two raters are used to assign scores, or when one rater assigns a score twice. When more than two raters are used, or when one rater assigns scores more than twice, coefficient alpha may be used (Padilla, 1990).

Stability refers to the implementation of the same measurement tool over a period of time, where testing intervals occur long enough apart to eliminate the practice effects but close enough so that the steady-state assumption of the sample is not violated. A Pearson product moment coefficient is used to calculate measures using interval or ratio level scales (Padilla, 1990).

Statistics used to determine stability can also be used to determine equivalence as long as two parallel forms are used prior to calculating an equivalence of alternate forms of an instrument. Internal consistency is the measure of reliability most often used for psychometric measures. It is used for norm-referenced measures only; it shows the agreement of performance of a subject across items or subsets of items of an instrument. Item homogeneity is indicated by consistent subject performance across items (Padilla, 1990).

Integrated Approaches

Hybrid Model

The modified hybrid model and triangulation are useful approaches that integrate qualitative and quantitative methods for nursing diagnosis validation research. The original hybrid model (Schwartz-Barcott & Kim, 1986) interfaces theoretical analysis with empirical observation. It involves identifying, analyzing, and refining concepts in the initial stage of theory development. This approach draws heavily on insights generated in clinical practice.

The hybrid model is composed of three

phases: the theoretical phase, the fieldwork phase, and the analytical phase. Although it draws heavily on experiences from clinical practice, the first phase is highly theoretic; it involves a literature search and the analysis and selection of a working definition of the concept. The fieldwork phase uses field research methods to collect qualitative data for further analysis and development of the selected concept. The analytical phase is the final step in interfacing the initial theoretical analysis with insights gained from the empirical observations.

The original hybrid model stems primarily from a social-psychologic perspective, which is qualitative in nature. The modified hybrid model is proposed here in order to include the dimension of biophysical phenomena of concern to nursing, which are quantitative in nature. It is reasoned that principles of the original hybrid model can be easily applied to the development and validation of biophysical clinical problems (i.e., nursing diagnoses) as well. For instance, biophysical concepts with the characteristics of quantitative as well as qualitative data can be identified, analyzed, and refined during the theoretical phase. During the fieldwork phase, field research methods can be used to collect both qualitative and quantitative data for further analysis of the selected concept. Insights gained from the empirical observations/measurements made during the field work are integrated with the results of the initial theoretical analysis made during the analytical phase.

Triangulation

The term triangulation has two distinct applications—one that focuses on convergence function, and one that focuses on attaining completeness (Knafl & Breitmayer, 1990). The triangulation approach that is relevant for nursing diagnosis validation research tends to fall in the former application: that is, to confirm or establish convergent va-

lidity of defining characteristics of a given nursing diagnosis.

According to Creason (1990), triangulation, particularly methodologic triangulation, is a way to combine qualitative and quantitative research methods in a single study. This approach comes from the social science research literature. Campbell and Fiske (1959) described the strategy as convergent methodology, while Denzin (1970) defined it as "the combination of methodologies in the study of the same phenomenon" (p. 291). This approach allows qualitative research to complement quantitative research or vice versa. Hence, the tools used for data collection in the triangulation approach must have known strengths and weaknesses that can be counterbalanced in order to minimize threats to validity (Knafl & Breitmayer, 1990).

Denzin (1970) identified four types of triangulation:

1. *Data triangulation* has three subtypes (time, space, and person), which in turn have three levels (aggregate, interactive, and collective).
2. *Investigator triangulation* has multiple rather than single observers of the same object.
3. In *theory triangulation* multiple theoretical perspectives are used, not a single perspective of the same set of objects.
4. *Methodologic triangulation* can be broken down into within-method and between-method triangulation.

For nursing diagnosis validation research, methodologic triangulation would be the most relevant, although other types of triangulation could be employed.

Summary

An integrated approach for validation of nursing diagnoses entails using both quantitative and qualitative methods. By doing so, the holistic essence/nature of nursing can be studied appropriately. In addition to the use of varying degrees of both methods for individual nursing diagnosis validation research, two other integrated approaches—modified hybrid model and triangulation—are sound mechanisms for integrating validation methods for the study of nursing diagnosis.

References

Allen, D., Benner, P., & Diekelmann, N. L. (1986). Three paradigms for nursing research: Methodological implications. In P. L. Chinn (Ed.), *Nursing research methodology: Issues and implementation* (pp. 23–38). Rockville, MD: Aspen.

Alexander, C. (1990). Epidemiological approaches to validation of nursing diagnosis. In *Monograph of the invitational conference on research methods for validating nursing diagnoses* (pp. 121–136). St. Louis, MO: North American Nursing Diagnosis Association.

Campbell, D. T., & Fiske, D. W. (1959). Convergent and discriminant validation by the multitrait-multimethod matrix. *Psychological Bulletin, 56,* 81–105.

Chinn, J., & Jacobs, M. (1987). *Theory and nursing: A systematic approach* (2nd ed.). St. Louis, MO: Mosby.

Creason, N. S. (1990). Clinical validation of nursing diagnoses. In *Monograph of the invitational conference on research methods for validating nursing diagnoses* (pp. 278–304). St. Louis, MO: North American Nursing Diagnosis Association.

Denzin, N. (1970). *The research act: A theoretical introduction to sociological methods.* Chicago: Aldine.

Dreher, M. (1990). Ethnographic methods as differentiated from phenomenology. In *Monograph of the invitational conference on research methods for validating nursing diagnoses* (pp. 78–97). St. Louis, MO: North American Nursing Diagnosis Association.

Fitzmaurice, J. (1990). Tool development: Validity related to nursing diagnosis. In *Monograph of the invitational conference on research methods for validating nursing diagnoses* (pp. 166–176). St. Louis, MO: North American Nursing Diagnosis Association.

Knafl, K. (1990). Concept development. In *Monograph of the invitational conference on research methods for validating nursing diagnoses* (pp. 37–63). St. Louis, MO: North American Nursing Diagnosis Association.

Knafl, K., & Breitmayer, B. (1990). Triangulation in qualitative research: Issues of conceptual clarity and purpose. In J. Morse (Ed.), *Qualitative nursing research, a contemporary dialogue.* Rockville, MD: Aspen.

Marshall, C., & Rossman, G. B. (1989). *Designing qualitative research.* Newbury Park, CA: Sage.

Munhall, P. L. (1986). Methodological issues in nursing research: Beyond a wax apple. *Advances in Nursing Science, 8*(3), 1–5.

Padilla, G. (1990). Tool development: Reliability and related statistics. In *Monograph of the invitational conference on research methods for validating nursing diagnoses* (pp. 177–195). St. Louis, MO: North American Nursing Diagnosis Association.

Rodgers, B. (1989). Concept analysis and the development of nursing knowledge: The evolutionary cycle. *Journal of Advanced Nursing, 14,* pp. 330–335.

Schroeder, M. (1990). Tool development: Validity related to nursing diagnosis. In *Monograph of the invitational conference on research methods for validating nursing diagnoses* (pp. 147–165). St. Louis, MO: North American Nursing Diagnosis Association.

Schwartz-Barcott, D., & Kim, H. S. (1986). A hybrid model for concept development. In P. L. Chinn (Ed.), *Nursing research methodology: Issues and implementation* (pp. 23–38). Rockville, MD: Aspen.

Walker, L. E., & Avant, K. (1988). *Strategies for theory construction in nursing* (2nd ed.). Norwalk, CT: Appleton and Lange.

Specialty Organizations: Nursing Diagnosis Use and Issues— A Panel Presentation

American Association of Critical-Care Nurses

Rebecca C. Kuhn, MS, RN, CCRN

Weaving nursing diagnosis into the fabric of professional nursing practice requires the efforts of multiple groups and individuals within the nursing profession. Specialty organizations can provide an important avenue for valuing nursing diagnosis and demonstrating opportunities for translating the use of nursing diagnosis into practice. Using nursing diagnosis as a framework for outcome standards is one way in which the American Association of Critical-Care Nurses (AACN) has demonstrated how nursing diagnosis is implemented in the practice setting.

In 1986, the AACN Board of Directors approved the AACN Outcome Standards Task Force, which I was asked to chair. The task force was charged with designing an approach for identifying and measuring outcomes for critical care nursing practice. At that time, the profession was beginning to appreciate the need for evaluating patient outcomes, in addition to structure and process criteria, within a quality-assurance framework. Developments within the health care environment, including recent initiatives by the federal government and the Joint Commission on Accreditation of Healthcare Organizations, have reinforced the need to look at patient outcomes.

When the Outcome Standards Task Force convened, one of the first tasks undertaken was adoption of an overall framework for the outcome standards document. The task force determined that the organizing framework should be one that reflected nursing, rather than medical, practice and that nursing diagnostic labels would be used to describe the patient problems addressed.

To strengthen the integrity of the document, the task force convened a consensus panel, a group of 25 critical care experts from both practice and education, representing various clinical specialties across the age continuum. The group was charged with coming to consensus on which nursing diagnoses should be included in the document. On the first day of the consensus conference, held in January 1988, the participants were provided an overview of the outcome standards project and then divided into four groups. Each group was given a preliminary list of 46 nursing diagnoses that had been generated by the Outcome Standards Task Force after a review of the current literature. The groups were first asked to determine which of the diagnoses were not relevant to critical care nursing and should be deleted. The entire participant group then reconvened and came to consensus on which diagnoses were to be deleted; there was lengthy debate on some of the diagnoses. For example, though its relevance was recognized, the experts agreed that *knowledge deficit* should be deleted and recommended that each diagnosis in the document, if appropriate, should include content to be taught to the patient or family. The small groups then discussed diagnoses that needed to be added to the list. After consensus was reached on the additions, the final list consisted of 30 nursing diagnoses.

On day two of the consensus conference, Dr. Carolyn Murdaugh consulted and assisted in determining priorities. Two different methods were used by the participants to rank order the list of nursing diagnoses according to frequency and importance. Frequency was defined as "how often, at a given point in time"; importance was defined as "how life-threatening or critical." The first method used was Likert-type scaling. Two Likert scales were constructed, one for rating frequency and one for rating importance. Instructions on the frequency scale asked the experts to rate each nursing diagnosis on "how frequently the diagnosis is seen in patients in the Intensive Care Unit"; instructions on the importance scale asked the experts to rate each nursing diagnosis on "how important the diagnosis is for nurses to make in the Intensive Care Unit." The participants were asked to rate each nursing diagnosis on a scale of 1 to 6, with 1 being least frequent/important and 6 being most frequent/important.

Magnitude estimation scaling, the second method of prioritizing the nursing diagnoses, was used to validate the Likert-scale results and increase confidence in the validity of the results. Magnitude estimation is defined as "the process of assigning numbers proportionally to social stimuli that reflect the intensity of a person's subjective response" (Sennott-Miller, Murdaugh, & Hinshaw, 1988). In other words, while the Likert scale requests a linear response, magnitude estimation records the exponential relationship among the scaled items. Magnitude estimation scaling requires that the participants be experts in the question to be studied. In this case, the participants were experts in a clinical field of critical care and had an understanding of nursing diagnosis. Also required is that the items on the scale must vary on the major concept dimensions to be scaled. Through the discussion, we knew that the nursing diagnoses varied considerably with regard to frequency and importance.

The participants underwent a training session to prepare them for magnitude estimation. First, the participants were asked to think of numbers proportional to the number 10 (e.g., one third as large, twice as large, etc.) to prepare them to think proportionally. Each participant was then given a list of food items commonly found in the home, such as cookies, bread, liver, wine, milk. Each participant was asked to select an item as a standard or average and assign a point value to it (e.g., 10, 50, 100). Participants then estimated the frequency with which each item would be found in their home on a given day and assigned the item a proportional point value. Participants then assigned points based on the importance of each food item to their physical or mental well-being.

After training was completed, the participants used this technique to assign point values to each of the 30 nursing diagnoses in terms of both frequency and importance. Each participant worked individually, assigning points on the basis of personal experiences in critical care units in their own fields of expertise. For example, an expert in pediatric critical care nursing judged the items in terms of caring for pediatric patients.

The results of the Likert scaling and MES initially were analyzed separately. The 10 diagnoses judged by the participants to occur most frequently by Likert scaling are displayed in Table 1. Table 2 reflects the 10 least frequently occurring diagnoses. The 10 diag-

Table 1: Most Frequently Occurring Nursing Diagnoses by Likert Scaling (n = 25)

Rating/Diagnosis	$\bar{X}$ (range 1–6)
1. Altered comfort	5.48
2. Potential for infection	5.48
3. Altered tissue perfusion	5.40
4. Altered fluid volume/dynamics	5.28
5. Impaired physical mobility	5.12
6. Altered nutrition	5.00
7. Potential for injury	4.96
8. Activity intolerance	4.96
9. Self-care deficit	4.96
10. Impaired gas exchange	4.80

Table 3: Most Important Nursing Diagnoses by Likert Scaling (n = 25)

Rating/Diagnosis	$\bar{X}$ (range 1–6)
1. Altered fluid volume/dynamics	5.68
2. Impaired gas exchange	5.68
3. Altered tissue perfusion	5.64
4. Potential for injury	5.32
5. Ineffective airway clearance	5.24
6. Potential for infection	5.12
7. Altered nutrition	5.08
8. Ineffective thermoregulation	4.60
9. Impaired skin integrity	4.56
10. Altered comfort	4.52

noses judged most important are displayed in Table 3. Table 4 lists the 10 least important diagnoses.

The 10 most frequent diagnoses judged with the magnitude estimation scale are displayed in Table 5. Of note is that although the magnitude estimation priority differed from the Likert scaling, all the top 10 diagnoses, with two exceptions, were the same for the two methods. Table 6 reflects the top 10 most important diagnoses judged by magnitude estimation. With the exception of one diagnosis, all 10 were the same 10 diagnoses rated by the Likert scale.

Using both the Likert and MES results, the diagnoses were categorized based on high or low frequency and high or low importance (see Table 7). Twelve items were classified as high frequency and high importance; all were physiologic in nature. Three diagnoses were considered low frequency and high priority; again, they were physiologic diagnoses. Seven diagnoses classified as high frequency and low priority included diagnoses more psychosocial in nature. *Alteration in elimination* did not fall neatly into one category and was classified as borderline. Low-frequency and low-priority diagnoses were

Table 2: Least Frequently Occurring Nursing Diagnoses by Likert Scaling (n = 25)

Rating/Diagnosis	$\bar{X}$ (range 1–6)
20. Grieving	3.84
21. Altered urinary elimination	3.83
22. Ineffective thermoregulation	3.80
23. Powerlessness	3.76
24. Altered bowel elimination	3.64
25. Disturbance in self-concept	3.63
26. Decreased adaptive capacity	3.40
27. Impaired breathing pattern	3.00
28. Spiritual distress	2.92
29. Altered growth and development	2.32
30. Noncompliance	2.00

Table 4: Least Important Nursing Diagnoses by Likert Scaling (n = 25)

Rating/Diagnosis	$\bar{X}$ (range 1–6)
20. Altered urinary elimination	3.56
21. Altered bowel elimination	3.48
22. Powerlessness	3.40
23. Grieving	3.36
24. Disturbance in self-concept	3.28
25. Altered role performance	3.28
26. Altered family process	3.24
27. Self-care deficit	3.20
28. Spiritual distress	3.00
29. Altered growth and development	2.96
30. Noncompliance	2.36

Table 5: Most Frequently Occurring Nursing Diagnoses by Magnitude Estimation Scaling (*n* = 25)

Rating/Diagnosis	$\bar{X}$	Median	Geomean
1. Potential for infection	2.583	300	13
2. Altered comfort	2.479	300	12
3. Altered fluid volume/dynamics	2.435	240	11
4. Altered tissue perfusion	2.362	180	11
5. Impaired gas exchange	2.310	180	10
6. Altered nutrition	2.251	180	10
7. Sensory/perceptual alteration	2.185	120	9
8. Anxiety	2.140	100	9
9. Self-care deficit	2.139	120	9
10. Potential for injury	2.127	120	8

mainly psychosocial in nature. Although the Outcome Standards Task Force decided to write outcome standards for all the diagnoses, this priority listing served as a guide for determining the order in which the diagnoses were developed.

Table 6: Most Important Nursing Diagnoses by Magnitude Estimation Scaling (*n* = 25)

Rating/Diagnosis	$\bar{X}$	Median	Geomean
1. Impaired gas exchange	2.646	300	14
2. Impaired tissue perfusion	2.624	300	13
3. Altered fluid volume/dynamics	2.573	300	13
4. Potential for infection	2.519	300	12
5. Ineffective airway clearance	2.504	240	12
6. Potential for injury	2.295	120	10
7. Altered nutrition	2.212	120	9
8. Ineffective thermoregulation	2.155	120	9
9. Impaired breathing pattern	2.118	120	8
10. Impaired skin integrity	2.080	120	8

Table 7: Categories of Nursing Diagnoses

High Frequency, High Priority (Importance)
- Altered fluid volume/dynamics
- Impaired gas exchange
- Altered tissue perfusion
- Potential for injury
- Ineffective airway clearance
- Potential for infection
- Altered nutrition
- Impaired skin integrity
- Altered comfort
- Activity intolerance
- Sensory/perceptual alteration
- Impaired physical mobility

Low Frequency, High Priority (Importance)
- Ineffective thermoregulation
- Impaired breathing pattern
- Decreased adaptive capacity

High Frequency, Low Priority (Importance)
- Anxiety
- Ineffective communication
- Ineffective coping
- Self-care deficit
- Fear
- Altered family process
- Altered role performance

Borderline
- Altered urinary elimination
- Altered bowel elimination

Low Frequency, Low Priority (Importance)
- Powerlessness
- Grieving
- Disturbance in self-concept
- Spiritual distress
- Altered growth and development
- Noncompliance

Given that the environment under consideration was the critical care unit, it is not surprising that all the high-frequency and high-importance diagnoses were physiologic in nature. Recognizing that these diagnoses, whether called physiologic or collaborative nursing diagnoses or whatever, often require both independent and interdependent interventions, the task force deliberated how to develop these diagnoses. Only the independent nursing interventions associated with these nursing diagnoses were addressed. Thus it was possible to articulate nursing's unique contribution to patient outcomes and to narrow the broad scope of the document. We were pleased with the significant number of independent nursing interventions that can be utilized in the critical care unit for a nursing diagnosis considered physiologic in nature.

There was much discussion at the eighth conference regarding the role of physiologic diagnoses, particularly those often found in critical care nursing. AACN found a rich body of knowledge in nursing regarding independent nursing interventions for physiologic nursing diagnoses. For example, nurses care for patients with *impaired cerebral tissue perfusion* related to increased intracranial pressure by providing independent interventions such as patient positioning, noise control, and timing of activities such as endotracheal suctioning. We believe that physiologic nursing diagnoses are valid and useful for the nurse practicing in critical care.

Do nurses have complete control over outcomes achieved relative to physiologic nursing diagnoses? Often not. However, few outcomes in hospitalized patients are attributable solely to the nurse. In the hospitalized patient, a variety of members of the health care team contribute to patient outcomes. Considering this reality, should nursing diagnoses exclude those patient problems not in the exclusive domain of nursing? The nursing diagnosis purist may say yes. If the concept of nursing diagnosis is narrowed, the problem arises when nursing leaders then attempt to use a nursing diagnosis framework to define the scope of nursing practice, such as has been mentioned in discussion of the World Health Organization's proposed 10th revision of the International Classification of Diseases (ICD-10) and development of patient acuity systems based on nursing diagnosis. If nursing diagnoses are used to define the scope of nursing practice, they must be broad and reflect both physiologic and psychosocial aspects of nursing practice.

We think that the next step in the evolution of outcome standards development within the context of a quality-assurance framework should be a collaborative effort joining nursing, medicine, and other health care professionals in determining patient outcomes toward which we all strive and contribute.

Because nursing diagnosis was used as a framework in AACN's development of outcome standards, it may be helpful to summarize how each standard is organized. The nursing diagnosis is followed by a definition, defining characteristics, and etiologies/related factors. The next component is the outcome standard, a statement of quality that reflects the desired result. Each outcome standard is accompanied by outcome criteria that are the key physiologic and psychosocial measures to determine if the outcome standard has been met. For each outcome standard, nursing interventions specifically designed to achieve the desired patient outcome are listed. Interventions for which scientific support is available are referenced to specific research publications so that the nurse is alerted to those interventions that reflect tested nursing practice. Monitoring activities, which determine the status of the nursing diagnosis and evaluate the effect of the interventions, are listed separately in a section on monitoring.

Since consensus was achieved on the 30 nursing diagnoses two years ago, there has been much progress in developing the outcome standards. The wording of the nursing diagnostic label has been changed to reflect the NANDA taxonomy prepared for inclusion in ICD-10. Although three of the diagnoses were not developed into standards, the remaining 27 diagnoses were expanded into 43 outcome standards by addressing diagnoses such as *altered fluid volume* separately in terms of excess and deficit.

The standards, as well as chapters on use of the standards by nurses practicing in various roles and in quality-assurance activities, were published in May 1990 as *Outcome Standards for Nursing Care of the Critically Ill* (AACN, 1990).

We are very excited about the potential for the *Outcome Standards* to positively influence the nursing care and subsequent outcomes of critically ill patients and their families. The nursing framework, operationalized through nursing diagnosis, provides an approach to articulating patient outcomes that will effectively serve patients and con-

tribute to the advancement of professional nursing practice.

References

American Association of Critical-Care Nurses. (1990). *Outcome Standards for Nursing Care of the Critically Ill.* Newport Beach, CA: Author.

Sennott-Miller, L., Murdaugh, C., & Hinshaw, A. S. (1988). Magnitude estimation: Issues and practical applications. *Western Journal of Nursing Research, 10,* 414–424.

Nurses' Association of the American College of Obstetrics and Gynecology

Angela Nicoletti, MS, RN, C

Like other nursing specialty groups, the obstetric, gynecologic, and neonatal (OGN) nursing community is working to adapt and integrate nursing diagnosis into professional practice. Toward this end, the Nurses' Association of the American College of Obstetrics and Gynecology (NAACOG) published a practice resource for OGN nurses, *OGN Nursing Diagnosis* (Nicoletti, 1989). It is intended to be a practical, handy resource for clinical staff to facilitate the integration of nursing diagnosis into OGN nursing practice.

In preparation for this presentation, I surveyed the NAACOG membership through the NAACOG Newsletter to get a sense of the use of nursing diagnosis and relevant issues. Three issues emerged: wellness, patient education, and physiologic diagnoses.

Wellness

OGN nurses keenly feel the lack of terminology to describe wellness issues. Pregnancy and the birth of a child are replete with issues of normal growth and development, which are neither comfortably nor accurately described as *knowledge deficit* or potential problems. For example, a positive maternal-infant interaction is probably the single most important outcome of childbirth that is entirely within the realm of nursing expertise. It is the cornerstone of healthy parenting and intrafamilial relationships. Though it is a natural process, it is also complex. The synchrony that develops between mother and infant, particularly in the early postpartum period, can easily become asynchronous with a negative interpretation of subtle cues from the infant by the new mother who is vulnerable in her new role. Nurses facilitate this process, but are loathe to describe it in negative terms (e.g., *potential for dysfunction of . . .*), as the basis for success is a positive attitude on the part of both the nurse and the new mother. The negative terminology is particularly problematic if one values the sharing of diagnoses with the client. Stolte (1986) suggests some terminology—progressive acquisition of . . . , maternal role behaviors, and beginning maternal acquaintance related to early contact with the newborn. The label *healthy maternal attachment process* also reflects change and growth in a positive direction. Interventions focus on reinforcing the mother's positive behaviors toward her infant to promote the development of synchrony and positive interaction between mother and infant.

J. S. Starn and V. Niederhauser (personal communication, 1989) from the University of Hawaii at Manoa are using an approach to diagnostic labeling that includes both adaptive and maladaptive diagnoses. They use an organizing framework that delineates stages of life into modes. Modes are further delineated as either psychosocial or physiologic. Each mode has associated developmental tasks, and clients are described as having adaptive or maladaptive responses. Though some of their diagnoses are problematic, the concept has potential for addressing wellness issues. Stevens (1988) also supports the use of the terms adaptive and maladaptive to capture what have been described as wellness issues.

The controversy in the diagnostic community about the inclusion of "wellness" terminology into the taxonomy may be inadvertently fueled by using the word wellness to describe issues of normal growth and maturation. Wellness connotes the absence of disease or dysfunction. It is an end point, a goal, which is why it may be difficult to consider the need for a diagnosis: If you are well, what more needs to be done? We are trying to describe a whole range of adaptive human responses—physical, emotional, psychosocial—to normal growth, within which there is a range of behaviors. Families may cope effectively, but within that adaptive response is a range of behaviors that result in grades of effectiveness. Using maternal-infant interaction as an example, a healthy beginning maternal-infant interaction process is not an end point but only the beginning of a relationship that the OGN nurse has a pivotal role in promoting. Promoting greater or higher levels of adaptation may make more sense than promoting higher levels of wellness. It seems much more useful to describe nursing's area of expertise as both the adaptive and maladaptive responses of the unitary being. The definition of a nursing diagnosis must reflect that concept.

Erickson, Tomlin, and Swain (1983) have proposed a theory and paradigm for nursing called Modeling and Role-Modeling. The concepts of Modeling and Role-Modeling are a realistic and valid theoretical framework for nursing. The theory provides a basis for adopting a classification system that accommodates both adaptive and maladaptive responses. Modeling and Role-Modeling use concepts from Maslow, Erikson, Piaget, Bowlby, Lindemann, and Engel/Selye. A major concept of the theory is that growth or responses at any given point can be adaptive or maladaptive. It fits very nicely with the belief that nursing is helping people to get better when they are ill, to adjust to chronic illness or disability when necessary, and to help them grow to their fullest potential.

Patient Education

Patient-education issues are most frequently dealt with, albeit not always comfortably, with the diagnoses *knowledge deficit* or *potential alteration in health management*. *Health-seeking behaviors* is being tried by a few agencies.

Knowledge deficit as a diagnosis has been called into question recently; there are many who question how validly it is used. Most often it is simply used to document patient education in instances when the need for it is assumed by the nurse because of the circumstances, rather than arrived at through a process of data collection and synthesis. At this point I do not believe it should be discarded completely, but we should face the fact that some of the patient education we do is not the result of a demonstrated knowledge deficit. That does not preclude demonstrable, positive outcomes from patient education. *Knowledge deficit* has become a catch-all diagnosis and is used without the data to support it; in many instances education is not effective in changing behavior because a knowledge deficit is not the problem. It is too easy to tack this diagnosis on to, for instance, the woman who comes for her annual gyn exam who does not perform monthly breast exams. Very often the failure to do breast self-exam is not related to lack of knowledge but to lack of motivation to do it or fear of finding a lump. Discussing it will remind her to do it, but her behavior is not likely to change unless the real reasons she does not do it are addressed. The indiscriminate use of *knowledge deficit* obscures the need to develop other methods of changing behavior for the purpose of health promotion when education is not the sole answer.

Physiologic Diagnoses

The issue of the appropriateness of some of the so-called physiologic diagnoses touches the OGN community as well. High-risk obstetrics and neonatal intensive care units are medically intensive areas where the nurse/physician roles seem to overlap to some extent. Quick responses to rapidly changing patient conditions are necessary and have resulted in nurses assuming responsibilities for which they are not primarily accountable. It is a mistake to think we have to legitimize these activities with nursing diagnoses. They are legitimate nursing actions to support the medical diagnosis. Professional nursing is not limited to the treatment of nursing diagnoses, and we must discard the notion that only those nursing activities that treat nursing diagnoses are important. There is a constellation of nursing actions that are expected for patients with particular medical problems, such as preeclampsia and preterm labor; however the *primary* intervention for the treatment of preeclampsia and preterm labor must be physician initiated. The asso-

ciated nursing diagnosis for which the nurse may independently treat the patient may be *anxiety* related to the survival or safety of the infant, or *altered role performance* or *impaired physical mobility*. Potential for infection related to premature rupture of membranes (PROM) has similar limitations as a nursing diagnosis. Monitoring the patient for infection is part of the medical treatment for PROM and the nurse acts as an extension of the physician in the monitoring activities. It may be considered a collaborative problem. *Anxiety* related to the infant's safety or to parenting a preterm infant is a more accurate nursing diagnosis. Some of the diagnoses that are being used for the patient with preeclampsia are *fluid volume deficit, altered cardiac output, potential/actual impaired fetal gas exchange, altered renal tissue perfusion,* and *potential for maternal injury.* Preeclampsia is still preeclampsia, even though we give it the nursing diagnoses of *fluid volume deficit* and *altered cardiac output.*

It is clear that although some of the words are different, OGN nurses are grappling with some of the same issues that confound the nursing profession as a whole.

References

Erickson, H., Tomlin, H., & Swain, M. (1983). *Modeling and role-modeling: A theory and paradigm for nursing.* Englewood Cliffs, NJ: Prentice-Hall.

Nicoletti, A. (1989). *OGN nursing diagnoses.* Washington DC: Nurses' Association of the American College of Obstetrics and Gynecology.

Stevens, K. A. (1988). Nursing diagnoses in wellness childbearing settings. *JOGNN, 17,* 329–336.

Stolte, K. M. (1986). Nursing diagnosis and the childbearing woman. *MCN: Journal of Maternal Child Nursing, 11,* 13–15.

The Society for Education and Research in Psychiatric Nursing

Marga Simon Coler, EdD, RN, CS, CTN

The Society for Education and Research in Psychiatric/Mental Health Nursing (SERPN) is an outgrowth of the Council of Directors of Graduate Programs in Psychiatric/Mental Health Nursing. Because of this, its membership consists mostly of academics. The mission of SERPN is to promote high standards in psychiatric nursing education and research, and to influence national policy toward that end. The focus of this presentation, therefore, is on the impact of nursing diagnosis on psychiatric nursing from an educational and research perspective.

As has been reported at the annual SERPN meetings, some members are presently doing research on the application of the NANDA Taxonomy to the psychiatric/mental health clinical specialty in assessment and intervention. There have been validation studies of diagnoses based on the Taxonomy (Coler et al., 1989; Coler, da Nobrega, Perez, & de Farias, 1990); nursing care plans based on NANDA nursing diagnoses (Doenges, Townsend, & Moorehouse, 1989); a book on psychiatric nursing interventions, which is NANDA-based (McFarland & Wasli, 1986); and the utilization of the Taxonomy as a basis for group therapy (Coler, 1989). The NANDA Taxonomy is also being used as a

framework for psychiatric graduate course syllabi, and there are models for psychiatric nursing assessment (Coler & Vincent, 1987) and interventions. Two SERPN members have coauthored a textbook (Stuart & Sundeen, 1987) that utilizes the NANDA Taxonomy and one member has been instrumental in the development of the American Nurses' Association (ANA) *Standards of Practice for Substance Abuse Nursing* (1989), which utilizes NANDA diagnoses in its framework. The evidence of bonds between NANDA and SERPN is not lacking.

NANDA provides stability and cohesiveness for the nursing profession because its Taxonomy has the potential to extend into any specialty. NANDA's criteria for the acceptance of new diagnoses are rigorous, and the subsequent classification of new labels is becoming increasingly accountable. The NANDA Taxonomy is being utilized internationally and has been submitted to the World Health Organization (WHO) for consideration for inclusion in the *International Classification of Diagnoses, 10th edition* (ICD-10). NANDA has been empowered by ANA as the diagnostic clearinghouse. The NANDA Taxonomy is the preferred diagnostic system of many members. However, there are other systems that are equally appealing, and therein lies the diagnostic dilemma of many psychiatric nurses.

ANA Taxonomy

The ANA Phenomena Task Force of the Council of Psychiatric Nursing was conceived as an ad hoc committee to address the need to identify generic and specialty phenomena to implement the ANA's *Social Policy Statement* (1980). It was created following the 1982 revision of ANA's *Standards of Psychiatric Mental Health Nursing Practice*. Its members consisted of psychiatric/mental health nursing specialists in specific age groups. It attempted to develop a classification with an atheoretical perspective (O'Toole & Loomis, 1989).

Members of the task force began by analyzing the profession's phenomena of concern: "human responses to actual or potential health problems" (ANA, 1980, p. 9). A preliminary look at these phenomena led the group to identify them as categories for en-compassing biologic, cognitive, affective, and motor behaviors. The task force also identified target populations (individual, family, community) as recipients of nursing intervention. The first draft of the proposed classification system designated the individual responses under six main categories. There were plans for subsequent refinement of the other two population classes, family and community. However, it became cumbersome to separate an individual from the family, especially when developmental groups were also of prime consideration. Consequently the second draft integrated the population classes into one, the individual. In this revision by O'Toole (representing the ANA task force) and Phyllis Kritek (representing NANDA), developed for submission to WHO for inclusion in ICD-10, the six response patterns became nine processes.

In the third draft, produced in March 1987, the nine processes were relabeled as human response patterns in one of eight processes (see Table 1). A human response pattern was defined as "a reliable sample of traits, acts, or other observable features characterizing an

Table 1: DSM-III-R Classification Axis IV: Severity of Psychosocial Stressors Scale: Adults

Code	Term	Examples of Stressors	
		Acute Events	**Enduring Circumstances**
1	None	No acute events that may be relevant to the disorder	No enduring circumstances that may be relevant to the disorder
2	Mild	Broke up with boyfriend or girlfriends; started or graduated from school; child left home	Family arguments; job dissatisfaction; resident in high crime neighborhood
3	Moderate	Marriage; marital separation; loss of job; retirement; miscarriage	Marital discord; serious financial problems; trouble with boss; being a single parent
4	Severe	Divorce; birth of first child	Unemployment; poverty
5	Extreme	Death of spouse; serious physical illness diagnosed; victim of rape	Serious chronic illness in self or child; ongoing physical or sexual abuse
6	Catastrophic	Death of child; suicide of spouse; devastating natural disaster	Captivity as hostage; concentration camp experience
0	Inadequate information, or no change in condition		

NOTE: From "Diagnostic and Statistical Manual III—Revised" (p. 11). Washington, DC: American Psychiatric Association.

individual" (O'Toole & Loomis, 1989, p. 290). The third draft was alphabetically arranged, giving the classification a sense of direction. Three subcategories were added:

1. *Not otherwise specified,* a category that can be used for processes that are not as yet classified. These will become sources of new data as the classification system evolves.
2. *Undeveloped,* a designation that should be used when a stage of development represented by a process has not yet been reached by a client (O'Toole & Loomis, 1989).
3. *Potential for* indicates, as in many of NANDA's explorations, that a person is at risk for the alteration.

The task force's fourth draft (1988) retained the eight basic processes. New diagnoses have been added, and some have been recategorized. Parenthetically, the NANDA Mental Health Special Interest Group, in its March 1988 meeting, declared the need for clinical validation of the ANA diagnoses for submission and subsequent incorporation into the NANDA system.

At present the ANA task force is recommending a move in the direction of becoming a subset of a generic system, or a move toward a classification system that represents the whole of nursing. O'Toole and Loomis (1989) describe the recommendation as analogous to that of the *Diagnostic and Statistical Manual-III-Revised (DSM-III–R)* (American Psychiatric Association, 1987), fitting into the ICD-9 medical diagnostic system. The task force has incorporated all the NANDA diagnoses into its classification and continues to collaborate with NANDA representatives. Updates of the jointly submitted diagnostic system for ICD-10 have evolved.

Meanwhile SERPN finds itself somewhere in the middle. Although there has been overwhelming support for endorsing the NANDA system by the SERPN board, some board members had been individually approached by members of the task force to elicit support for their system. Perhaps the dilemma of the two systems will be resolved as the task force continues to collaborate further with NANDA.

Third-Party Payment

A further dilemma that impacts on psychiatric/mental health nursing is third-party reimbursement. At present a vendor is required to use diagnoses within the DSM-III-R system of the American Psychiatric Association (APA) (see Table 2). Psychiatric/mental health nursing has traditionally operated under DSM-III-R classification, and many graduate programs continue to highlight this diagnostic system for teaching psychiatric content. Within it students learn how to assess and diagnose schizophrenia, bipolar mood disorder, borderline personality disorder, and how these conditions are impacted by medical states of illness (DSM-III-R, Axis III). Many psychiatric/mental health nurses are more adept at rating stressors on DSM-III-R Axis IV (see Table 3), and at assessing a client's functional level through the Global Assessment Scale on DSM-III-R Axis V (see Table 4), than they are at making psychiatric nursing assessment leading to nursing diagnoses. Few practitioners (if any) get third-party reimbursement for treating a diagnosis

Table 2: Classification of Human Responses of Concern for Psychiatric Mental Health Nursing Practice (ANA, Phenomena Task Force, 1988)

Human Response Patterns in Activity Processes
Human Response Patterns in Cognition Processes
Human Response Patterns in Ecological Processes
Human Response Patterns in Emotional Processes
Human Response Patterns in Interpersonal Processes
Human Response Patterns in Perception Processes
Human Response Patterns in Physiological Processes
Human Response Patterns in Valuation Processes

Table 3: DSM-III-R Classification: Axes I and II Categories

Disorders usually first evident in infancy, childhood, or adolescence
Developmental disorders
Organic mental disorders
Psychoactive substance use disorders
Schizophrenia
Delusional (paranoid) disorders
Psychotic disorders not elsewhere classified
Mood disorders
Anxiety disorders
Somatoform disorders
Dissociative disorders
Sexual disorders
Sleep disorders
Factitious disorders
Impulse control disorders not elsewhere classified
Adjustment disorders
Psychological factors affecting physical condition
Personality disorders
Codes for conditions not attributable to a mental disorder that are focus of attention of treatment

NOTE: From "Diagnostic and Statistical Manual III—Revised" (pp. 3–9). Washington, DC: American Psychiatric Association.

Table 4: DSM-III-R Classification Axis V: Abbreviated Global Assessment of Functioning (GAF) Scale

Consider psychological, social, and occupational functioning on a hypothetical continuum of mental health–illness. Do not include impairment in functioning due to physical (or environmental) limitations.

NOTE: Use intermediate codes when appropriate.

Code	
90	Absent or minimal symptoms (e.g., mild anxiety before an exam), good functioning in all areas, interested and involved in a wide range of activities, socially effective, generally satisfied with life, no more than everyday problems or concerns (e.g., an occasional argument with family members).
81	
60	Moderate symptoms (e.g., flat affect and circumstantial speech, occasional panic attacks) OR moderate difficulty in social, occupational, or school functioning (e.g., few friends, conflicts with co-workers).
51	
10	Persistent danger of severely hurting self or others (e.g., recurrent violence) OR persistent inability to maintain minimum personal hygiene OR serious suicidal act with clear expectation of death.
1	

NOTE: From "Diagnostic and Statistical Manual III—Revised" (p. 12). Washington, DC: American Psychiatric Association.

of *self-esteem disturbance, social isolation, defensive coping,* or any of the other almost 100 NANDA labels. Nurses get paid for diagnosing and treating disorders of schizophrenia and mood disorders, not for treating alterations in Perceiving or Choosing. Many nurse clinicians therefore survive by promoting the medical diagnosis system as they communicate and collaborate with other members of the mental health team. At present some clinicians are attempting to intervene with the third-party payment system so that psychiatric nurse clinical specialists will get paid for nursing practice and diagnoses rather than being coerced into making medical diagnoses. "The debate over the utilization of the medical model versus a nursing model is not an empty exercise in rhetoric. Rather its resolution will inform the direction we take in [molding the psychiatric nurse of the future]" (Taylor, 1986–1987, p. 8).

Slowly, however, nurses such as those on the ANA task force using their system and nurses using the NANDA system are meeting together as scholars in SERPN, whose mission is to meet the *nursing* care needs of a variety of population groups. Psychiatric nursing must look beyond the traditional institutional walls and deliver holistic care "that addresses clients' dysfunction in a setting that will be community-based without the professional support systems which are present in institutional settings. [This care must be delivered] in a cost-effective manner that is still clinically effective" (Taylor, 1986–1987, p. 9). Through a sound system of nursing diagnoses, we have to continue developing new roles for the psychiatric nurse, and we have to give up old ones (Slavinsky, 1984).

In keeping with a philosophy of evolution within the specialty, SERPN supports a diagnostic classification system that

1. Is built on the nursing paradigm.
2. Is consistent with the ANA *Social Policy Statement.*
3. Conforms to the ANA *Standards of Psychiatric/Mental Health Nursing Practice.*
4. Permits nurses to communicate with nurses in other clinical specialties in the terminology of the profession so that they may continue holistic intervention.
5. Permits nurses to communicate with nurses in other cultures and countries regarding the recipients of psychiatric/mental health nursing care.

DSM-III-R also is part of the gestalt of psychiatric/mental health nursing and some clinicians have developed unique ways of integrating this medical-based system into a nursing paradigm. The axial system of DSM-III-R (see Table 5) has been adapted for use with nursing modification. Coler and Vincent (1987), members of SERPN, have developed a model that uses Axes I and II for prioritizing NANDA nursing diagnoses—Axis I for those diagnoses having high intervention priority; Axis II for NANDA diagnoses having lower intervention priority. In their system, Axis III lists all medical (including psychiatric) diagnoses, while Axes IV and V are used, as in DSM-III-R, to indicate stressor and functional status. SERPN represents colleagues who continue to find the NANDA diagnoses inadequate to describe the phenomena addressed by psychiatric/mental health nurses as well as clinicians who practice only within the NANDA system. Therefore even though SERPN represents educational concerns, it must deal with the moral, ethical, and professional dilemmas in the area of diagnostics.

In summary, then, a dilemma of psychiatric nursing is that there are three diagnostic systems at its disposal. All the systems have something to contribute concerning communication within nursing and other disciplines. Autonomous practice does not preclude throwing the baby out with the medical bathwater, for the baby is swaddled in the clothing of holistic, intraprofessional, and interprofessional communication. The generic NANDA system seems to be the one that will eventually gain foothold, while the others will likely become incorporated into the NANDA system in creative ways.

References

American Nurses' Association. (1980). *Nursing: A social policy statement.* Kansas City, MO: Author.

American Nurses' Association. (1989). *Standards of practice for substance abuse nursing.* Kansas City, MO: Author.

American Nurses' Association. (1982). *Standards of psychiatric/mental health nursing practice.* Kansas City, MO: Author.

American Psychiatric Association. (1987). *Diagnostic and statistical manual III—Revised.* Washington, DC: Author.

Coler, M. (1989, October). *A nursing paradigm for group therapy.* Paper presented at the meeting of the Society for Education and Research in Psychiatric Nursing, Washington, DC.

Coler, M., da Nobrega, M., Perez, V., de Farias, J. (1990,

Table 5: DSM-III-R Multiaxial System

Axis I	Clinical syndromes
	V codes
Axis II	Developmental disorders
	Personality disorders
Axis III	Physical disorders and conditions
Axis IV	Severity of psychosocial stressors
Axis V	Global assessment of functioning

NOTE: From "Diagnostic and Statistical Manual III—Revised" (p. 10). Washington, DC: American Psychiatric Association.

March). *A Brazilian study of two diagnoses in the NANDA Human Response Pattern, Moving: A transcultural comparison.* Poster presented at the ninth biennial meeting of the North American Nursing Diagnosis Association, Orlando, FL.

Coler, M., Johnson, T., Amaro, A., Johnson, B., Snayd, J., Wiedliger, C., Caplan, C., Dodge, J., Lee, Y., & Thayer, K. (1989). NANDA Taxonomy I: A preliminary validation/invalidation study. In R. M. Carroll-Johnson (Ed.), *Classification of nursing diagnoses: Proceedings of the eighth conference* (pp. 141–151). Philadelphia: Lippincott.

Coler, M., & Vincent, K. (1987). Psychiatric/mental health assessment: A new look at the system. *Archives of Psychiatric Nursing, 1*, 258–263.

Doenges, M., Townsend, M., & Moorehouse, M. (1989). *Psychiatric care plans. Guidelines for client care.* Philadelphia: Davis.

McFarland, G., & Wasli, E. (1986). *Nursing diagnoses and process in psychiatric mental health nursing.* Philadelphia: Lippincott.

North American Nursing Diagnosis Association. (1989). *Taxonomy I revised.* St. Louis, MO: Author.

O'Toole, A., & Loomis, M. (1989). Revision of the phenomena of concern. *Archives of Psychiatric Nursing, 3*, 288–299.

Slavinsky, A. (1984). Psychiatric nursing in the year 2000: From a nonsystem of care to a caring system. *Image: The Journal of Nursing Scholarship, 16*, 17–20.

Stuart, G., & Sundeen, S. (1987). *Principles and practice of psychiatric nursing.* St. Louis, MO: Mosby.

Taylor, C. (1986–1987). Challenges and constraints in designing the educational blueprint for psychiatric-mental health nursing education: Climbing the down staircase. *Psychiatric-mental health nursing. Educational blueprint in the 21st century. Proceedings of regional conferences in curriculum development.* Washington, DC: U.S. Department of Health and Human Services.

American Society of Post Anesthesia Nursing

Maria T. Zickuhr, BS, RN, CPAN

This paper describes a method of implementing nursing diagnosis and nursing process in a rapid care setting. The American Society of Post Anesthesia Nursing (ASPAN) developed *Standards of Nursing Practice* (1986) in the format of the nursing process. At that time, the recovery room, as it was called in earlier years, was considered a "ship them in/ship them out" type of nursing. The rapid changing of patient conditions and quick turnover of patients provided the professional postanesthesia nurse with problems of documenting assessments, nursing diagnoses, and plans of care.

As Chairperson of ASPAN's Standards of Nursing Practice Committee at that time, I wanted to develop a documentation format that could utilize the Standards of Nursing Practice as a structure for documenting professional nursing care in the postanesthesia care units (PACUs) across the country. So in 1985 the Cleveland Clinic Foundation PACU implemented a mechanism to (1) provide planned care for and (2) document each prevalent postanesthesia nursing diagnosis. It was named the PES-EO-IO system.

The PES-EO-IO Charting System

The record, a foldout flow sheet, was developed to simplify charting all aspects of the nursing process. The front page consists of a data-collection portion and initial physical assessment. Each component is taken directly from the Standards of Nursing Practice. The second page lists the 12 most prevalent postanesthesia nursing diagnoses, also taken directly from the Standards and numbered 1 through 12 (see Figure 1). Note that *respiratory dysfunction* is a clustering of the multitude of respiratory problems we diagnose in the PACU of (1) *ineffective breathing pattern,* (2) *impaired gas exchange,* and (3) *ineffective airway clearance.* Also note that nursing diagnosis #1, *altered level of consciousness,* is utilized 100% of the time for each patient in PACU, but needs more research and study before it receives official NANDA approval.

Charting is then done using the following initials:
P = Problem
E = Etiology
S = Symptoms

NURSING DIAGNOSIS

1. altered level of consciousness
2. respiratory dysfunction
3. alterations in comfort
4. anxiety
5. alterations in cardiac output
6. abnormal tissue perfusion
7. alterations in fluid volume
8. alterations in urinary elimination
9. impairment of mobility (this includes decrease in muscle strength)
10. potential for injury
11. impairment of skin integrity
12. alterations in body temperature
13.
14.
15.

TEMP q _____

TURN q _____

INCENTIVE SPIROMETRY q _____

_____

SUCTION & SIGH q _____

_____

MOUTH CARE q_____

FOLEY CARE q _____

TREATMENTS _____

_____

_____

_____

Time		NURSING ASSESSMENT/INTERVENTIONS	Time		NURSING ASSESSMENT/INTERVENTIONS
9:00 a.m.	P	Alterations in comfort (or#3)			
	E	Anxiety, surgical procedure			
	S	Restlessness, tachycardia			
	EO	STD.*			
	I	Pain medication as needed, posi-			
		tion of comfort, turn of 2 hrs.,			
		provide emotional support,			
		provide PACU visitation with			
		family support member.			
	O	Patient resting comfortably with			
		family member present at 11:00a.m.			
		*Standard may be individualized			

FIGURE 1 The PES-EO-IO Charting System. Source: The Cleveland Clinic Foundation. Used with permission.

EO = Expected Outcome

I = Interventions

O = Outcome.

Because structurally nursing diagnosis consists of three elements—problem, etiology, and signs and symptoms—all three aspects are charted in this system.

The problem is documented using either the number of the nursing diagnosis on the record or by writing it out. If more than one nursing diagnosis (e.g., *impairment of mobility* and *potential for injury*) uses the same symptoms, etiology, and interventions, the problems can be clustered. Standards of care have been developed for each of the 12 nursing diagnoses. These are posted and are provided in the horizontal format. The expected outcome for each nursing diagnosis is documented. The nurse can use the standard of care and document "Std," or can individualize the standard. For example, the standard expected outcome (Std) for *alterations in comfort* may be "The patient will experience a decrease in pain sensation or freedom from pain." Or the standard expected outcome may be individualized to say "The patient's pain will be decreased from a severe level to a moderate level." More expert nurses are expected to individualize the expected patient outcomes on a routine basis.

Interventions are planned and listed to meet the expected outcome. Routine treatments such as temperature taking, turning, incentive spirometry, suctioning and sighing, mouth care, Foley catheter care, and treatments are listed and signed off on the treatment section, which is also found on the same page (Figure 1). The patient outcome is then charted when it is achieved. The goal is to meet all the expected outcomes prior to discharge. See Figure 1 for completed PES-EO-IO note.

Upon discharge, a PACU Discharge Summary is completed to communicate major treatments and unresolved nursing diagnoses to the patient care units (Figure 2). The primary care nurse then signs that the postanesthesia standards of care were met, with date and time.

The Cleveland Clinic Experience and Results

The PACU Practice Committee, whose members were all advanced postanesthesia nurses, monitored the charting system in 1985. Advanced postanesthesia nurses are so designated by the PACU's specifically designed clinical ladder, which includes a knowledge base and skill level for four levels of practice. The four levels of practice are based on the Benner (1984) model.

ASPAN's *Standards of Nursing Practice*

PACU DISCHARGE SUMMARY

Communicate major treatments and unresolved nursing diagnosis to patient care unit.

1. altered level of consciousness: _____
2. respiratory dysfunction. _____
3. alterations in comfort: _____
4. anxiety: _____
5. alterations in cardiac output: _____
6. abnormal tissue perfusion: _____
7. alterations in fluid volume: _____
8. alterations in urinary elimination: _____
9. impairment of mobility (this includes decrease in muscle strength): _____

10. potential for injury: _____
11. impairment of skin integrity: _____
12. alteration in body temperature: _____
13. _____
14. _____
15. _____
Dressing(s) _____
Drain(s) _____
IV(s) - Site(s) _____
Family Interaction _____

FIGURE 2 The PACU discharge summary. Source: The Cleveland Clinic Foundation. Used with permission.

(1986) were utilized as the basis for evaluation. Each standard and aspect of the nursing process was evaluated. Thirty charts were reviewed. Scores were consistently low with the exception of assessment, leading the Committee to conclude that the mechanism for documentation was inadequate. A new PACU record was developed based on the AS-PAN *Standards* and the nursing process. The PES-EO-IO charting system was developed by the author in order to implement planned care for each prevalent nursing diagnosis and as a mechanism for documenting care in a rapid care setting.

The PACU Practice Committee provided each staff member with a 2-hour inservice and practice session. A documentation reference book provided chart examples for several types of patients. Education included review of the Standards of Nursing Practice and emphasis on the relationship between the nursing process and PES-EO-IO charting. The goal was to teach nurses to evaluate the outcomes based on nursing diagnosis and to communicate this to the patient care unit upon discharge.

After implementation of the new record, the PACU Practice Committee reevaluated the charting system in 1988. The same number of charts were reviewed using the same criteria. The results of the second evaluation showed 90% to 100% compliance with all the standards (see Table 1).

Advantages of the PES-EO-IO System

Advantages of documentation using the PES-EO-IO system are many:

1. Nursing process and nursing diagnosis are utilized 100% of the time.
2. It provides a care plan without duplication of documentation.
3. Etiology, symptoms, and expected outcomes are documented in a time-saving method.

Table 1: Analysis of the Content of PACU Nurses' Notes Before and After Implementation of PES-EO-IO Charting and the New PACU Flow Sheet (n = 30)

	Before [%]	After [%]
Data collected and documented	30	99
Assessment completed	90	100
Nursing diagnosis present and based on data collected and assessment phase	25	100
Plan of care is formulated in conjunction with pre/intra/post-anesthesia health status assessments and involvement of family	46	99
Plan is implemented, altered, documented to achieve goal including family, planned intervention, routine care	50	90
Plan is evaluated and current assessment is collected and recorded to evaluate patient status for discharge	66	100
Patient is safely discharged in accordance with the ASPAN *Standards of Nursing Practice*, including communication to family member	70	100

4. It promotes follow-up on the patient care units on any unresolved nursing diagnoses.
5. It assists patient care units to develop their plan of care.
6. It incorporates the most prevalent nursing diagnoses in the postanesthesia care specialty, but leaves room for additional nursing diagnoses.
7. Addenda can be utilized in emergency situations such as when a patient comes into PACU in respiratory distress.
8. In their last two reviews of the Cleveland Clinic, the Joint Commission on Accreditation of Healthcare Organizations has been extremely positive regarding this method of charting, as patient expected outcomes and patient actual outcomes are documented.

9. Possibly the most important advantage is that it facilitates the development of a quality-assurance program utilizing prevalent nursing diagnoses. This can be achieved by
   a. Using each nursing diagnosis as the important aspect of care.
   b. Monitoring both process standards and outcome standards that were developed based on nursing diagnosis.
   c. Utilizing the flow sheet for retrospective monitoring by peers.
   d. Utilizing a concurrent method to monitor patients' actual outcomes.
   e. Utilizing initial reports and status reports to provide ongoing information of progress on each of the most prevalent patient problems and the current status of meeting patient needs.

The PES-EO-IO system can be adapted to any unit, but is especially helpful in any nursing area that has a rapid turnover of patients (e.g., emergency room, outpatient surgery areas, PACUs, and surgical intensive care areas) where patient status changes so rapidly that before the plan can be documented the problem changes. Therefore a time-saving method of documenting care is very desirable.

Integration of Nursing Diagnosis into Practice

The PES-EO-IO charting system is only a portion of the program to implement and integrate nursing diagnosis and nursing process into daily practice. The levels of the nursing professionals working on the particular unit can influence the program. The more advanced and senior the nurses are, the less time it will take to integrate nursing diag-

nosis. The entire program at Cleveland Clinic includes seven steps:

Step 1: Increase the staff's knowledge of the ASPAN *Standards of Nursing Practice* and nursing process.

Step 2: Decide on which nursing diagnoses are the most prevalent for a particular population.

Step 3: Develop process and outcome standards based on those nursing diagnoses.

Step 4: Develop a plan of care for each nursing diagnosis including etiology, symptoms, expected outcome, interventions, and deadline for achieving goals.

Step 5: Develop a documentation tool that augments all aspects of the nursing process.

Step 6: Develop a quality-assurance program based on each nursing diagnosis.

Step 7: Monitor the care based on both process and outcome standards for each nursing diagnosis.

Conclusion

The above seven-step program utilizes the ASPAN *Standards of Nursing Practice* and nursing diagnosis as the structure for the development of outcome and process standards and plans of care, and provides a basis for a unit-based quality-assurance program. This program can be utilized in all areas of nursing. It provides a cost-effective method of providing professional nursing care.

References

American Society of Post Anesthesia Nurses. (1986). *Standards of nursing practice.* Richmond, VA: Author.
Benner, P. (1984). *From novice to expert.* Norwalk, CT: Appleton-Century-Lange.

Association of Rehabilitation Nurses

Catherine A. Tracey, MS, RN, CRRN

The healthy function of the human body is dependent, in part, on a minimum level of activity. Many body systems are greatly affected when for any reason both healthy and ill individuals are immobilized. It has been noted in clinical practice and in the literature that symptoms related to prescribed or unavoidable immobilization appear in clusters (Asher, 1947; Beland & Passos, 1981; Carroll-Johnson, 1989; Dietrick, Whedon, & Shorr, 1948; Lentz, 1981; Levy & Talbot, 1983; Nicogossian & Parker, 1982; Olsen, 1967). Nurses observing the phenomena resulting from disuse have tended to list each component separately when in fact they occur as a cluster or syndrome. The nursing diagnosis of *potential disuse syndrome* assists nurses to identify and label the many potential complications of immobilization.

Immobilization is a condition that presents itself in many clinical areas of nursing. In fact most hospitalized patients are immobilized to some degree. The clinical specialty of rehabilitation nursing focuses on individuals with disabilities or changes in functional status. Immobilization is present in nearly 100% of this population, making *potential disuse syndrome* both common and useful in describing an important aspect of rehabilitation nursing. Also, interventions to treat *potential disuse syndrome* emphasize the preventive aspects of all nursing including rehabilitation.

Because the diagnosis is complex, requiring many interventions, it is very conducive to the development of standard process and outcome criteria. Through a standard plan of care, clinical specialty areas of nursing can develop interventions and outcomes that match their patient populations. Individual needs can then be added or deleted from the standard care plan. An example of a standard criteria set for rehabilitation is found in Table 1. It is a generic plan of care for the rehabilitation patient. It could be made more specific to address a designated population such as spinal cord injury or stroke patients.

Through the development of standard process and outcome criteria, quality-assurance monitors can be established. Review of both process and outcomes will reveal important data on the prevention and treatment of the complications of immobilization. Adjustments in treatment can then be recommended to assure more positive outcomes. Comparison of these data and associated costs in length of hospital stay, dollars, and patient discomfort or inconvenience can further outline the severity of the complications of immobilization.

Immobilization presents a unique challenge to rehabilitation nurses. The use of *po-*

Table 1: Potential Disuse Syndrome: Process and Outcome Criteria

Potential Disuse Syndrome: A state in which an individual is at risk for the complications of immobilization.
Risk factors: Paralysis, mechanical or prescribed immobilization, severe pain, altered level of consciousness

Complication	Process Criteria	Outcome Criteria
Pressure sore	Reposition 2–3x/shift. Relieve pressure qh when OOB. Initiate use of pressure-reducing devices. Reduce shearing forces. Monitor skin over bony prominences. Initiate bowel/bladder training programs. Monitor nutritional intake. Teach client rationale for above measures.	Intact skin
Constipation	Obtain bowel history. Plan bowel program to include when able: • Maximum mobility • Adequate fluid intake (2 liters/day) • Balanced diet (including fiber, fruit, vegetables). Assess need for stool softeners/peristaltic stimulators. Provide consistent implementation of bowel program. Schedule bowel program based on preillness pattern. Provide sitting position for bowel care when able. Dcument effectiveness of program. Teach rationale for interventions. Maximize client participation in program.	Regular, planned bowel movements
Urinary retention/ infection	Observe and assess for presence of retention/infection. Provide adequate fluid intake (2,400 cc/day, unless restricted). Space fluid to prevent distention. Monitor urine output. Provide sitting toileting position when able. Monitor retention with postvoid residuals. Collaborate with MD for management of retention. Teach rationale for interventions. Maximize participation in process.	Effective bladder emptying
Stasis of secretions/ pneumonia	Maximize mobility when able. Reposition, cough, and deep breathe 2–3x/shift. Institute incentive spirometry. Maintain adequate fluid intake (2,400 cc/day). Limit secretion-producing food and fluids. Institute pulmonary toilet. Provide aerosol treatment if necessary. Monitor breath sounds and change in volume/color of secretions. Discourage smoking. Teach rationale for interventions. Maximize participation in program.	Effective airway clearance
Thrombus formation/ pulmonary embolus	Maximize mobility when able. Utilize pressure boots when ordered (neg. PRG prior to application). Institute use of elastic stockings/wraps when OOB. Measure and record leg circumference at 6 in. and 9 in. above knee and 6 in. below knee qd; report differences greater than 2 cm.	Absence of thrombus/embolus

(continued)

Table 1: (*Continued*)

Complication	Process Criteria	Outcome Criteria
Decreased strength and endurance Muscle atrophy	Monitor legs for pain, heat, and redness. Monitor for SOB, ABG changes: • Decrease in PD^2 • Increased secretions • Cyanosis • Change in mental status • Change in breath sounds • Chest or referred pain • Splinting • Use of accesssory muscles • Shoulder pain Discourage smoking. Teach rationale for interventions. Maximize participation in program. Maximize mobility when able. Maximize involvement in self-care. Involve client in muscle-strengthening exercises in collaboration with PO/OT. Encourage/perform ROJM. Pace activities to increase endurance.	Maintenance of muscle strength and mass
Orthostatic hypotension	Teach rationale for interventions. Maximize involvement in preventive measures. Maximize mobility when able. Institute measures to increase vascular support (e.g., elastic stockings/wraps). Gradually raise head of bed to tolerance. Provide reclining chair and elevating leg rests if necessary for OOB activities. Monitor BP before and after activity.	Activity tolerance
Decreased ROJM/con-tracture	Teach rationale for interventions. Maximize involvement in preventive measures. Monitor for changes in ROJM. Encourage ROJM exercises. Consult PO/OT for interventions. Evaluate presence of spasticity. Apply positioning splints as needed.	Functional ROJM
Confusion/disorientation	Teach rationale for interventions. Maximize involvement in preventive measures. Assess baseline sensory/perceptual function. Provide for orienting devices (e.g., calendar, clock, TV, radio). Encourage client/family to obtain personal/familiar items. Orient client to person, place, and time if necessary. Orient client to seasons, weather, time of day. Provide diversional/recreational activities. Change position for environmental stimulation. Maximize involvement in self-care. Explain all procedures, treatments, tests. Introduce all caregivers/wear name tags. Institute measures to promote normal sleep/rest schedule.	Lack of confusion

(*continued*)

Table 1: (*Continued*)

Complication	Process Criteria	Outcome Criteria
Powerlessness	Teach rationale for interventions. Maximize involvement in preventive measures. Assess client's knowledge and involvement in self-care. Explain all care, procedures, tests. Provide for mutual goal setting for care. Plan team meetings to provide feedback and goal-setting opportunities. Provide for consistent caregivers. Provide means for calling for assistance. Teach method and rationale for all care, problem-solving skills, and methods of directing others to provide care. Maximize involvement and independence in self-care.	Expressed feeling of control
Body-image disturbance	Encourage verbalization of feelings. Offer choices for food, clothing, activities, schedule. Maximize mobility when able. Encourage peer interaction. Assess body-image perception. Encourage verbalization of feelings. Maximize independence in self-care. Encourage normalization activities (e.g., involvement with family and friends, client-initiated activities). Orient client to body changes through verbal description, reading material, mirrors. Teach rationale for interventions. Maximize client's involvement in preventive measures.	Expressed adjustment to body changes

tential disuse syndrome can assist the nurse to clearly identify a course of action to prevent the serious and life-threatening complications of immobilization.

References

Asher, R. (1947). Dangers of going to bed. *British Medical Journal, 2,* 967.

Beland, I. L., & Passos, J. Y. (1981). *Clinical nursing.* New York: Macmillan.

Carroll-Johnson, R. M. (Ed.). (1989). *Classification of nursing diagnoses: Proceedings of the eighth conference.* Philadelphia: Lippincott.

Dietrick, J. E., Whedon, D., & Shorr, E. (1948). Effects of immobilization upon various metabolic and physiologic functions of normal men. *American Journal of Medicine, 4,* 3–34.

Lentz, M. (1981). Selected aspects of deconditioning secondary to immobilization. *Nursing Clinics of North America, 16,* 729–737.

Levy, T., & Talbot, J. (1983). *Research opportunities in cardiovascular deconditioning* (Contract No. NASA 3616). Washington, DC: National Aeronautics and Space Administration.

Nicogossian, A., & Parker, J. (1982). *Space physiology and medicine* (NASA SP-447). Washington, DC: National Aeronautics and Space Administration.

Olsen, E. (1967). The hazards of immobility. *American Journal of Nursing, 67,* 780–797.

V

Poster Presentations—Abstracts

Validation Studies

Falls in the Elderly: Clinical Validation of Nursing Diagnoses and Defining Characteristics

Chanda Harrison, RN, CEN

The purpose of this study was to validate the defining characteristics of selected nursing diagnoses that might occur in the elderly client who has fallen and presented to the emergency department (ED). This descriptive study used the nursing process and the clinical validation model as its conceptual framework.

A convenience sample consisted of 35 English-speaking elderly clients with fall injuries who were conscious on arrival and who presented to the ED within 72 hours of the reported fall. The participant observer utilized a systematic assessment tool developed for this study. Nursing diagnoses and defining characteristics included in the tool were selected from the working list approved by NANDA. Content validity of the tool was examined by a panel of experts in geriatric emergencies and nursing diagnosis.

The raw data were analyzed using the SPSS-9 statistical package to obtain frequencies and percentages of occurrences of defining characteristics and nursing diagnoses. Major findings for the sample revealed that the most frequent defining characteristics observed were from the physically impaired functions (e.g., musculoskeletal and integumentary systems), the self-care deficits, and the coping problem categories. A large number of defining characteristics were present in only a few cases or absent in all cases. No clusters of critical defining characteristics were identified in the data. Some defining characteristics were cues for more than one diagnostic label. Two labels, *anxiety* and *fear*, were found to be used as both defining characteristics and nursing diagnoses. The most frequently identified nursing diagnoses were *impaired physical mobility* and *self-care deficit*.

The results of these findings contribute to the body of knowledge of nursing diagnosis validation studies. Also, the results have implications for the development of the role of the ED nurse in the care of the elderly. The ED nurse can use those results to alter assessment expectations to include pathologies and symptomatologies unique to the elderly client. An assessment tool could be used to generate a database specifically tailored for elderly clients who suffer falls, with subsequent development of a standard care plan for these clients. A computer program could be designed from the assessment tool to pre-select nursing diagnostic labels based on the presenting signs and symptoms. Further research studies should be designed to define a method for identifying an effective means of determining the criteria for clustering categories.

Respiratory Nursing Diagnoses: Nurses' Ability to Select Their Defining Characteristics

Terry A. Capuano, MSN, RN
Kim S. Hitchings, MSN, RN
Sharon E. Johnson, BSN, RNC
Karen M. Schaefer, DNSc, RN

The proceedings of the Eighth National Conference on Nursing Diagnosis lists three respiratory nursing diagnoses (RND): *impaired gas exchange (IGE), ineffective airway clearance (IAC),* and *ineffective breathing pattern (IBP),* and the defining characteristics for each. Whether or not the defining characteristics listed for each diagnosis are mutually exclusive or valid has not been firmly established. This study was conceived as the first of a series of studies intended to validate the RNDs. The purpose of this research was to investigate whether professional nurses working in two comparable tertiary care settings in eastern Pennsylvania were able to select the defining characteristics associated with each RND as defined by NANDA.

A retrospective method design using a survey approach was used to determine if a convenience sample of 100 professional nurses employed in medical-surgical units at Lehigh Valley Hospital Center and Bryn Mawr Hospital during spring 1988 were able to select the defining characteristics associated with each of the RNDs. Each institution had formally introduced nursing diagnosis to all nurses and had integrated nursing diagnoses into their plans of care five years previously. The sample was limited to nurses who had been employed for more than one year and less than five years. A Respiratory Nursing Diagnosis Scale (RNDS) was developed for this study by the investigators. Major defining characteristics associated with the RNDs were listed alphabetically to avoid predetermined clustering of characteristics. Data collectors were three of the investigators who stayed with subjects during the data collection. Simple statistical analysis was used.

Findings indicated that the nurses were unable to select the defining characteristics associated with each RND on a consistent basis. Of the three RNDs, *IAC* had the highest percent agreement with NANDA. This occurred both when NANDA did and did not identify a characteristic as associated with an RND. When all three RNDs were considered, if NANDA identified a characteristic as such, there was a 45% to 99% range of agreement with a mean of 80.3%. When NANDA did not identify a characteristic, the range of agreement was 2% to 58% with a mean of 29.6%. For those defining characteristics NANDA associated with one RND and not the others, the percent agreement with NANDA did not approach 50%.

These findings have significance since nurses must be able to select and label respiratory problems correctly if desired interventions are to be implemented.

Toward a Model of Clinical Validation of Nursing Diagnoses: Developing Conceptual and Operational Definitions of *Impaired Physical Mobility*

Nancy S. Creason, PhD, RN

At the April 1989 NANDA Invitational Conference on Clinical Validation of Nursing Diagnoses, the need for ongoing development of models of validation and research to define diagnoses was emphasized. A comprehensive model that included as its first phase the operational and conceptual definition of specific diagnoses was proposed.

The goal of this study was to develop a prototype tool to be used in the conceptual and operational definition of nursing diagnoses. The specific focus of this project was to develop and test a tool to determine conceptual and operational definitions for the diagnosis *impaired physical mobility.*

Conceptual and operational definitions for the etiologies and defining characteristics of *impaired physical mobility* were developed, based on empirical data from experience and from the literature. These were incorporated into a tool that asked the respondent to agree or disagree with the definition and to provide suggestions for change. The tool was given to 10 nurses with expertise in the use of nursing diagnosis and in the care of patients with mobility problems. This multistep process involved three rounds to achieve consensus on definitions of etiologies and two rounds to achieve consensus on definitions of defining characteristics. A fairly comprehensive operational definition of *impaired physical mobility* has resulted from this work.

The next phase of this research, testing the definition with a larger group of nurses who work with patients with mobility problems but who do not necessarily have highly developed expertise in nursing diagnosis use or mobility care, is presently underway. After this broad consensual validity, the definitions can be used in clinical validation studies.

Validation of *Sleep Pattern Disturbance*

Samar N. Assousa, MSN, RN
Nina D. Wilson, RN

A study was conducted to validate the defining characteristics of *sleep pattern disturbance (SPD)*. The purpose of the study was to examine those defining characteristics and their frequency of occurrence, and to distinguish between *SPD* and *sleep deprivation (SD)*.

A sample of 60 registered nurses caring for hospitalized adult patients in two 800–1,000-bed, acute care facilities participated in this study. Each nurse assessed three written patient scenarios for the purpose of diagnosing *SPD*. Demographic data were collected on the experience of nurses in applying nursing diagnoses in their practice.

Thirty-three defining characteristics were analyzed using factor analysis and stepwise multiple regression to distinguish between *SPD* and *SD*, and to identify the critical defining characteristics that nurses used when making the diagnosis of *SPD*. Factor analysis produced two factors that were consistent with *SPD* and *SD*. Results from the stepwise multiple regression of the scenarios supported the proposition that *SPD* and *SD* are two separate, yet related, entities. In addition, these results suggested that *SD* may be the result of unrecognized or untreated *SPD*.

Validation of the Defining Characteristics of *Ineffective Airway Clearance*

Genee Brukwitzki, MSN, RN
Cynthia Holmgren, MSN, RN, OCN
Regina Maibusch, MS, RN

To build a scientific base for the use of nursing diagnosis, validation studies are needed. This study explored the question: What are the major and minor defining characteristics of the nursing diagnosis *ineffective airway clearance?* A total of 546 nurses (members of the nursing section of the American Thoracic Society, American Association of Critical Care Nurses, American Lung Association of the Wisconsin Nursing Assembly, or published authors in this area) who care for respiratory patients were sent the validation questionnaire. This instrument requested the respondent to rate the relevancy of 29 characteristics of the diagnosis on a five-point Likert scale. Using the Fehring formula of weighted ratios, characteristics rated as 0.8 or more were identified as major; characteristics rated as more than 0.5 but less than 0.8 were identified as minor. Those characteristics rated less than 0.5 were designated not relevant.

A three-round Delphi survey was used to gain consensus among respondents. The number of respondents totaled 183 (33.5%) in the first round, 88 (48%) in the second round, and 50 (56.8%) in the third round. Comments from participants were shared in the second and third rounds.

The typical respondent had a 90%+ caseload of respiratory patients, was a staff nurse or clinical nurse specialist, and was employed in a respiratory intensive care unit or respiratory outpatient service in an acute care hospital.

Frequency distributions of responses were done and descriptive statistics were calculated. One characteristic was rated as major: cough, ineffective (.905). Nineteen characteristics were rated as minor: sputum, tenacious (.790); subjective complaints of inability to cough up secretions (.770); sputum, copious (.750); rhonchi (gurgles) (.724); sputum, increased (.670); absent breath sounds (.670); decreased breath sounds (.600); air hunger (.597); tachypnea (.595); abnormal breath sounds (.575); abnormal respiratory pattern (.575); rhonchi (wheezes) (.570); cyanosis (.564); nasal flaring (.561); rales (crackles) (.560); anxiety (.560); dyspnea at rest (.535); sputum, change in color (.530); restlessness (.500). Nine characteristics were rated as not relevant: asymmetric chest excursion (.490); abnormal inspiratory to expiratory ratio (.465); dyspnea on exertion (.460); fever (.395); pain (.390); bradypnea (.367); diaphoresis (.350); sputum, decreased (.347); and cough, effective (.310).

Nurse Validation of Pressure Ulcer Risk Factors

Sheila M. (Cress) Sparks, DNSc, RN, CS

The management of skin integrity problems has traditionally been recognized as an independent nursing function. Human need theory considers maintenance of skin integrity to be a survival need; interruption of skin integrity poses serious and life-threatening consequences. A study was conducted to validate risk factors of patients with the nursing diagnosis of *potential impaired skin integrity: pressure ulcer.*

The purpose of this study was to (1) obtain expert nurse validation of risk factors present in patients with the nursing diagnosis of *potential impaired skin integrity: pressure ulcer,* and (2) compare these factors with the risk factors identified in the NANDA Taxonomy 1 and those identified by the investigator through a review of the pressure ulcer research literature.

Two investigator-developed instruments, the Diagnostic Content Validity Tool: Potential Impaired Skin Integrity (DCVT:PISI) and Q-Sort: Potential Impaired Skin Integrity (QS:PISI), were used. Demographic data about the subjects were collected on the Demographic Data Sheet. Initial content validity indices established the reliability of the DCVT:PISI to be 0.89 by coefficient alpha,

the diagnostic content validity score was 0.77; both tools were judged by a panel of 10 experts to be representative of the domain of interest (3.6 on a scale of 1 to 4).

Categories for items were drawn from risk factors identified by NANDA and those identified by the investigator through literature review. The diagnostic content validity model (DCV) described by Fehring and the Q-Sort methodology were used. Identification of major, minor, and unnecessary risk factors was made, and risk factors were ranked.

The sample consisted of 204 registered nurses identified by the director of nurses as being expert in the management of skin integrity problems and who responded to a mail survey sent to a geographically stratified random sample of 300 facilities drawn from 280 facilities with inpatient rehabilitation units and 172 VA facilities (68% return rate).

Major risk factors of the patient who develops a pressure ulcer were pressure, shearing forces, mobility status, incontinence, nutritional status, and friction. The diagnostic content validity score was 0.76; reliability was 0.8963 by coefficient alpha. Further analysis is being conducted.

Given the number of risk factors identified

by NANDA and the investigator, it is possible that nurses are not able to organize the data into retrievable clusters. The information-processing model may aid cluster formation. The knowledge gained about risk factors may assist nurses in preventing pressure ulcers, thus alleviating or minimizing human suffering.

Self-Care Deficit, Bathing/Hygiene: Defining Characteristics and Related Factors Utilized by Staff Nurses in an Acute Care Setting

Rosemary J. McKeighen, PhD, RN, FAAN
Peg A. Mehmert, MSN, RN, C
Carol A. Dickel, RN

The purpose of this descriptive study was validation and refinement of the nursing diagnosis *self-care deficit, bathing/hygiene.* Data from a computerized, NANDA diagnosis-based care planning program were used to examine the defining characteristics and related factors nurses chose to support this diagnosis in their clinical patient populations. The list of defining characteristics included those identified by NANDA plus inability to perceive need for hygienic measures. The related factors also contained the published NANDA list, as well as those inductively identified by the hospital nursing staff. They were (a) *ineffective coping*, (b) *knowledge deficit* regarding affected body parts, (c) *knowledge deficit* regarding spatial relationships, (d) *mobility impairment*, and (e) maturational factors.

The following research questions were generated: (1) Which defining characteristics are clinically assessed by staff nurses when diagnosing *self-care deficit, bathing/hygiene*? (2) Which related factors are selected by staff nurses that are antecedent to, contribute to, are associated with, or support the existence of the diagnosis? (3) What age groups are represented when the diagnosis is made? and (4) In what Diagnosis Related Groups (DRGs) is the diagnosis present? Orem's Self-Care Deficit Nursing Theory served as the theoretical framework.

Computerized reports that listed utilization of diagnostic labels, defining characteristics, related factors, as well as patient expected outcomes and nursing orders for all inpatients became accessible to the division of nursing in May 1989. The sampling frame consisted of those patients with this diagnosis who were discharged subsequent to the availability of these reports. This convenience sample consisted of 124 subjects discharged between May 16 and July 31, 1989.

Data were retrospectively abstracted by electronic data retrieval and reports were analyzed to determine the presence or absence of defining characteristics and the frequency of each factor associated with the presence of the diagnosis. Age and DRG were examined to determine heterogeneity/homogeneity of the diagnosis across the sample.

Descriptive summary statistics, Chi-Square, and Fisher's One Factor ANOVA were applied to the data. Some of the defining characteristics and related factors were affirmed. Major support was found for inability to wash body or body parts (84%) and minor support for inability to obtain/access water source (77%). The third NANDA defining characteristic, inability to regulate temperature or flow, was supported by only 0.8% of respondents. A refinement of the diagnostic process would be enhanced with the addition of another characteristic, inability to perceive need for hygienic measures, which garnered 9% support across the sample and was demonstrated in 100% ($n = 3$) of the psychiatric subset.

Decreased activity tolerance (intolerance to activity) was shown to be the strongest related factor (40%). Pain and musculoskeletal impairment were each supported by 19% of the subjects, followed by neuromuscular impairment (9%), perceptual or cognitive impairment (4%), and anxiety (.8%). No support was shown for depression. *Mobility impairment* demonstrated the strongest support (24%). The maturational factor yielded 2% and the remaining two, *ineffective coping* and *knowledge deficit*, were each supported by 0.8%. Support for these refinement factors suggests a need for inclusion of these as criteria to be used for accurate assessment of *self-care deficit, bathing/hygiene*. The diagnosis appeared across all age groups (range 9 to 29 years) and demonstrated heterogeneity among DRGs ($n = 80$). The use of Orem's Self-Care Deficit Nursing Theory as explication of nursing practice adds to second-level theory building.

Diagnostic Content Validity of *Impaired Gas Exchange:* A Construct Replication

Joan Love, MS, RN
Marie Cox, MSN, RN
Joseph Molinatti, BSN, RN
Carol Ann Mitchell, EdD, RN

Many nurses in acute and critical care settings are believed to diagnose and treat signs, symptoms, and medical diagnoses of patients, but other studies are finding that nurses are increasingly using nursing diagnoses to organize their care. The complexity of the diagnostic process is increased because of the nature of critical care units (CCUs), the dynamic and often unreliable or unstable state of cues, and the rapidity with which diagnoses must be generated. Making nursing diagnoses and prescribing interventions without having established a valid research base make validation studies a research imperative. The purpose of this study was to determine the diagnostic content validity (DCV) of the diagnostic category *impaired gas exchange*, a frequently observed problem in CCUs. This study was part of a cluster study investigating tracer diagnoses in different patient populations.

A survey design was used for data collection. A convenience sample of 67 critical care nurses was obtained from a major metropolitan teaching/research hospital. Levin, Krainovich, Bahrenburg, and Mitchell's modification of Fehring's DCV model was used to determine validity of the defining characteristics. For this study, the New York State practice act was the first criterion for selecting RNs as expert, regardless of educational background, and the second was more than 6 months' experience in critical care units. A demographic form and a DCV rating scale for the diagnostic category under investigation were used to collect data. Content validity of the diagnostic category was determined by calculating an average for each defining characteristic and then obtaining a total DCV score by summing and averaging these subscores. Characteristics with a score of 4.1 to 5.0 are major indicators, 3.1 to 4.0 are minor indicators, while those below 3.0 are not considered relevant.

The total DCV score for this diagnosis was 4.02. Major and minor defining characteristics were identified; no characteristic scored below 3.5. The subscores for each characteristic were hypoxia (4.8); hypercapnea (4.7); confusion (3.9); restlessness (3.9); inability to move secretions (3.8); irritability (3.6); and somnolence (3.5). Many diagnoses in CCUs are physiologic in nature, requiring immediate expert attention. Not surprisingly, CCU nurses seem to prefer ratio-measurable data. Of note is that confusion scored 3.9, perhaps reflecting expert use of quantitative and qualitative data for inferences. Further study is indicated to differentiate confusional states observed in critical versus stable conditions.

Diagnostic Content Validity of *Fluid Volume Excess:* A Construct Replication

Elizabeth Sergent, BS, RN
Cathrine Strauss, BS, RN
Michelle Jaffe, BS, RN
Eleanor Majewsky, BS, RN
Carol Ann Mitchell, EdD, RN

Many nurses are currently using nursing diagnoses and prescribing interventions without having established a valid research base. Because organizations such as the Joint Committee for Accreditation of Hospital Organizations are requiring documentation of nursing diagnoses on care plans and the possibility that reimbursement for services will be based on nursing diagnoses make validation studies a research imperative. The purpose of this study was to determine the diagnostic content validity (DCV) of the diagnostic category *fluid volume excess*, a frequently observed problem in clinical practice. This study was part of a cluster study investigating tracer diagnoses in different patient populations.

A survey design was used for data collection. A convenience sample of 100 medical-surgical registered nurses was obtained from two teaching hospitals of approximately 500 beds each. Levin, Krainovich, Bahrenburg, and Mitchell's modification of Fehring's DCV model was used to determine validity of the defining characteristics. This model uses experts to establish the relevance of items of the concept being measured. For this study, the New York State nurse practice act was used to determine that a registered nurse working with a population of patients diagnoses and treats them and is therefore expert. A demographic form and a DCV rating scale for the diagnostic category under investigation were used to collect data. Content validity of the diagnostic category was determined by calculating an average for each defining characteristic and then obtaining a total DCV score by summing and averaging these subscores. Defining characteristics with a score of 4.1 to 5.0 are major indicators, 3.1 to 4.0 are minor indicators, while those below 3.0 are not considered relevant.

The DCV score for *fluid volume excess* was 4.29. Major and minor defining characteristics were identified; no characteristic scored below 3.0. The subscores for each characteristic were edema, effusion, anasarca (4.84); abnormal breath sounds (4.56); pulmonary congestion by chest x-ray (4.51); shortness of breath, dyspnea, orthopnea (4.50); sudden weight gain (4.41); intake greater than output, oliguria, urine specific gravity changes (4.40); blood, venous/pulmonary artery pressure changes (4.39); jugular vein distention, positive hepatojugular reflex, S_3 heart sound (4.35); altered electrolytes (4.16); restlessness, anxiety (3.83); decreased Hgb and Hct (3.82); and mental status changes (3.71). Physiologic indicators and those indicative of a more critical status were rated higher than psychologic and less serious indicators. An implication for further study would be temporal order of the characteristics to facilitate early intervention for this problem.

Nursing Diagnoses in Particular Settings, Places, Populations

A Brazilian Study of Two Diagnoses in the NANDA Human Response Pattern, Moving: A Transcultural Comparison

Marga Simon Coler, EdD, RN, CS, CTN
Maria Miriam Lima da Nobrega, BS
Vera Lucia de Almeida Peres, MS
Juracy Nunes de Farias, MS

The necessity to validate nursing diagnoses for use in other cultures is frequently addressed and emphasized in the scientific literature of the profession. The use of nursing diagnoses in the clinical area is a significant step for Brazilian nursing in its quest for professional autonomy. However, it is of utmost importance to validate them for use in the context of the Brazilian culture. The purpose of this study, therefore, was to begin the validation process of and within the NANDA human response patterns (HRPs) with the objective of validating and comparing the defining characteristics of two nursing diagnoses. *Diversional activity deficit* and *altered health maintenance*, both in the NANDA HRP Moving, were identified in a majority of nursing students in a study that later served to justify the establishment of a mental health center at the Federal University of Paraiba (Brazil). This mental health center, Centro de Atendimento de Saude Mental (CASM), inaugurated at the univer-

sity in August 1989, is based on a nursing paradigm. Its two objectives are to (1) assess and treat (via nursing diagnoses) nursing students during their academic life, and (2) serve as a center for research on nursing diagnoses.

This phenomenologic study began with an interview of a convenience sample of 34 undergraduate nursing students, using a translated version of the Coler and Vincent Comprehensive Assessment Tool: Individual. From this the investigators were able to isolate subjective and objective data in each category to facilitate the identification of diagnostic characteristics. These were clustered and ultimately pointed the way to diagnostic labeling. Each student emerged with at least one nursing diagnosis. The greatest frequency was found in the HRP Moving, in which the diagnoses *diversional activity deficit* ($n = 31$; 91.2%) and *alteration in health maintenance* ($n = 21$; 73.5%) were identified in the majority of subjects.

The data demonstrated that there is little

difference between the defining characteristics approved by NANDA for the two diagnoses, and that the characteristics were identified in the subjects. The significance of the study lies in the area of transcultural/international nursing. At this juncture, the taxonomy, based only on North American input, has been submitted by the NANDA Board of Directors and the Taxonomy Committee, with American Nurses' Association liaison, to the World Health Organization for inclusion in the ICD-10. It is important that diagnoses in the ICD represent all cultures.

High-Volume/High-Risk Nursing Diagnoses as a Basis for Priority Setting in a Tertiary Hospital

Joan B. Fitzmaurice, PhD, RN
Joseph Thatcher, BS, RN
Nancy Schappler, MSN, RN

Patient populations are often described using diagnosis related groups (DRGs), yet this classification may not adequately direct nursing activity. The purpose of this descriptive survey was to identify the high-volume/high-risk nursing diagnoses in a 1,000-bed tertiary hospital in order to guide standards development, quality-assurance programs, educational activities, and resource allocation. Because patient records were an unreliable or unavailable source of data at the time of the study, elected members of nine nursing practice committees were surveyed by mailed questionnaire. Eighty-five nurses (81% response rate) selected 10 high-volume/high-risk nursing diagnoses from a preprinted list for which nursing interventions would be expected to affect outcome during hospitalization (average length of stay less than 10 days).

The most frequent nursing diagnoses across all practice committees were *pain* (52%), *potential for infection* (43%), *potential impairment of skin integrity* (38%), *knowledge deficit* (38%), *impaired physical mobility* (35%), *constipation* (32%), *ineffective airway clearance* (28%), *nutritional deficit* (27%), *anxiety* (26%), and *potential for injury* (26%). Eight of these nursing diagnoses relate to a deviation of normal body functioning, while *knowledge deficit* and *anxiety* are known to be associated with hospitalization.

When the findings were examined according to nursing service, other nursing diagnoses were identified by more than 50% of the respondents in all but the Orthopedic (*n* = 5) and Psychiatric (*n* = 7) Nursing Practice Committees. They were Surgical (*n* = 23): *impaired skin integrity;* Medical (*n* = 15): *total self-care deficit;* Neuroscience (*n* = 10): *total self-care deficit, impaired thought processes, altered urinary elimination;* Pediatric (*n* = 6): *impaired gas exchange, decreased cardiac output;* Intensive Care (*n* = 8): *sleep pattern disturbance, decreased cardiac output, impaired gas exchange, excess fluid volume;* Operating Room (*n* = 8): *po-*

tential altered temperature; and Ambulatory (*n* = 3): *diarrhea.*

Within the broad scope of practice in a tertiary facility, a description of high-volume/high-risk nursing diagnoses will help delineate those areas in which professional nursing should assume accountability for outcomes of care. These nursing diagnoses can also provide a framework for recruiting clinically expert nurses.

Nursing Diagnosis–Nursing Process for the Group Client

Shirley M. Ziegler, PhD, RN
Wilda K. Arnold, EdD, RN
Rose M. Nieswiadomy, PhD, RN

The purpose of a large, ongoing study is to validate a developing nursing process model, generated by the investigators, that is designed to focus on the client "group" as an interactional whole. Three specific problems were identified for this step of the research: (1) evaluate the content validity of a developing Model of Nursing Process for the Group Client; (2) determine the extent to which selected group nursing diagnosis etiologies reflect the dimension of group process that each etiology was intended to reflect; and (3) determine the frequency of occurrence of selected group nursing diagnoses.

Fourteen nurse subjects experienced in working with groups of clients, but unfamiliar with the proposed model, were asked to indicate on a Likert scale the degree to which they viewed the validity of each of the 37 assumptions of the model. Sample nursing diagnoses were presented for each of the nine dimensions of groups (identified from the literature) that the model assumed should be assessed, diagnosed, and then serve as the focus of group nursing interventions. Subjects indicated the frequency with which they had observed each of the components of the diagnoses and the degree to which they believed each diagnosis reflected the dimension it was designed to describe.

Thirty-two of the 37 assumptions were viewed as valid, indicating the need to modify only five of the assumptions. Although all nursing diagnoses were observed at least occasionally, none of the diagnoses was observed frequently, indicating a need for generating more commonly occurring diagnoses. Because most of the sample diagnoses were judged to be representative of the dimension they were designed to represent, some content validity for them was established. More representative diagnoses for the developmental-phase dimension need to be generated. The model has potential usefulness for familiarizing the nurse with the use of nursing diagnosis and nursing process with the group client.

Preliminary work in describing a group nursing diagnosis and nursing process model has been partially validated. As nurses focus on groups of clients, the need to reframe a nursing diagnosis–nursing process format specific to the group client is imperative.

259

The Effects of Implementation of an Operational Definition and Guidelines for the Formulation of Nursing Diagnoses in a Critical Care Setting

Kay Knox Greenlee, MSN, RN, CCRN

The purpose of this study was to validate the findings of previous research on the use of nursing diagnosis in an acute care setting. Previous research indicated that with the implementation of an operational definition and guidelines for the formulation of nursing diagnoses, the critical care patient care area had a significantly increased mean score assigned to each diagnostic statement. The mean score was a determination of quality of the diagnostic statement as measured by five criteria that evaluated the relationship between the nursing diagnosis and the other steps of the nursing process. The eight other patient care areas included in the study did not have a significant change in the mean scores for the diagnostic statements. In this study the charts of 75 patients were reviewed to obtain a list of nursing diagnoses written one year before the implementation of a definition and guidelines (Group A), and 75 charts were reviewed one year after implementation (Group B). The 75 charts represent 25 charts from each of three different types of critical care units: intensive care, intermedi-

ate care, and telemetry. The review resulted in 120 nursing diagnoses in Group A and 106 nursing diagnoses in Group B. The diagnostic statements were evaluated and scored using evaluation forms designed for the initial study. The percentage of nursing diagnoses with a perfect score of 5 was 12% for Group A and 50% for Group B. The mean score for the entire sample significantly increased from 3.39 for Group A to 4.37 for Group B ($p < .001$). The mean scores for the individual units also significantly improved from Group A to Group B.

Three nursing diagnoses, *altered comfort, anxiety,* and *potential for injury,* were most frequently used in each group. *Knowledge deficit* and *impaired gas exchange* were the other nursing diagnoses used most frequently in Group A, and *activity intolerance, self-care deficit,* and *ineffective coping* were those used most frequently in Group B. A significantly greater number of nursing diagnoses could be categorized under one of Gordon's 11 Functional Health Patterns after the implementation of an operational definition and guidelines for the formulation of nursing diagnoses. The nursing diagnoses identified included diagnoses categorized in eight of the Functional Health Patterns. No nursing diagnoses were identified in either group for the Elimination, Sexuality-Reproductive, of Value-Belief Patterns.

The researcher concluded that the operational definition and guidelines for the formulation of nursing diagnoses provided the critical care nurse with a method to write higher quality nursing diagnoses. The guidelines also helped the nurse to write diagnostic statements that were in the realm of nursing. This is supported by the results that almost all the nursing diagnoses could be categorized under one of the Functional Health Patterns for Group B. In Group A

there were a number of general nursing diagnoses written that related to the medical diagnosis; only one such diagnosis was written for Group B.

The results of this study indicate the methods used to refine the use of nursing diagnosis in an acute care setting are most helpful to the critical care setting. Critical care has been one patient care area that has struggled with the use of nursing diagnosis since its inception. Further research on the use of nursing diagnosis in a practice setting is indicated. As organizations implement or refine the use of nursing diagnosis, it will be important to monitor and evaluate the changes that take place. The researcher recommends a replication of this study in an institution that has not implemented nursing diagnosis.

Utilization of Nursing Diagnosis in South Dakota

June Larson, MS, RN
Deborah Soholt, BSN, RN
Candice Friestad, MS, RN, CCRN, CNA
Marilyn Abraham, BSN, RN
Deb Fischer Clemens, BSN, RN
M. Kay M. Judge, EdD, RN
Phyllis Meyer Gaspar, PhD, RN
Donna Loy Ritter, MN, RN

The purpose of the South Dakota Nursing Association ad hoc Committee on Nursing Diagnosis is to promote the utilization of nursing diagnosis and to encourage research in all areas of nursing diagnosis. The committee views nursing diagnosis as a concept, a tool, and a documentation system whose time has come. A review of articles in current nursing journals and nursing texts published in the past five years confirms the impression that the issue is not whether to implement nursing diagnosis in a health care agency, but *how* to do so.

This research was conducted to determine (1) the utilization of nursing diagnosis by health care agencies in South Dakota and (2) what resources are needed to assist with utilization of nursing diagnoses. This descriptive study was carried out in the rural state of South Dakota. A questionnaire was mailed to the Director of Nursing or Administrator of 248 South Dakota health care facilities; 111 (44.8%) were returned. Two of the returned questionnaires were not usable and were not included in the data analysis. The questionnaire consisted of questions concerning the implementation of nursing diagnosis in that agency and addressed the need for further resources. The participants were asked to identify a contact person for nursing diagnosis in the agency. Fifty-three percent of the 111 responding agencies indicated that they have implemented nursing diagnosis using various implementation strategies. Eighty-two percent of the respondents indicated a need for additional resources.

The use of nursing diagnosis is a vital part of the advancement of the nursing profession. The survey results indicate a strong need for various educational resources to assist in the implementation of nursing diagnosis. As a result of this survey, the Committee for Nursing Diagnosis will develop resources and make these accessible to all nurses in South Dakota. This is necessary to assist nurses in developing or advancing their care planning skills utilizing nursing diagnosis.

Alteration in Self-Care: An Instance of Ineffective Coping in the Geriatric Patient

Christina Lewis, BSN, RN
Brooke P. Randell, DNSc, RN

Alteration in individual coping was one of the most frequently used NANDA diagnostic categories on adult and geriatric psychiatric inpatient units of a major university hospital. Analysis of the defining characteristics associated with this diagnostic category revealed that it was used to describe 17 different problems. Given the inconsistencies observed in the use of this and other NANDA labels, a diagnostic system was instituted that was derived from the Johnson Behavioral Systems Model, the basis for the provision of nursing care in the institution.

This study sought to identify the most frequently occurring Johnson-based diagnostic labels utilized in a population of hospitalized geropsychiatric patients. The defining characteristics and the related factors associated with these diagnostic labels were compared to those of NANDA diagnostic categories to determine areas of similarity and differences.

The study was descriptive and involved a retrospective chart review of 36 patient records. Sixty percent of the patients whose records were reviewed had a primary diagnosis of

depression. At admission, 85% of the 36 patients carried an additional medical diagnosis such as heart disease or diabetes. A total of 56 nursing diagnoses were identified. Five different Achievement System diagnoses were combined resulting in a total of 17 diagnoses (30%) reflecting patient problems with self and environmental mastery. Defining characteristics and related factors associated with these 17 Johnson-based diagnoses were compared with the NANDA diagnostic categories.

The study revealed that there were 10 different NANDA diagnostic categories that overlapped or were related to the five Johnson-based diagnostic labels. Based on a review of defining characteristics, all 17 diagnoses could be subsumed under the NANDA diagnostic category of Alteration in Individual Coping. Nine of the diagnoses could be included under the NANDA diagnostic category of Impaired Physical Mobility. An additional six Johnson-based achievement diagnoses fell under the diagnostic category of Alteration in Self-Care.

These findings suggest redundancy in the

264

NANDA diagnostic categories and offer support for consolidation. In addition, these data suggest an underlying problem with the taxonomy. If all the Johnson-based diagnoses were described by the defining characteristics and related factors associated with Alteration in Coping, a category under the taxonomic label of Choosing, how can we reconcile the fact that 75% of these diagnoses also included the defining characteristics and related factors associated with diagnostic categories under the taxonomic label of Moving?

Independent Nursing Diagnosis in Emergency Nursing

Kathleen M. Baldwin, PhD, RN

The problem of study was the validation, by emergency nurses, of investigator-generated nursing diagnoses occurring secondary to illness/injury in emergency nursing. The study's purpose was to delineate an area of independent practice within emergency nursing.

The research questions for this study were as follows:

1. What is the frequency of occurrence, as estimated by emergency nurses, of the investigator-generated (actual or potential) unhealthful responses of emergency patients that are secondary to injury/illness?

2. What is the frequency of occurrence, as estimated by emergency nurses, of the selected investigator-generated nursing diagnoses (selected investigator-generated responses plus selected investigator-generated etiologies) that reflect the independent nursing role in emergency patients secondary to injury/illness?

3. What additional etiologies are associated with the selected investigator-generated (potential or actual) unhealthful responses in emergency pa-

tients secondary to injury/illness as identified by emergency nurses?

4. To what extent are additional nursing etiologies (for the selected investigator-generated responses) identified by the emergency nurses associated with the independent or interdependent nursing role?

The nursing process model of Ziegler, Vaughan-Wroble, and Erlen was used as the theoretical framework for the study. A descriptive design was used in this national survey of emergency nurses, who were accessed through 59 local chapters of the Emergency Nurses Association. A total of 590 surveys were mailed; 254 (42%) were returned. Instruments used in the study were investigator-generated questionnaires. These had been submitted to three panels of experts to establish content validity. Reliability of the tools is unknown. Descriptive statistics were tabulated and presented.

The major findings included: 40% of the sample had never been taught to write nursing diagnoses; none of the unhealthful responses were seen in more than 50% of patients, by more than 50% of nurses; none of the complete diagnoses were seen in more than 20% of patients, by more than 50% of nurses; and subjects generated 887 etiologies, 311 of which represented independent role. Conclusions from the date were that a variety of nursing diagnoses that address nursing's independent functions were observed; combining the response with an etiology increased the specificity of the diagnosis and limited the scope; the sample had difficulty separating independent from interdependent functions; and there is interest among emergency nurses in the use of nursing diagnosis, although many have had little exposure to it.

Relationships among Community Health Nursing Diagnoses, Interventions, and Outcomes

Karen Martin, MSN, RN, FAAN

What are the relationships among client problems/nursing diagnoses, nursing interventions, and client outcomes in the community health setting? A research study designed to address that question was initiated in January 1989 and will continue in progress until December 1991. Participating in the study are nurses at four community health nursing agencies, representing diverse geographic locations.

The purpose of the research study is to build upon work begun during three previous research projects. During these projects, language or tools were developed that are referred to as the Omaha System and that consist of the Problem Classification Scheme, Problem Rating Scale for Outcomes, and Intervention Scheme.

The prospective design of the research study is organized to include three phases. During a nine-month preparation phase, data-collection instruments were pilot tested and completed, and data analysis was planned involving discriminant analysis. A time study was conducted and nurses were oriented at the beginning of the 18-month implementation phase. The agency nurses used the Omaha System to document client care. Client record data generated by nurses will be abstracted by project staff. Before the implementation phase is completed, a 15-month evaluation phase will be initiated. The final phase will include data assessment and analysis activities.

The research study has the potential to establish a descriptive client database, project resource utilization, and predict client outcomes. The study will increase the model's potential generalizability and utility for community health agencies through the United States.

Funded by National Center for Nursing Research, National Institutes of Health, Grant #1 R01 NR02192-01.

Human Response Patterns and Outcomes of the Critically Ill Patient

Mary E. Kerr, MN, RN
Ellen B. Rudy, PhD
Barbara J. Daly, MSN, RN

In the critical care environment, as a result of the interdependent nature of patient care, it is difficult to extract nurses' contribution to patient outcomes. Nursing diagnosis and the NANDA taxonomic structure of nine human response patterns (HRPs) represent the basis for independent nursing actions and provide a method for identifying nurses' contribution to patient outcomes. Study aims were to identify (1) trends in the nine HRPs during hospitalization of the critically ill person and (2) relationships among the nine HRPs and outcomes of the critically ill person. The independent variables were the nine HRP scores and a total human response pattern (THRP) score. The dependent variables were length of stay, functional health status, and patient's satisfaction with outcomes of care.

Patients were randomly selected from the surgical intensive care unit (SICU). Nursing diagnoses were identified daily by the nurses and categorized into the nine HRPs as designated by the NANDA taxonomy. HRP scores were calculated by summing patients' nursing diagnoses within each HRP. The Functional Health Status (FHS) instrument,

adapted from the Katz Daily Activities Index, measured the patients' functional health upon admission and discharge. A Satisfaction with Outcome (SO) tool, investigator developed and content validated by clinical experts, measured patients' satisfaction with outcome on the day before discharge. The alpha coefficients of the FHS and SO instruments were .91 and .95 respectively. Length of stay consisted of both the number of days spent in the SICU and the total number of days spent in the hospital. The sample of 38 patients (210 women and 28 men) ranged in aged from 21 to 85 ($\bar{X}$=55.8), with an acuity (APACHE II) from 2 to 36 ($\bar{X}$=17.3). The patients' prehospital admission FHS ranged from 16 to 21 ($\bar{X}$=20.7) and discharge FHS ranged from 14 to 21 ($\bar{X}$=20). The SICU length of stay ranged from 1 to 57 days ($\bar{X}$=7.8) with a median of 4 days. Total hospital stay ranged from 3 to 72 ($\bar{X}$=18.8) with a median of 12 days. Patient satisfaction with outcomes ranged from 13 to 28 ($\bar{X}$=24.1).

The results of this study document what nurses already know occurs during the hospitalization of the critically ill patient. Graphic analysis revealed that all HRP scores, except

269

Knowing and Feeling, increased as the patient entered the SICU, decreased as the patient transferred from SICU, and were lowest the day before discharge. The HRP score on the day before discharge showed the best relationship with outcomes. A high Choosing score (coping, denial, or conflict) was negatively related to patient satisfaction with outcome ($r=.64$, 27, $p=.000$). High Exchanging scores (physiologic conditions) were positively related to the number of days spent in the SICU ($r=.71$, 28, $p=.000$). The THRP was negatively related to discharge FHS ($r=.53$, 27, $p=.004$) and positively related to total hospital days ($r=.67$, 28, $p=.000$). In other words, patients with the most nursing diag-

noses on the day of discharge had the most difficulty with FHS and the longest length of stay.

This study represents a first step to document HRPs across the hospitalization experience of the critically ill patient and to validate that nurses' judgment is related to outcomes. It is exciting that the demonstrated relationships substantiate that the knowledge embedded in practice is related to the outcomes of care. Human response patterns have potential for identifying areas that nurses can influence and lay the groundwork for future research for intervention and change.

Taxonomy

A Validation Study of NANDA's Taxonomy I

Cathy Aden, BSN, RN
Judith Warren, PhD, RN

Taxonomy I was developed by NANDA to classify and organize nursing diagnoses. The basic structure of the Taxonomy is the nine Patterns of Unitary Person. This organizing structure needs to be tested for validity and consistency.

The purpose of this exploratory study was to determine if practicing nurses classify nursing diagnoses similarly to NANDA's Taxonomy I. The 42 original nursing diagnoses from 1980 were used by the nurse theorists to derive the Patterns of Unitary Person, upon which Taxonomy I is based.

Fourteen registered nurses employed in the school health program of the Visiting Nurse Association (VNA) of Omaha were selected as a convenience sample. All had experience using nursing diagnosis in practice, and all were over 30 years old. The 42 diagnoses were placed on individual cards and the subjects were requested to sort them according to perceived similarity. Successive pile-sort technique was utilized. Cluster analysis and multidimensional scaling were then used to analyze the data.

The diagnoses were grouped into three clusters: (1) physiologic diagnoses that are also grouped in the Exchanging pattern, (2) diagnoses concerning activities of daily living that closely parallel the diagnoses grouped in the Moving pattern, and (3) psychosocial diagnoses that parallel the diagnoses grouped in the remaining seven Patterns of Unitary Person. The nurses demonstrated two different intermediate clustering behaviors. Nine nurses clustered similarly while five nurses had more successive sorting rounds. The second group consisted of five nurses with supervisory experience, which may account for the fact that they used more successive sorts. The three final clusters were the same for all 14 nurses. The final taxonomic groupings were very similar to the organization of the documentation system of the agency.

This pilot study indicates that the relationship between agency documentation systems and nursing diagnosis grouping may influence the similarity of perceptions of nurses more than the formal structure of NANDA's Taxonomy I. Replication in other geographic and clinical sites is needed. Because nursing diagnosis is fairly new, studies with nurses younger than 30 also may yield significant information.

Construction and Content Validity Testing of a Comprehensive Taxonomy of Diagnoses for Pediatric Nurse Practitioners

Catherine E. Burns, PhD, RN, PNP

Pediatric Nurse Practitioners (PNPs) need an integrated, comprehensive classification system including nursing, disease, and developmental diagnoses with minimal overlaps to describe their scope of practice in a conceptually sound manner. No single classification system available meets these needs. Further, there are no methodologic studies evaluating the content validity of any taxonomy in the nursing literature. The goal of this study was to develop such an integrated classification for PNPs. A secondary goal was to explore a method to test the content validity of the classification constructed.

A conceptual framework was derived from theories of nursing. It identified three domains of diagnoses: Developmental Problems, Disease, and Daily Living Problems. All diagnoses from the NANDA 1986 list and selected diagnoses from the *International Classification of Diseases* and *Diagnostic and Statistical Manual, 3rd Revision* were listed alphabetically with definitions. The diagnoses were sorted into the three domains using scores of 1 (not related) to 4 (highly re-

lated) assigned by a panel of eight expert nurses. Diagnoses assigned to the Daily Living Problems domain were then sorted by the same panel into the 11 Functional Health Patterns described by Gordon. Reliability was measured using Proportions of Agreement and Kappas for all pairs of judges on test and retest. The content validity of the groups created was measured using Indices of Content Validity and Average Congruency Percentages.

The experts sorted the diagnoses in a new way that decreased overlap among the domains. The Developmental and Disease domains were judged reliable and valid. The Daily Living domain of nursing diagnoses demonstrated marginally acceptable validity with acceptable interrater and intrarater agreement. On the second sort, six Functional Health Patterns were judged reliable and valid; mixed results were found for four categories. The coping/stress tolerance category was reliable but not valid using either test. Twenty-six of the nursing diagnoses currently classified in the NANDA Exchanging ca-

274

tegory were assigned to the Disease domain. There were considerable differences between the panel's and Gordon's assignment of NANDA diagnoses into Functional Health Patterns.

The study represents an attempt to define the diagnostic practice of nurses from a holistic, patient-centered system perspective. It is believed to be the first study to use quantitative methods to test a diagnostic classification system for nursing. It is assumed that the classification model could be adapted to other types of practices by substituting other diseases and developmental problems.

Field Testing of a Comprehensive Taxonomy of Diagnoses for Pediatric Nurse Practitioners

Catherine E. Burns, PhD, RN, PNP

Pediatric Nurse Practitioners (PNPs) need an integrated, comprehensive classification including nursing, disease, and developmental diagnoses to describe their scope of practice in a conceptually sound manner. Such a classification was constructed and then field tested to identify gaps and to evaluate its usefulness in practice. A secondary goal was to describe the clinical practice of PNPs using the diagnostic system.

A conceptual framework was derived from theories of nursing. It identified three domains of diagnoses: Developmental, Disease, and Daily Living. All the NANDA diagnoses from 1986 as well as selected disease and developmental diagnoses were sorted into the three domains by a panel of experts. Diagnoses assigned to the Daily Living Problems list were then sorted into the 11 Functional Health Patterns of Gordon. The system, except for one Functional Health Pattern category, was judged reasonably reliable and valid using several tests.

Six PNPs working in general primary health care settings in Oregon achieved inter-rater agreements above .80. Each then used the classification to code diagnoses they identified and managed for 240 consecutive cases. They added new diagnoses if unable to find suitable listed diagnoses. Finally, they evaluated the system for usefulness.

The PNPs identified 3,361 diagnoses with 1,450 cases. Their diagnostic scope of practice included 1% Developmental Problems; 72% Pediatric Diseases, which included 51% illnesses and 21% preventive diagnoses; and 27% Daily Living Problems (often referred to as nursing diagnoses). The most common diagnoses were otitis media, *potential for infection*, acute nasopharyngitis, *knowledge deficit: nutrition*, *knowledge deficit*, *development*, and *altered comfort: pain*. The open numbers were used in less than 2% of the total diagnoses, indicating few gaps in the system. The system was rated quite positively by the PNPs.

Nurses in independent roles need a comprehensive system for documentation of their diagnostic practices. This study developed and field tested a system that was conceptually sound, adequately tested for reliability and validity, and relatively complete. Further, it was quickly learned, easily understood, and useful to the PNPs who applied it to their practices. It is assumed that the classification model could be adapted to other types of practices by substituting other diseases and developmental problems.

Comparison of Nursing Diagnostic Statements Using a Functional Health Pattern and a Health History/Body Systems Format

Marilyn Henning, MSN, RN

The purpose of this study was to compare the nursing diagnostic statements generated by registered nurses (RNs) using a Functional Health Pattern admission assessment format and a Health History/Body Systems admission assessment format.

Data for this study were obtained from the charts of an accessible population of 100 adult medical patients in two metropolitan medical hospitals. The charts were reviewed to obtain the diagnostic statements written by RNs. Fifty charts were obtained from the medical unit in Hospital A, whose RN staff had received preparation in the use of a Functional Health Pattern admission data-collection format and used it on a daily basis. The second group of 50 charts was obtained from the medical unit in Hospital B, whose RN staff had received preparation in the use of a Health History/Body Systems admission assessment format and used it on a daily basis. The review resulted in 51 nursing diagnoses from Hospital A (Group A) and 64 nursing diagnoses from Hospital B (Group B).

The diagnostic statements were evaluated using the Analysis of Diagnostic Statements Form developed and tested by Greenlee and revised for this project. Reliability and validity of this tool were established by Greenlee and further testing of the revised tool was done prior to this study.

Using a Mann-Whitney U test, a significant difference was found between the mean ranks of scores from Hospital A and Hospital B ($U = 722$, $z = 5.40$, $p = .01$), indicating that there is a difference between the nursing diagnostic statements generated from assessment data gathered by the RN using a Functional Health Pattern admission assessment format and a Health History/Body Systems admission assessment format.

Anxiety, activity intolerance, and *altered comfort* were the most frequently used diagnoses in Hospital A, and *altered comfort, potential for injury,* and *altered elimination* were the most frequently used diagnoses in Hospital B. All the nursing diagnoses from Hospital A could be categorized under one of the 11 Functional Health Patterns, while 16% of those nursing diagnoses written at Hospital B could not be categorized under one of the Functional Health Patterns. No nursing diagnoses were identified for either group for the Value-Belief, Sexuality-Reproduction, or Sleep-Rest patterns.

The researcher concluded that the admission assessment format organized under Functional Health Patterns assisted nurses to generate diagnostic statements that were more in the realm of nursing. This is supported by the results that indicate a significant difference between the ranks of scores between Group A and Group B. The conclusion is further supported by the results that all the nursing diagnoses could be categorized under the Functional Health Patterns for Group A. A large number of the nursing diagnostic statements generated from the Health History/Body Systems admission assessment format at Hospital B related to a body system or medical model. The results of this study provided implications for nursing practice, nursing education, and further nursing research.

Diagnostic Reasoning

The Relationship between Nursing Diagnostic Reasoning and Reimbursement in Home Health Care

Jesse Earl Greene, MSN, RN

Use of nursing diagnostic reasoning by nurses practicing in home health care settings has been reported to improve documentation for third-party payers. Reimbursement, however, as an outcome of improved documentation for third-party payers and as a result of the use of nursing diagnostic reasoning has been neglected by researchers in the past.

The use of nursing diagnostic reasoning by nurses practicing in a home health care agency and the reimbursement of those nurses' visits to patients were measured in this study. Use of nursing diagnostic reasoning was measured as a proportion of total clinical inferences, documented by agency nurses on the nursing care plans, that qualified as nursing diagnoses using NANDA's 1987 list. Reimbursement of nursing visits was measured as a proportion of total nurse visits. Nurse demographic data (age, experience, and educational level) were collected by means of a questionnaire that was administered to each nurse who qualified for inclusion in the study ($n = 48$). Two patient records were randomly selected from each qualifying nurse's patient caseload, resulting in a patient record sample

of 96 patient records. Nurses' clinical inferences and associated reimbursement data were collected from the patient record sample by the researcher.

Observed sample proportions were transformed into their corresponding logits using the logit transform developed by Haldane. Using these logits, Pearson correlation coefficients were computed to test the hypothesis that when a greater proportion of total clinical inferences that are nursing diagnoses is used to establish the nursing care plan, a greater proportion of nursing visits will be reimbursed. No significant relationship was found between the use of nursing diagnostic reasoning and reimbursement of nursing visits. Because the majority of the patient record sample received 100% reimbursement, secondary analysis of the hypothesis was performed using only data from those patient records that had received less than 100% reimbursement ($n = 11$). Using linear regression analysis, the use of nursing diagnostic reasoning explained 70% of the variation in reimbursement of the nursing visits, indicating that greater use of nursing diagnostic reasoning was associated with greater reim-

283

bursement of nursing visits in this small sample of patient records.

Further research is needed to determine if the tendency for greater use of nursing diagnostic reasoning to be associated with greater reimbursement of home health nursing vis-

its can be found in a larger sample of patients' records where reimbursement is less than 100%. This knowledge could be helpful in improving reimbursement rates in units where low rates are a problem.

An Exploration of the Relationships Between Diagnostic Reasoning Ability and Learning Style in Undergraduate Nursing Students

Rita J. Olivieri, PhD, RN

This study was undertaken to describe and explore the relationships between diagnostic reasoning ability and learning style in undergraduate nursing students. These variables were examined with reference to the role of the nurse in making clinical judgments and the related need to assist the student nurse in his/her learning. The theoretical bases for the study were Elstein's theory of medical problem solving and Kolb's experiential learning theory.

The sample for this study was comprised of 126 upper-division baccalaureate nursing students at one university in the northeastern United States. The subjects had completed their first semester of clinical nursing. Data were collected by self-completed questionnaires that included (1) Gordon's Diagnostic Reasoning Tool (DRT) and (2) Kolb's Learning Style Inventory (LSI).

In the analysis of the data the following procedures were performed: means, ANOVA, and t-tests for examining differences among groups, and Pearson correlations for exploring the relationship between the variables.

Undergraduate nursing students exhibited a diversity of learning styles. The preferred styles were assimilator and diverger, equally represented with 29.5%. Accommodator and converger styles were less preferred. This group was characterized as slightly more concrete than abstract and more reflective than active.

In relation to the DRT, the sample scored high on diagnostic recognition, cue interpretation, and hypothesis generation abilities, and moderately well on the concept characteristics and data interpretation tests. There were no significant differences among learning style groups on the DRT or the subtests of concept recognition, concept characteristics, or data interpretation. A low but significant correlation was found between the abstract conceptualization stage and the number of correct cues used. There was a similar correlation between the number of correct hy-

285

potheses generated and the abstract conceptualization stage.

The ability to determine learning style and its relationship to diagnostic reasoning may assist nursing students in coping with the demands of the nursing curriculum and separate the fear of developing the nursing care plan from the experience of implementing nursing care in the clinical setting.

Nursing Diagnosis by Neural Networks: A New Aid for Nursing Practice

Rose Mary Harvey, DNSc, RN

The purpose of this pilot study was to apply neural networks, a new and developing computer technology, to aid the decision-making process in nursing diagnosis. ART-2, a type of neural network, enables the computer to learn by example, that is, the computer programs itself to make decisions.

To apply this technology to a specific example, an assessment tool was constructed based on NANDA diagnoses and defining characteristics as they appear in Gordon's Manual of Nursing Diagnosis. The bowel elimination categories within the Functional Health Pattern of Elimination were used in the study. Assessment questions were answerable by yes/no or numerical scores. Answer sheets were used to produce diagnostic "patterns" that were then taught to the ART-2.

Real and fictitious case descriptions were used to sufficiently test the ART-2. The diagnoses made by the ART-2 agreed with those made by the researcher based on the NANDA defining characteristics and diagnostic labels.

There are advantages and disadvantages to this approach. Compared to other computer-based approaches, neural networks are a "natural" for making nursing diagnoses. They can handle probabilistic, fuzzy, and ill-defined data in a simple manner. They can be taught by example only: that is, no programming is required to enable decision making. They can incorporate new data and experiences and can make diagnoses based on new characteristics not seen during training. A disadvantage is that at least one case example for each diagnostic category must be available for teaching the neural network.

Diagnosis Development/Identification

Investigation of a New Diagnostic Label—*Impaired Resource Management: Time*

Noreen Frisch, PhD, RN
Janet Weber, MSN, RN

The presenters investigated the utility of a new diagnostic category, *impaired resource management: time,* after practicing nurses suggested that a diagnosis having to do with resource management might describe an important nursing function. After reviewing relevant literature, a tentative definition was suggested, along with defining characteristics. Next, the presenters assessed if the diagnosis could be made in two distinct populations.

The working definition of *impaired resource management: time* is the situation where the client demonstrates inability to manage or structure time. Nursing literature indicates that nurses frequently observe clients who are not accomplishing tasks related to daily living or expected social roles, and encounter clients who verbalize that they are not satisfied with their own time management. These conditions were taken as the defining characteristics of the diagnosis. Available research on the concept of time provided background into etiology that led to the following related factors: inability to plan and manage personal activities; external locus of control; lack of social support; unrealistic time demands; discrepancy between subjective time experience and objective time; loss of time perspective, sense of tempo, or personal meaning for time; and obsessive-compulsive disorders.

Two populations were surveyed using the above criteria. Population 1 was a randomly selected sample of university students living at a campus residence hall ($n = 93$) who were participating in a study of health needs on campus. Data obtained revealed that 19 (20.4%) exhibited the major defining characteristics. Population 2 was a small sample ($n = 16$) of hospitalized psychiatric patients receiving care at a state mental health facility. Nurses caring for these patients assessed these clients on one day and reported that none of these patients exhibited the defining characteristics. There were two of the 16 that the nurses judged to be having difficulty with managing time, but they felt that *diversional activity deficit* was a more appropriate label. The nurses suggested other psychiatric patients for whom they judged the diagnosis to be useful, but these patients were not part of the study population.

These findings and ideas were presented at a regional nursing diagnosis conference and generated much interest among nurses from a variety of practice settings. Further study is indicated, particularly in long-term care facilities, psychiatric units, critical care, and community health.

In Search of Perioperative Nursing Diagnoses: A Preliminary Study

Susan V. M. Kleinbeck, MS, RN, CNOR

Perioperative nursing standards and recommendations for practice advocate the identification of nursing diagnoses for patients undergoing intraoperative procedures and the integration of those diagnoses into perioperative documentation. Research data substantiating the appropriateness or the incidence of particular nursing diagnoses in the perioperative patient population are not available in the literature. The purpose of this exploratory study was to identify the prevalent preoperative, intraoperative, and postoperative nursing diagnoses among surgical patients in one large midwestern medical center.

Twenty-five adult surgical patients were assessed and nursing diagnoses formulated before admission to the operating room. Patients were then followed intraoperatively and postoperatively by a senior baccalaureate nursing student enrolled in a perioperative clinical management course. The diagnoses were updated as the patient progressed through each surgical phase. A total of 479 individual nursing diagnoses were generated for an average of 19.16 diagnoses per patient. Most patients had more preoperative (8), about the same number of intraoperative (7), and fewer postoperative nursing diagnoses

(5). Because the data were analyzed by phases, it was possible for any one patient to have the same diagnostic label counted once in the preoperative phase, once in the intraoperative phase, and again in the postoperative phase (e.g., *potential for infection*). The majority ($n = 44$) of the intraoperative nursing diagnoses were directed toward the prevention of injury. Almost two-thirds (63%) of the preoperative and nearly half (49%) of the postoperative nursing diagnoses were written only once, while more than three-quarters (77%) of the nursing diagnoses listed for the intraoperative period were repeated 52% of the time. These data would seem to support the appropriateness of a generic intraoperative plan.

The nursing diagnoses with the highest frequencies (8 operative, 11 intraoperative, and 7 postoperative) served as the basis for a standardized generic plan of care that could be computerized and later individualized for each surgical patient. This exploratory study begins the process of identifying nursing diagnoses appropriate for perioperative practice. Further study with a larger sample is needed before the information can be applied more widely.

Testing of *Alteration in Potassium Balance: Hypo-* and *Hyperkalemia* as Nursing Diagnoses

Norma Metheny, PhD, RN
Sharon Merritt, EdD, RN
Judith Myers, MSN, RN

The existing NANDA taxonomy lacks nursing diagnoses that deal with electrolyte disturbances. Yet nurses in both acute and long-term care settings must deal with these physiologic derangements on an almost daily basis. According to Kim, a physiologic nursing diagnosis is defined as an inferential statement made by a professional nurse that describes physiologic disturbances that impede optimum functioning and then directs the nurse to specific interventions both independent and interdependent. The purpose of this study is to propose two new nursing diagnoses: *alteration in potassium balance: hypokalemia,* and *alteration in potassium balance: hyperkalemia.*

In order to test the two proposed nursing diagnoses, a clinical study was undertaken in which subjects with laboratory-documented hypo- or hyperkalemia were assessed for etiologic factors and defining characteristics of the imbalances. Tools used in the study were developed by Metheny by means of an extensive literature review. Over a 16-month period, 210 subjects reviewed for entry into a clinical study to assess feeding tube placement served as potential subjects for testing of the proposed nursing diagnoses. If a subject's serum potassium level was abnormally high or low a clinical assessment and chart review were done to complete the appropriate tool. Forty-eight subjects with hypokalemia and nine subjects with hyperkalemia were identified.

Of the subjects with hypokalemia, the most commonly associated etiologic factors included administration of potassium-losing diuretics, presence of diarrhea, history of poor dietary intake, and administration of steroids and insulin. Other less frequently associated factors included recent gastric suction, aggressive refeeding, and administration of antibiotics known to cause renal potassium wasting. Identified defining characteristics included presence of anorexia, nausea, and vomiting; fatigue; muscle weakness; slowed gastrointestinal motility; and ECG changes. A substantial number of subjects (73%) also had mild to moderate hyperglycemia. It is not known if this phenomenon was causative in nature or an aftermath of hypokalemia—it could have been either.

Approximately two thirds of the subjects with hyperkalemia were in renal failure. The other third were found to have artifactual readings or metabolic acidosis not associated with renal failure. Other than evidence of ECG tracing changes, there were no discernible symptoms. Probably the reason other clinical indicators were not present is that (1) none of the subjects had markedly elevated potassium levels, and (2) those with true hy-

perkalemia had suffered the condition over a prolonged period of time and had built up a tolerance to the potassium elevation.

The present study can serve as an initial phase of the evaluation of the two proposed nursing diagnoses. Refinement of the data-collection tools needs to be accomplished before further testing of the diagnoses is attempted. Both independent and interdependent nursing interventions are available for these proposed nursing diagnoses and can be instituted when deemed appropriate by the nurse, based on a meaningful assessment.

The Preliminary Delineation of a New Nursing Diagnosis, *Terminal Syndrome* Related to the Dying Process

Deborah Caswell, MN, RN, CCRN
Anna Omery, DNSc, RN

The patient for whom death is imminent presents special challenges for the nurse. It is nursing care that gives the dying patient dignity and comfort as the patient moves toward the end of the life process. The purpose of this exploratory, descriptive study was to determine if the complex care often required by the dying patient could be organized under a single diagnostic label. Specifically, this study sought to determine if there was a common core of defining characteristics, nursing goals, and nursing interventions that could be catalogued under a single diagnostic label, *terminal syndrome*.

The nonprobability sample consisted of 25 "Do Not Resuscitate" patients in a surgical, critical care setting. Data were collected via a retrospective chart review, using an investigator-developed questionnaire that documented both quantitative and qualitative data to measure or describe demographics, defining characteristics, nursing goals, and interventions. Content validity and interrater reliability coefficients (.98 to 1.00, $p < 0.05$) were established for the questionnaire prior to and during data collection. Quantitative data were analyzed using descriptive statistics. Qualitative data were analyzed using content analysis. Categories for this analysis were established from the data, not from a presupposed theoretical framework.

Findings supported the identification of the diagnosis. A core group of physiologic and psychosocial defining characteristics were identified. The physiologic characteristics included an increase in cardiac output, a decrease in blood pressure, and decreased level of consciousness. Psychosocial characteristics included imminent death as a medical prognosis and patient's or family's documented request for all medical treatments to cease. The major nursing goal was to maintain comfort and dignity to the conclusion of the life process. Four detailed patient outcomes were categorized under this major goal. Organized under these outcomes were 287 possible nursing interventions. These nursing interventions were collapsed into 19 physiologic and seven psychosocial interventions. All the physiologic interventions were patient focused. Three of the psychosocial interventions focused on the care of the patient; four guided the nurse in the care of the patient's family.

Recommendations include the validation of these findings in a larger, more diverse sample and cohort studies to demonstrate that the diagnosis is indeed specific to the patient for whom death is impending. It is nursing care that gives life honor and succor in its final stages. The development and use of the diagnosis *terminal syndrome* can enable the nurse to assist the patient to maintain comfort, quality, and dignity until the life process is complete.

Conception of a Nursing Diagnosis— Decision Making, Family: Required

Mary Beth Myers, MS, RN

This descriptive study, utilizing the Delphi technique and an expert group of nurses, identifies 49 defining characteristics of families faced with the required decision of organ donation. While nurses are cited as a vital link in the organ-donation process, there is currently no nursing diagnosis to identify and guide care in this situation. The purpose of this study was to generate characteristics of the proposed nursing diagnosis *decision making, family: required* related to the potential for organ donation.

The expert groups utilized in generating and identifying the characteristics included general, pediatric, and neurologic intensive care nurses, emergency nurses, and transplant coordinator nurses. Characteristics were generated through a literature review and survey of intensive care and emergency nurses. The generated characteristics were then refined by a group of 47 emergency, neurologic intensive care, and transplant coordinator nurses utilizing two Likert scale tools. Survey response rates were 87.2% and 88.9% on these two scales. All characteristics with a mean score greater than 3.00, indicating approximately a 50% chance of observation, were retained. The retained characteristics indicate an intense need for support by the family network, support from the health professional, and a negative effect on cognitive processing during this process.

Identifying this group to nursing as a whole will assist in the correct nursing diagnosis being made. Specific intervention for this group may then be derived and instituted. These interventions would be directed at facilitating and enhancing the decision-making process while the family's normal problem-solving skills are blunted by crisis. The study findings would suggest the need for sensitive guidance by a knowledgeable professional familiar with crisis theory, and inclusion of the family network during the process.

SECTION

VI

Business Meeting

Minutes of the NANDA General Assembly, Orlando Marriott Hotel, Orlando, Florida, March 19, 1990

I. Welcome and Call to Order

K. Cianfrani welcomed the Assembly and introduced J. Lancour, President. J. Lancour called the meeting to order at 8:10 A.M.

II. Establishment of a Quorum

J. Lancour announced that a quorum was established. K. Cianfrani, Program Chairperson, made several announcements related to the program.

III. Rules for Business

J. Lancour reviewed the rules for business and added two rules.

IV. Approval of Minutes

S. Popkess-Vawter moved that the minutes of the March 15, 1988 General Assembly Meeting be approved as printed. Seconded. Passed.

V. Report of the President, J. Lancour

J. Lancour overviewed the President's report. (Note: Officer and Committee reports follow on page 309.)

VI. Report of the Treasurer, M. Briody

M. Briody highlighted the Treasurer's report.

VII. Committee Reports

A. Publications Committee, D. Jones

D. Jones reviewed the Publications Committee report. She noted that the new journal *Nursing Diagnosis* is in print and now available for each member attending the Conference. She expressed appreciation to the Publications Committee, Editorial Advisory Board, and Rose Mary Carroll-Johnson, Editor, for their outstanding work on the Journal. Rose Mary Carroll-Johnson also will edit the Ninth Conference Proceedings.

B. Public Relations/Membership Committee, J. McCloskey

J. McCloskey overviewed the Public Relations/Membership Committee report. She noted several promotional items that can be purchased at the NANDA booth in the exhibit hall.

C. Diagnosis Review Committee, L. Carpenito

L. Carpenito highlighted the Diagnosis Review Committee report. She noted the revised Review Guidelines that will be explained at the Conference. Also she reported that an ad hoc translation committee will be established to translate diagnoses and related information into other languages.

P. Kucharski inquired whether there would be a membership vote to accept the proposed guidelines. L. Carpenito explained that the guidelines never had been voted upon by the membership in the past. These guidelines have been approved by the Board.

D. Research Committee, E. McFarlane

E. McFarlane highlighted the Research Committee report. She announced that the monograph of the Invitational Research Conference held in Palm Springs last April will be available for purchase at the NANDA booth.

E. Finance Committee, M. Briody

M. Briody presented the Finance Committee report. This new committee was established to assist in monitoring and strategizing for financial growth of the Association.

F. Program Committee, K. Cianfrani

K. Cianfrani presented the Program Committee report. J. Lancour thanked Ken and the committee for a very fine program.

G. Taxonomy Committee, J. Fitzpatrick

J. Fitzpatrick presented the Taxonomy Committee report.

H. Regional Affairs Committee, M. A. Kelly

M. A. Kelly highlighted the Regional Affairs Committee report. She noted the Bylaws changes that will be discussed later in the meeting to provide for reconstitution of the Regional Affairs Committee.

I. International Affairs Committee, A. Becker

A. Becker presented the International Affairs Committee report. She recognized the large number of international attendees at the Conference.

New Business

A. Proposed Amendments to the Bylaws, A. McLane

A. McLane directed the Assembly to the proposed Bylaws changes. She made motions for each proposed change and J. Lancour asked for seconds to the motions so that discussion could ensue.

Article VI, Section 2, Item J

A. McLane moved that this article regarding the International Committee be changed as submitted. Seconded. Passed.

Article XII, Section 1

A. McLane moved that this article regarding amendments be changed as submitted. Seconded. Passed.

Article II, Section 3

A. McLane moved that this article regarding membership be moved to Section 4 and replaced by the new section as submitted. Seconded. Passed.

Article II, Section 4

A. McLane moved that this article regarding membership year be moved to Section 7 and be replaced by the new section as submitted. Seconded. Passed.

Article II, Section 5

A. McLane moved that this new section regarding affiliate association membership be added as submitted.
(Parliamentarian informed the President that a second to the motion was not needed for these changes.)

J. Lancour called for discussion. J. Shoemaker commented that the proceedings were moving so rapidly that she had concerns about whether members were fully aware of the changes for which they were voting. She encouraged more discussion on the related issues.

J. Shoemaker moved that Article II, Section 3 be reconsidered. Seconded. Passed.

M. A. Kelly overviewed this proposed Bylaws change related to the Regional Affairs Committee and the rationale for the proposed changes. She read aloud the states and provinces that were temporarily assigned to each of the proposed seven Districts referred to in Article II, Section 3.

In opposition to the proposed Bylaws change: J. Shoemaker raised questions about benefits and costs related to the change and believed that more than one model for change should be presented. J. Warren shared concerns about the costs of such a change. M. Magnan was unclear about the long-term mission of regional groups in forwarding the work of the Association.

In favor of the proposed Bylaws change: B. Mottet summarized reasons for using the proposed structure to facilitate grassroots involvement. L. Carpenito discussed how creation of Districts would provide a liaison between grassroots and the Board. L. Rossi believed that this change will improve communication among members.

C. Baer called the question. Seconded. Passed.

Article II, Section 3 passed.

Article II, Section 5

A. McLane moved that this article regarding affiliate membership be changed as submitted. Discussion.

In opposition to the proposed Bylaws change: B. Ross expressed concerns about implications for regional groups regarding item c), "criteria as shall be determined by the association," being too restrictive for regional groups. V. Aukamp had concerns that the addition of the district strata would increase the distance from regional groups and the Board.

In favor of the proposed Bylaws change: M. Gordon believed that this change may even allow for existing specialty organizations (such a neuroscience nurses) within a district to become a regional group.

M. A. Kelly was asked to answer several questions related to the difference between districts and regional groups and how members know to which regional group they belong.

B. Ross moved that c) be deleted from Article II, Section 5. Seconded. Discussion. Failed.

After further discussion related to the relationship between regional groups and districts,

S. Weber moved that Article II, Section 5 be amended to read: "affiliate organization membership is granted to organizations who apply for membership and" and continue as proposed in a), b), and c). Seconded. Discussion.

C. Baer called the question. Seconded. Passed.

Voted. Failed.

B. Lyon moved to take 5-minute recess to

give the people involved with this motion time to confer and present a revised motion. Second. Passed.

(Whereupon, a brief recess was taken at 9:40 A.M., after which the following proceedings transpired.)

B. Ross moved that the content of the Bylaws be referred back to the committee for input from local and regional member groups for revision and resubmission. Seconded. Discussion.

E. Borkowski called the question. Seconded. Passed.

Voted. Failed.

C. Pinkley moved that Article II, Section 5 read: "affiliate NANDA membership is granted to regional organizations" and a), b), and c), will remain as is proposed. Seconded.

M. J. Kim amended the amendment to read: "affiliate *regional* NANDA membership." Seconded. Discussion. Voted. Passed.

J. Lancour announced a 15-minute recess; proceedings resumed at 10:45 A.M.

Article II, Section 6

A. McLane moved that this article regarding membership application and fees be changed as submitted. Seconded.

M. A. Kelly noted the editorial changes needed in this article to be consistent with the other changes previously adopted.

P. Wetsch moved that the following be incorporated into Section 6: "Affiliate membership with the association may be established by application to the Regional Affairs Committee. Approval of the application is made by the Association Board. Benefits for affiliate membership and membership fees required will be established by the Regional Affairs Committee and approved by the Association Board." Seconded. Passed.

A. McLane noted that for former Article II, Section 4 becomes Section 7 as previously discussed.

Article VI, Section 1

A. McLane moved that this section regarding committee appointments be changed as submitted. Discussion.

M. A. Kelly moved that this proposed section be amended to read: "Committee *selection*. The Association may have standing committees. Each committee shall be chaired by a NANDA member, as appointed by the President. Committee members shall be *elected or appointed* with attention to geographic and clinical practice distribution. The size of the committee shall be determined by the Board unless otherwise stated by the Bylaws. Committees shall report to the Board and to meetings of the Association as requested or as required by these Bylaws."

L. Mondoux asked for clarification regarding the phrase "concurrence by the President," which was omitted in the proposed amendment since some members will be elected.

A. Becker moved that Article VI, Section 1 be amended to read: "Committee members shall be elected or appointed *by the committee chairperson* with attention to geographic and . . . ." Seconded. Voted. Passed.

Article VI, Section 2, Item h

A. McLane moved that this section regarding regional affairs be changed as submitted. Discussion.

M. A. Kelly noted that implications of this section change for several members who had concerns regarding international countries being excluded by this amendment.

M. Wyman moved that the terms "regional affairs" be changed to "district affairs." Seconded. Discussion. Voted. Passed.

B. Bartlett asked for differentiation between the terms "selected" and "elected," in reference to committee member appointments. W. Mills voiced that the international enlargement is difficult to picture without a visual model to show the relationships among individual members, regions, districts, Board, etc. . . . L. Rossi suggested that some mechanism, e.g., the Journal, be used to clarify the district configuration.

J. Shoemaker amended the motion so that "elected" be substituted for "selected" in Article VI, Section 2, item h). Seconded. Passed.

Article VI, Section 2, item h) was voted upon. Passed.

D. Ver Steeg asked that editorial changes be made to consistently use newly adopted terms and language throughout the revised Bylaws.

J. Lancour asked for a motion to pass the Bylaws as amended by 2/3 majority vote.

A. McLane moved that Bylaws as amended be accepted. Seconded. Passed.

Miscellaneous Bylaws Motions

H. Cox moved that reconsideration be given to Article XII, Section 1, regarding Board endorsement of Bylaws changes 120 days prior to submission to the membership. Seconded.

H. Cox moved that Article XII, Section 1 be changed to read: "Amendments to these Bylaws must be submitted to the Board (*for their endorsement—omitted*) 120 days prior to submission to the membership." Seconded. Discussion. Passed.

D. Moritz moved that the organization be called the International Nursing Diagnosis Association, under Article I, Section 1.

J. Fitzpatrick recommended that we support the motion in concept and that it be taken to the International Committee for in-depth consideration.

It was moved that the proposed amendment regarding changing the organization name be referred to the International Committee for consideration and be brought back to the Assembly with future recommendations. Seconded. Voted. Passed.

D. Moritz moved that the conventions be held on years alternating with the ANA convention. Seconded.

D. Moritz agreed that this convention tim-

ing issue should be referred to the Program Committee.

D. Moritz moved to amend Article V, Section 1, regarding Board composition, to read: "That the Board of Directors of the Association shall be officers plus seven Directors who shall be elected as hereinafter provided and should be comprised of 50 percent Master's prepared clinicians/practitioners and 50 percent academicians/researchers." Seconded. Discussion.

In opposition to the proposed Bylaws change: C. Baer asked how this proposal is different from the situation that presently exists. J. Maklebust thought that designated distribution runs the risk of not finding sufficient numbers of specified persons to run in future elections. J. Mirkin emphasized the need for nurse administrators to be equally represented.

In favor of the proposed Bylaws change: S. Weber believed that even though this distribution of Board members may exist now, the Bylaws should specify this distribution to assure a balance among research, education, and clinical practice.

The question was called. Seconded. Passed. Voted. Failed.

V. Aukamp requested that a Forum be established at the next Conference to review proposed changes before the Business Meeting to expedite the business of the Association. J. Lancour referred this recommendation to the Program Committee.

M. Tyler moved that Article VI, Section 1, item d) read: "d) Diagnosis Review Committee. The Diagnosis Review Committee shall designate the format for submission of proposed diagnoses or changes to existing diagnoses; and following meetings of the General Assembly shall prepare proposed diagnoses in final form as recommended for membership voting." Seconded. Discussion.

In opposition to the proposed Bylaws change: K. McGilton and C. Peltier-Coviak believed that the review tasks implied by this motion would be completely unwieldy for a large group to manage. L. Carpenito and L. Mondoux spoke to the lack of scholarly and scientific review that this recommended process implies.

In favor of the proposed Bylaws change: M. Lunney supported the proposed change in concept since she has concerns about the gatekeeping function of the DRC Committee.

Voted. Failed.

Definition of Nursing Diagnosis

A. McLane moved the proposed nursing diagnosis definition be accepted as stated. Seconded. Discussion.

In favor of the proposed definition: B. Wesorick supported the new definition but asked what the difference was between this definition and a scope of practice. K. Sheppard asked for clarification regarding accountability implied in the definition.

B. Lyon moved that the proposed nursing diagnosis be changed to read: "A nursing diagnosis is a clinical judgment about an individual, family, or community response to actual or potential health problems/life processes. It provides the basis for initiation of nursing interventions that lead to outcomes for which the nurse is accountable." Seconded. Discussion. Voted. Failed.

C. Dougherty moved to omit the last part of the proposed definition (ending with the word processes and striking remaining words) to read: "A nursing diagnoses is a clinical judgment about an individual, family, or community response to actual or potential health problems/life processes." Seconded. Discussion. Voted. Failed.

V. C. Schonlau Meissner, representing the Wellness Special Interest Group, proposed that the definition be revised to read: "A nursing diagnosis is a clinical judgment about an individual, family, or community response to life processes and at high risk/actual health problems which provides the basis for definitive actions toward achievement of outcomes for which the nurse is accountable." Seconded. Discussion. Voted. Failed.

L. Boles moved that the original definition remain but should end with "which provides the basis for therapeutic interventions." and strike the remainder of the proposed definition. Seconded. Discussion. Voted. Failed.

J. O'Neil moved that the definition be retained as stated but end after "basis" to read: ". . . basis for nurses' accountability for predicting outcomes and designing interventions to achieve these outcomes." Seconded. Discussion. Voted. Failed.

C. Pinkley moved that the definition be amended to read: "Nursing diagnosis is a clinical judgment about individual, family, or community responses to actual and potential health problems/life processes. Nursing diagnoses provide the basis for selection of interventions to achieve outcomes for which the nurse is accountable." Seconded.

B. Lyon moved to withdraw her amended definition if C. Pinkley agreed to add "nursing" to interventions. C. Pinkley agreed and the amended definition reads: "Nursing diagnosis is a clinical judgment about individual, family, or community responses to actual or potential health problems/life processes. Nursing diagnoses provide the basis for selection of nursing interventions to achieve outcomes for which the nurse is accountable."

D. Moritz called the question. Seconded. Passed.

Voted. Passed.

Resolutions

M. Lunney moved that "Whereas the NANDA system for nursing diagnosis has broad organizational and professional support, and whereas nurses rely on diagnostic labels in the NANDA system for the implementation of nursing diagnoses in their practice, and whereas additional diagnoses are needed to reflect the complexity and diversity of nursing, therefore be it resolved that: 1. NANDA adopt an approach of openness and inclusiveness in the acceptance of nursing diagnoses for clinical testing, and 2. the NANDA system for nursing diagnosis will include all concepts submitted as criteria for submission accepted by the membership." Seconded. Discussion.

L. Carpenito spoke against the motion in support of the current review process. J. Dungan and J. Jenny spoke in favor of the motion since it supports the development of nursing science.

Voted. Failed.

K. Vincent moved that the NANDA Board of Directors send a letter to the Board of ANA with copies to the Cabinet of Nursing Practice and the Council of Psychiatric-Mental Health Nursing within the ANA, recognizing and commending the work of the Phenomena of Concern Task Force but asking again for the group to submit their work through the formal structure of NANDA. We appreciate the ANA's efforts to date to accomplish this. Seconded.

The motion could not be acted upon due to quorum no longer being present.

At 1:05 P.M. quorum was no longer in attendance and therefore the meeting was adjourned.

Business Referred to Committee

Issues, listed below, not presented while a quorum was present at the meeting were referred to the Board for consideration and referral to the appropriate committee.

The following issues were referred to the Taxonomy Committee

K. Sheppard moved that the Taxonomy Committee continue work on Taxonomy II using the model/structuring of Taxonomy I Revised and ICD-10 pattern composition (e.g.,

definitions and rearrangement of diagnoses in different patterns) at this time.

S. Weber presented this resolution: Whereas transitions from one taxonomy to a successor taxonomy necessitates development of different coding and record-keeping systems, with rules for transition from one to the other, and, Whereas the widespread distribution of NANDA Taxonomy I (including the ICD submission) means that many institutions and nurses would have major transition steps to implement any successor Taxonomy II, and, Whereas, debate and consideration of the merits of any successor taxonomy should be informed by *both* the soundness of the taxonomy *and* the associated transition process, Therefore be it resolved that the Taxonomy Committee be directed by the Board that any Taxonomy II brought forward for debate and adoption be accompanied by a written rationale for changes *and* guides for transition from Taxonomy I (i.e., terms coded XX will now be coded YY).

The following issues were referred to the Taxonomy, Research, and DRC Committees

D. Jakob moved that the Board provoke critical exploration for developing more and improved diagnoses of communities which might take the form of (1) a call for conceptual papers to stimulate critical mass in the literature, (2) a review and listing of existing diagnoses for applicability to the community unit-of-analysis, e.g., groups, subpopulations, (3) a call for case studies that include community health diagnostic formulations, and (4) a clarification by the DRC of particular criteria and guidelines for nursing diagnosis submission as they relate to community as client.

The following issues were referred to the DRC Committee

E. Miller moved that NANDA develop and implement a two-phase process for the identification and classification of nursing diagnoses, where Phase I consists of screening and presentation of proposed nursing diagnoses to the NANDA membership and the nursing community for the purpose of clinical testing and research, and Phase II consists of a rigorous scientific review of the proposed nursing diagnoses from Phase I for the purpose of acceptance/modification or rejection. Following final acceptance, the nursing diagnoses will be placed into the NANDA Taxonomy.

M. Pullen recommended that consideration be given to publishing a summary in the NANDA Biennial Business Meeting book of reports of the rationale(s) for acceptance, rejection, hold, or return of each nursing diagnosis submitted [to the DRC] so that NANDA members and future and past nursing diagnosis submitters be aware of this process.

The following issue was referred to the Program Committee

B. Lyon suggested that consideration be given to have a meeting *next year* to deal with the conceptual, theoretical, structural issues via e.g., position papers, debates, etc. . .

Respectfully submitted,
Sue Popkess-Vawter, PhD, RN
Secretary

President's Report

Submitted by Jane Lancour, President

The Board of Directors extended appreciation to Marjory Gordon (Massachusetts) for her years of service as the first NANDA President. Her second term expired June 30, 1989. Appreciation was also extended to Directors Gertrude McFarland (Virginia) and Mi Ja Kim (Illinois), whose terms also expired in 1989. Congratulations were given to Lynda Carpenito (New Jersey) and Ann Becker (Missouri) for their re-election as Directors. Lynda Carpenito's term is successive. Ann Becker served as a Director from 1983 to 1987. New members welcomed to the Board are Ken Cianfrani (Illinois), Director, and Sue Popkess-Vawter (Kansas), Secretary. The Board of Directors held five meetings during this biennium.

I commend Debi Folkerts, Executive Director, for her expertise in directing the operations of the organization. Her continual availability, responsiveness, creativeness, and ability to maximize limited resources serve the best interest of NANDA.

Organizational Affairs

Committee composition and structure changed with implementation of the 1988 change in Bylaws. Committees are now com-posed of 50% elected members and 50% appointed members. Three committees are chaired by non-Board members: Research Committee—Elizabeth McFarlane (Virginia); Regional Affairs Committee—Mary Ann Kelly (North Carolina); and Nominating Committee—Joyce Shoemaker (Ohio).

Beginning July 1, 1989, the membership year and fiscal year coincide with the same 12 consecutive months: July 1 to June 30. A biennial budget was initiated July 1989 and is reviewed and revised on a quarterly basis. See *Treasurer's Report.*

At this Conference, we were proud to present the first issue of *Nursing Diagnosis,* The Official Journal of the North American Nursing Diagnosis Association. This is a refereed, quarterly publication, the cost of which is included in membership dues. Praise is given to Dottie Jones, Publications Committee Chair; Members of the Publications Committee; Rose Mary Carroll-Johnson, Editor; and the Editorial Board for this accomplishment.

An Invitational Conference on Research Methods for Validating Nursing Diagnosis was held in Palm Springs, California, April 23–30, 1989. A monograph of this conference is available for purchase.

The Board unanimously agreed to change

the election process from a mail ballot to an in-person vote to take place at the biennial conference beginning in 1992. Individuals not able to attend the conference can participate in the election process by obtaining an absentee ballot. To accommodate this transition the Board extended all present terms by one year.

The Board established priorities for the 1990–1991, 1991–1992, and 1992–1993 fiscal years at their January 1990 Board meeting. See Figure 1. Accountability for attainment of these priorities was designated and communicated.

Classification of Diagnoses

A joint meeting of the Board and the Taxonomy Committee was held January 28 and 29, 1989. The combined group accepted the Proposed NANDA Taxonomy I Revised—Proposed ICD-10 version. This document is a translation of Taxonomy I Revised that meets ICD coding requirements. ANA and NANDA submitted the NANDA Taxonomy I Revised—Proposed ICD-10 Version to the World Health Organization (WHO) in April 1989 for acceptance in the 1993 publication of the International Classification of Diseases (ICD-10). We await WHO's decision on this matter.

The joint meeting of the Board and the Taxonomy Committee also resulted in approval of a working definition of "nursing diagnosis" to be submitted to the General Assembly 1990 and to be reviewed in 1992. The definition is as follows:

A Nursing Diagnosis is a clinical judgment about an individual, family, or community response to actual or potential health problems/life processes which provides the basis for definitive therapy toward achievement of outcomes for which the nurse is accountable.

International Affairs

NANDA presented a special session program at the International Congress of Nurses (ICN) Quadrennial, Seoul, Korea, Summer 1989. See *International Committee Report*.

Inter-Organizational Affairs

NANDA continues collaborative relationships with ANA in keeping with shared interest in classifying nursing diagnoses and ANA's interest in intervention and outcome classification. ANA recognizes NANDA as the body to be utilized by ANA Practice Councils for the development, review, and approval of nursing diagnoses. ANA endorses the NANDA taxonomy as the ANA nursing diagnosis taxonomy.

A joint NANDA-ANA program was held at the 1988 Biennial Convention in Kentucky. This year NANDA will again present a program in Boston at the 1990 ANA Convention. Sue Popkess-Vawter, Secretary, serves as NANDA's representative to the ANA Nursing Organizations' Liaison Forum (NOLF).

The Public Relations Committee has worked to establish a liaison relationship with specialty organizations. To date, NANDA has formal relationship with 40 specialty groups. See *Public Relations/Membership Committee Report*.

In January 1990, Jane Lancour, President, represented NANDA as a member of the Nursing Advisory Panel on Guideline Development, Medical Treatment Effectiveness Program (MEDTEP), Agency for Health Care Policy and Research (AHCPR), Department of Health and Human Services. Joanne McCloskey, Director, also served on this panel.

MEDTEP will be implemented through four sets of activities: (1) database development, (2) effectiveness and outcome research, (3) dissemination of research findings, and (4) guidelines development. See pages 313–315 for more detailed information about MEDTEP and specific information about research proposals.

By January 1, 1991, the Forum for Quality and Effectiveness in Health Care of AHCPR must assure the development of an initial set of guidelines, standards, performance measures, and review criteria for three clinical treatments or conditions. The legislation gives AHCPR authority to contract with public and nonprofit private organizations to develop guidelines and to convene expert panels to review the guidelines. The guidelines must (1) be based on the best available research and professional judgment regarding the effectiveness and appropriateness of health care services and procedures; (2) be presented in formats appropriate for use by physicians, other health care providers, educators, review organizations, and consumers of health care; and (3) be treatment/condition-specific, reflecting the needs and priorities of the program under Title XVIII.

To help AHCPR meet the legislative responsibilities outlined above, the Nursing Advisory Panel on Guideline Development was convened to provide professional nursing assistance and advice in six major areas:

1. Discussion of nursing issues relative to guidelines
2. Attributes of guidelines, substantive and procedural
3. Consumer involvement in guideline development
4. Recommendations for assuring nursing input in practice guideline development
5. The recommended process for formulating a nursing research agenda in relationship to guideline development
6. The recommended process for providing continual nursing advice to the AHCPR.

Four nursing work groups provided recommendations in the six major areas identified. Among other recommendations, the work groups recommended that guidelines be developed by nursing for "clinical conditions" that are either medical diagnoses, nursing diagnoses, or combinations. An executive summary of this convened panel is available from AHCPR Publications and Information Branch, 18–12 Parklawn Bldg., Rockville, MD 20857, (301) 443-4100.

The involvement of nursing and, specifically, NANDA in fulfillment of this legislative mandate is a giant leap forward. Individuals who have made this possible are Clinton Jarrett, MD, Acting Director of the AHCPR; Kathleen Hastings, RN, C, JD, MPH, Senior Health Policy Analyst/AHCPR, Forum for Quality and Effectiveness in Health Care; and Norma Lang, PhD, RN, FAAN, Panel Chairperson.

Conclusion

I extend appreciation to the Executive Committee, Directors, Committee Chairs and Members, Diagnostic Reviewers, and the Editorial Board for many hours of work given to fulfill the mission of NANDA. Special thanks to those members who matched their dues or worked to increase the membership of the organization. I thank the membership for commitment to NANDA's focused endeavor of developing the scientific basis of nursing. Finally, thanks to Debi Folkerts, Executive Director, and Diane Wainwright, Office Secretary, for graciously, efficiently, and effectively serving NANDA.

ATTACHMENT A: NORTH AMERICAN NURSING DIAGNOSIS ASSOCIATION STRATEGIC PLAN: 1990–1993

Priorities to Be Completed by June 30, 1993

Prepared by NANDA Board, January 1990.

1. Increase the economic base of the organization by 25%.
   a. Stabilize membership to 1500.
   b. Increase regional group membership by 25%.
   c. Provide NANDA-endorsed programs at specialty meetings.
   d. Program one income-generating conference during the off-conference year with special attention to underserved areas.
   e. Explore the establishment of a Nursing Diagnosis Foundation.
2. Develop and disseminate Taxonomy II.
   a. Convene the Taxonomy Committee for work sessions two times per year.
   b. Commission taxonomy papers to be published in a monograph or proceedings from the 1990 Conference.
   c. Develop a model for validation of Taxonomy II.
   d. Insert definitions and new diagnoses into the working document.
   e. Publish and disseminate Taxonomy II.
3. Provide direction for the development and refinement of new and existing nursing diagnoses.
   a. Develop and disseminate the "to be developed (TBD)" listing.
   b. Develop a mechanism for joint membership work on TBDs.
   c. Establish a diagnostic review board of approximately 100 individuals.
   d. Develop educational materials/program to guide submission of new diagnoses.
   e. Develop a mechanism for evaluating the translation of nursing diagnoses into other languages.
   f. Review the mechanism for revision/deletion of previously accepted diagnoses.
4. Continue to refine the diagnostic labels and components through research.
   a. Evaluate the approved diagnoses for consistency and accuracy according to NANDA's nursing diagnosis definition.
   b. Identify gaps in defining characteristics that require further development.
   c. Evaluate developed diagnoses and components in relationship to changes inherent in Taxonomy II, e.g., axes.
   d. Generate research questions for proposal and facilitate focused research groups.
   e. Establish a plan for the development of a research data bank.
   f. Direct research activities for validation of approved diagnoses.
   g. Disseminate monograph of 1989 research conference. Consider a plan for a 1991 conference in combined effort with DRC, Taxonomy, and Research.

(continued)

(Continued)

    h. Develop a plan to facilitate NANDA's involvement in integration of nursing diagnoses into information systems with retrieval capabilities.

5. Participate with key health care policy-making bodies and nursing organizations.

    a. Establish formal linkages with American Nurses' Association (ANA), Canadian Nurses' Association (CNA), and Quebec Nurses' Association (QNA). Schedule NANDA presentations on a regular basis at meetings of these organizations and International Council of Nurses (ICN).

    b. Expand participation in Nursing Organization Liaison Forum (NOLF).

    c. Develop a plan to interface with federal agencies that have a health care focus to delineate priorities that are consistent with the NANDA mission.

    d. Continue to develop linkages with international groups.

    e. Interface with Joint Commission for Accreditation of Healthcare Organizations (JCAHO) as advisors to the standards.

6. Promote networking and education of professional nurses about the integration of nursing diagnosis into practice.

    a. Develop position papers on issues surrounding nursing diagnosis.

    b. Develop educational videos about nursing diagnosis.

    c. Expand the circulation of the *Nursing Diagnosis Journal* by 25%.

    d. Implement formal relationship with regional groups.

    e. Increase the visibility of NANDA through targeted activities with other professional organizations.

    f. Evaluate a mechanism for developing a distinguished speakers bureau.

    g. Plan to organize the documents of the organization for development of the archives.

Figure 1   List of priorities to be completed by June 30, 1993.

Program Note
Agency for Health Care Policy and Research, Medical Treatment Effectiveness Program, January 1990

The Department of Health and Human Services established in FY 90 the Medical Treatment Effectiveness Program (MEDTEP).

The Agency for Health Care Policy and Research (AHCPR) (formerly the National Center for Health Services and Health Care Technology Assessment (NCHSR)) has primarily implementation responsibility for MEDTEP ensuring a broadly based research and dissemination effort through collaborative activities with other components of the Public Health Service and the Health Care Financing Administration (HCFA). Approximately $32 million may be available for MEDTEP activities in FY 90.

MEDTEP's purpose is to improve the effectiveness of health care services through better understanding of the effects of health care practices on patient outcomes. The central questions of this program are:

- What treatments work best?
- Has the patient's functional status improved?
- According to whose viewpoint?

MEDTEP will be implemented through four sets of activities:

- Database development
- Effectiveness and Outcomes Research
- Dissemination of research findings
- Guidelines development

Database Development

This activity will expand the databases available for analysis and improve linkages among them. Emphasis will be placed on improving Medicare databases and linking these with other databases available on patient populations. Much of this work will be undertaken by HCFA. Both AHCPR and HCFA will provide grants and contracts to facilitate various aspects of database development.

Effectiveness and Outcomes Research

AHCPR will expand the earlier work undertaken in health services research generally and the Patient Outcome Assessment Research Program specifically in establishing an effectiveness and outcomes research program for the evaluation of the outcomes of preventative, diagnostic, and treatment strategies available for medical disorders.

In FY 87 and FY 88, AHCPR funded studies of the treatment of prostatism, heart disease, hypertension, diabetes, and rheumatoid arthritis. In FY 1989, AHCPR supported four assessment teams, each funded at approximately $1 million per year for five years, to evaluate the treatment of cataracts, myocardial infarction, prostatism, and back pain. Small awards were provided to consider assessment team research on the management of peripheral vascular disease, cerebral vascular disease, hip disease, colon cancer, gall bladder disease, and coronary artery disease.

Research proposals should consider the controversies regarding alternative treatments for common conditions, the volume of cases and treatments in the population, and total cost or charges per treatment and the amount of unexplained variation in medical practice for the particular practice or condition.

Research proposals may focus on three major components of research: evaluation of current treatment strategies, synthesis of findings, and demonstration of the effectiveness of dissemination efforts. Alternatively, proposals may focus on a subset of these components for a given condition.

Research proposals may also focus on methodological issues underpinning MEDTEP, such as improved measures of patient outcomes, dissemination methodologies and examinations of factors associated with variations in medical practice patterns.

Dissemination of Findings

In addition to dissemination research noted above, grants and contracts will be awarded to organizations for proposing innovative and effective programs to translate research findings into educational curricula for physicians and demonstrable practice assimilation. Proposals to educate nonphysician members of the health care team also will be considered, as will those for education of patients.

Guidelines Development

ACHPR will provide support to professional organizations to develop guidelines for physicians and other health care providers, to assist in the prevention, diagnosis, and treatment of medical conditions. Standards, review criteria, and performance measures also will be developed to assess and assure quality of care.

Further Information

Further information on MEDTEP program activities may be obtained from:

Database development: J. Michael Fitzmaurice, Ph.D. (301-443-5650)

Effectiveness and outcomes research: Fitzhugh Mullan, M.D. (301-443-2345) or Norman Weissman, Ph.D. (301-443-2345)

Dissemination: Z. Erik Farag, Ph.D. (301-443-2904)

Guidelines development: Stephen King, M.D. or Kathleen E. Hastings, R.N.C., J.D. (301-443-8754)

For information on other programs of the AHCPR, contact: Publications and Information Branch, 18-12 Parklawn Bldg., Rockville, MD 20857 (301-443-4100).

Treasurer's Report: March 1988–March 1990

Submitted by Margaret Briody, Treasurer

1. The organization is financially stable. Many of the financial strategies proposed by the previous Ad Hoc Finance Committee have been implemented and have contributed significantly to the achievement of this financial stability. The two most noteworthy strategies were the change in the membership year to be consistent with the fiscal year (July–June) and the approval of the dues. A heartfelt THANK YOU is extended to the membership for approving these changes.

2. The Treasurer's Report includes Table 1—"Statement of Revenue, Expense, and Changes in Fund Balance—Cash Basis for Years Ended June 30, 1989 and 1988."

3. The books and records have been examined by Betty Sano, CPA. A copy of her report is available for your inspection, if desired.

4. The Treasurer's Report includes Table 2—"Budgeted Income and Expenditures for Fiscal Years 1988–1989 and 1989–1990."

5. For information purposes, the Treasurer's Report includes Table 3: "Revenues and Expenditures, Six Months Ending December 31, 1989." The fund balance on December 31 was $95,737.

Table 1

Statement of Revenue, Expense, and Changes in Fund Balance—Cash Basis Years Ended June 30, 1989 and 1988

Income:	1989	1988
Membership Dues	$ 38,036	$ 43,472
Newsletter	2,600	3,613
Contributions	1,530	2,450
Royalties	3,120	8,278
Conference Registration	1,390	139,487
Interest	1,921	2,573
Miscellaneous	0	15
Mailing Lists	566	636
International Conference	0	9,776
In-House Publications	10,432	6,193
Newsletter Sponsorship	100	500
Sales of Promotional Items	2,283	0
Advertising—Newsletter	0	0
TOTAL REVENUE	$ 61,978	$216,993

Expenses:	1989	1988
Program Services Conference Expenses	$ 0	$ 63,620

(continued)

Table 1 (*Continued*)

Expenses:	1989	1988
Newsletter	11,851	4,217
Proceedings	5,000	0
Marketing	533	444
In-House Publications	8,495	4,442
General Assembly Expense	0	8,134
Membership Expense	5,537	0
Research Models Conference	1,507	0
Taxonomy Think Tank	3,597	0
Promotional Items Expense	2,070	0
Sub-Total	38,590	80,857
Board Expense	14,105	19,087
Committee Expense		
Diagnosis Review	$ 100	8,068
PR/Membership	53	348
Master Planning	0	58
Program	4,276	654
Publications	1,634	1,114
Research	3,203	374
Taxonomy	3,959	5,116
Nominating	288	149
Regional Affairs	12	2,641
International	291	2,064
Finance	0	0
Bylaws	0	0
Sub-Total	13,816	20,581
Management and General		
Salaries	32,285	29,848
Payroll Taxes	2,886	2,632
Telephone	1,419	1,109
Postage	1,997	2,433
Miscellaneous	245	224
Office Supplies	1,540	1,042
Printing	2,000	1,687
Office Services	0	96
MC/Visa Fees	296	1,606
Professional Services	1,978	1,565
Executive Director Expense	575	537
Medical Insurance	1,619	999
Association Travel	523	741
Interest Expense	0	704
Scholarship Fund	3,000	0
Equipment Repairs	507	0
Sub-Total	$ 50,870	$ 45,223
Equipment Purchases	250	0
TOTAL EXPENSES	$117,631	$165,748
EXCESS REVENUE OVER/ UNDER EXPENSE	$ (55,653)	$ 51,245
FUND BALANCE, BEGIN- NING OF YEAR	58,716	7,471
FUND BALANCE, END OF YEAR	$ 3,063	$ 58,716

Table 2

Budgeted Income and Expenditures for the Fiscal Years 1988–1989 and 1989–1990

Income:	1988–89	1989–90
Membership Dues	$ 45,000	$ 75,000
Newsletter	3,500	4,500
Contributions	0	0
Royalties	8,000	8,000
Penny Schoenmehl Fund	0	0
Conference Registration	0	150,000
Pre-Conference Registration	0	5,000
Interest	0	0
Miscellaneous	0	0
Mailing Lists	500	1,000
In-House Publications	3,000	15,000
Exchange Fees	0	0
International Conference	0	0
Newsletter Sponsorship	0	0
Journal Revenue	0	25,750
Sales of Promotional Items	0	6,000
Advertising—Newsletter	0	0
From Reserves	57,681	0
TOTAL BUDGETED IN- COME	$117,681	$290,250

Expenses:	1988–89	1989–90
Program Services		
Conference Expenses	$ 0	$82,025
Pre-Conference Expenses	0	2,500
Newsletter	8,500	4,400
Proceedings	5,000	0
Research Grants	2,462	0
Marketing	1,250	2,700
In-House Publications	2,300	10,500
General Assembly Expense	0	5,000
Membership Expense	3,500	3,500
Journal Expenses	0	23,407
Research Models Conference	2,500	0
Taxonomy Think Tank	5,000	0
Promotional Items Expense	0	2,500
Sub-Total	30,512	136,532
Board Expense	14,500	30,000
President's Expense	1,500	1,500
Committee Expense		
Diagnosis Review	$ 3,350	8,000
PR/Membership	450	2,800
Program	3,500	3,000
Publications	700	1,500
Research	3,500	3,000
Taxonomy	3,450	10,000
Nominating	600	200

(*continued*)

Table 2 (*Continued*)

Expenses:	1988–89	1989–90
Regional Affairs	450	3,500
International	200	1,200
Finance	0	600
Bylaws	0	900
Sub-Total	16,200	34,700
Management and General		
Salaries	31,860	39,374
Payroll Taxes	4,000	4,500
Telephone	1,500	2,000
Postage	3,000	3,300
Miscellaneous	200	300
Office Supplies	1,500	1,750
Printing	2,000	2,500
Office Services	500	0
MC/Visa Fees	500	1,800
Professional Services	2,300	2,500
Executive Director Expense	700	700
Board Liaison Expense	500	0
Medical Insurance	1,600	2,300
Association Travel	1,000	1,500
Interest Expense	0	0
Equipment	0	3,200
Equipment Repairs	728	600
Sub-Total	$ 51,888	$ 66,324
Scholarship Fund	3,000	3,000
TO RESERVES	81	10,000
TOTAL BUDGETED EXPENDITURES	$117,681	$282,056
TO OPERATING ACCOUNT		$ 8,194

Table 3

Revenues and Expenditures, Six Months Ending December 31, 1989

Revenues:	Actual for 6 months ending Dec. 31	Budget 1989–90
Membership Dues	61,255	75,000
Newsletter	3,802	4,500
Contributions	701	0
Royalties	4,704	8,000
Penny Schoenmehl Fund	55	0
Conference Registration	58,120	150,000

Table 3 (*Continued*)

	Actual for 6 months ending Dec. 31	Budget 1989–90
Pre-Conference Registration	2,750	5,000
Interest	807	0
Miscellaneous	0	0
Mailing Lists	100	1,000
In-House Publications	13,869	15,000
Exchange Fees	(158)	0
Journal Revenue	19,712	25,750
Sales of Promotional Items	6,185	6,000
Advertising—Newsletter	0	0
TOTAL REVENUES	171,902	290,250

Expenditures:	Actual for 6 months ending Dec. 31	Budget 1989–90
Program Services		
Conference Expenses	10,321	82,025
Pre-Conference Expenses	0	2,500
Newsletter	1,748	4,400
Proceedings	0	0
Research Grants	0	0
Marketing (ex. ANA)	2,870	2,700
In-House Publications	7,984	10,500
General Assembly Expense	0	5,000
Membership Expense	3,447	3,500
Journal Expenses	1,042	23,407
Research Models Conference	(672)	0
Taxonomy Think Tank	0	0
Promotional Items Expense	2,667	2,500
Sub-Total	29,407	136,532
Board Expense	8,314	30,000
President's Expense	298	1,500
Committee Expense		
Diagnosis Review	2,648	8,000
Membership/PR	82	2,800
Program	528	3,000
Publications	167	1,500
Research	76	3,000
Taxonomy	6,272	10,000
Nominations	178	200
Regional Affairs	49	3,500
International	37	1,200
Finance	0	600
Bylaws	0	900
Sub-Total	10,037	34,700

(*continued*)

(*continued*)

Table 3 (*Continued*)

Expenditures:	Actual for 6 months ending Dec. 31	Budget 1989–90
Management and General		
Executive Director Salary	13,068	26,136
Secretary Salary	5,570	13,238
Payroll Taxes	1,512	4,500
Telephone	1,104	2,000
Postage	1,222	3,300
Miscellaneous	172	300
Office Supplies	1,148	1,750
Printing	1,629	2,500
Office Services	0	0
MC/Visa Fees	370	1,800
Professional Services	1,000	2,500
Executive Director Expense	157	700
Board Liaison Expense	0	0
Medical Insurance	632	2,300
Association Travel	431	1,500
Interest Expense	0	0
Equipment	3,156	3,200

(*continued*)

Table 3 (*Continued*)

Expenditures:	Actual for 6 months ending Dec. 31	Budget 1989–90
Equipment Repairs	0	600
Sub-Total	31,172	66,324
Scholarship Fund	0	3,000
TO RESERVES		10,000
TOTAL EXPENSES	$ 79,228	$282,056
FUND BALANCE BEGIN-NING OF YEAR	$ 3,063	
TOTAL REVENUES	171,902	
Sub-Total	$174,965	
LESS TOTAL EXPENDI-TURES	(79,228)	
FUND BALANCE, END OF PERIOD	$ 95,737*	
TO OPERATING AC-COUNT		$ 8,194

*This fund balance consists of Cash of $96,379, Prepaid Postage of $823 and Taxes Payable of ($1,465).

Executive Director's Report

Submitted by Debi Folkerts, Executive Director

Inquiries

An average of 300 inquiries are addressed per month. Requests consist of membership information, conference information, in-house publications, bookmarks, and other miscellaneous items.

Administration

The *Taxonomy I Revised* (1989) booklet has been available since March 1989. Approximately 2,928 copies have been sold.

Approximately 6,211 nursing diagnosis bookmarks have been sold since April 1989.

The *Taxonomy I Revised* (1990) booklet estimated publication date is Summer 1990.

The monograph for the Invitational Conference on Research Methods for Validating Nursing Diagnoses is an in-house publication and will be available for purchase March 1990.

Personnel/Equipment

NANDA employs two full-time people, the Executive Director and a secretary.

A laptop computer was purchased to ac-commodate increased demands. It provides a work station in the office, and allows for entry of Board/General Assembly minutes and changing of documents at on-site meetings.

A fax machine is now available in the office to allow for rapid transmission/reception of information.

Site Visits/Future Biennial Conferences

Several site visits have been made for future conference planning. By contacting convention bureaus of cities that have potential, familiarization trips are arranged at no cost to the Association. This enables us to compare possible future meeting locations on cost, safety, tourist attractions, and accommodations.

- The Tenth NANDA Conference will be held April 25–29, 1992, at the Sheraton on Harbor Island in San Diego, California.
- The 11th NANDA Conference will be held March 26–30, 1994, at the Stouffer Hotel in Nashville, Tennessee.
- Various locations in Canada are being explored for the 1996 Conference.

Program Committee Report

Submitted by Kenneth Cianfrani, Chairperson
Linda Cooper
Peggy Lindsay
Kathy Bloom
Elizabeth Hiltunen
Ann Kelly
Sharon Summers
Jane Lancour, Board Liaison, November 1988–July 1989
Debi Folkerts, Executive Director, Ex-Officio

The Program Committee met November 1988 to plan the 1990 Conference. Materials considered to determine the theme included the goals of NANDA, participants' evaluations of the 1988 Conference, titles and topics of all previous conferences, results of a NANDA Board survey, and suggestions from the Committee members.

The theme, objectives, and conference schedule were identified and approved by the Board. Suggestions for speakers were considered from the Board, Program, Taxonomy, and Diagnosis Review Committees.

Program Committee members volunteered for various tasks. A conference call in April 1989 finalized plans. A meeting to operationalize last-minute details will be held immediately prior to the conference.

Abstract Review

The abstract review process has been completed. The call for abstracts went out Spring/Summer 1989. Reviewers were contacted and sent abstracts for a blind review with sheets for scoring. Each abstract was read by five reviewers. Ninety-eight (98) abstracts were received.

For final selection, an Abstract Review Subcommittee was formed with two members of the Program Committee and two members of the Research Committee. Linda Cooper (doctoral student, Ontario, Canada), Ken Cianfrani (IL), Elizabeth McFarlane (Washington, DC), and Jacqueline Fortin (RI) selected twelve (12) papers for presentation and thirty-one (31) abstracts for poster presentations.

Each member of the subcommittee was responsible for tallying the reviewers' scores for each abstract. The final decisions were based on scores, abstract content, recommendations by reviewers, and the author's preference for paper or poster presentation.

Fifty-five (55) papers were rejected. One reason for this number of rejections was the

27 requests for "paper only." The "paper only" scores ranged from 1.34 to 3.53. Eight of these papers scored 3.00 or more. One author accepted for paper presentation declined and a runner-up was selected. The final number of presentations is 12 and for poster presentations it is 30.

The Program Committee and the Board would like to acknowledge and thank those who participated as reviewers of abstracts for the 1990 Conference:

Carol Allen, BSN, RN
Virginia Aukamp, PhD, RN
Kay Avant, PhD, RN
Beverly Bartlett, PhD, RN
Doris E. Bell, PhD, RN
Andrea Bircher, PhD, RN
Eleanor Borkowski, BSN, RN
Lillian Bramwell, PhD, RN
Gloria Bulechek, PhD, RN
Shirley Burd, EdD, RN
Betty Chang, DNSc, RN
Marga Coler, EdD, RN
Nancy Creason, PhD, RN
Joan Crosley, PhD, RN
Richard Fehring, DNSc, RN
Mildred Fenske, PhD, RN
Joyce Fitzpatrick, PhD, RN
Sheila Fredette, EdD, RN
Sandra Frick, PhD, RN
Davina Gosnell, PhD, RN
June Gray, EdD, RN
Cathie Guzetta, PhD, RN
Elizabeth Hale, PhD, RN
Edith Hamilton, PhD, RN
Linda Harrington, PhD, RN
Pamela Hill, PhD, RN
Carole Hudgings, PhD, RN
Janice Janken, PhD, RN
Dorothy Jones, EdD, RN

Jane Kelley, PhD, RN
Mary Ann Kelly, EdD, RN
Mary Lou Kiley, PhD, RN
Nancy Lackey, PhD, RN
Carla Lee, PhD, RN
Rona Levin, PhD, RN
Margaret Lunney, PhD, RN
Suzanne MacAvoy, EdD, RN
Patricia Martin, PhD, RN
Carol McFadyen, PhD, RN
Audrey McLane, PhD, RN
Sharon Merritt, EdD, RN
Norma Metheny, PhD, RN
Christine Miaskowski, PhD, RN
Judith Miller, PhD, RN
Carol Ann Mitchell, PhD, RN
Derry Moritz, MSN, RN
Gail Mornhinweg, PhD, RN
Anne Neufeld, PhD, RN
Sue Popkess-Vawter, PhD, RN
Dee-J Putzier, PhD, RN
Brooke Randell, DNSc, RN
Evelyn Redding, EdD, RN
Carol Rossel, EdD, RN
Barbara Rottkamp, EdD, RN
Virginia Saba, EdD, RN
Maureen Shekleton, DNSc, RN
Elsie Shiramizu, EdD, RN
Mariah Snyder, PhD, RN
Carol Soares-O'Hearn, PhD, RN
Ruth Stollenwerk, DNSc, RN
Sharon Summers, PhD, RN
Roberta Thiry, PhD, RN
Rosemary Wang, PhD, RN
Judith Warren, PhD, RN
Sylvia Weber, MS, RN
Mary Louise Welch, MSN, RN
Georgia Whitley, EdD, RN
Barbara Whitmeyer, DNSc, RN
M. Anne Woodtli, PhD, RN
Kenneth Zwolski, EdD, RN

Publications Committee Report

Submitted by Dorothy Jones, Chairperson
Joan Fitzmaurice
Brenda Lyon
Joyce Shoemaker
Janet Weber

Meetings

There have been two meetings of the Publications Committee since the last General Assembly. Telephone conference calls and the mail were used to conduct the Committee's additional business.

Summary of Committee Activities

The major activities addressed by this Committee included

a. The continued publication of the Association's *Newsletter.*
b. Preparation of manuscripts for in-house publications.
c. Establishing *Nursing Diagnosis,* the Official Journal of the North American Nursing Diagnosis Association.
d. Creating a mechanism to preserve the Association's history.
e. The conference proceedings.

A. Newsletter

The *Newsletter* has continued to be published quarterly since the last General Assembly. The final copy of the *Newsletter* was printed with the Fall 1989 issue. Debi Folkerts, Executive Director of NANDA, served as Associate Editor and facilitated the production of this manuscript. Dorothy Jones served as Editor during the past two years. Mary Sampel (St. Louis) was Editor in previous years. The contents of the *Newsletter* will be incorporated into the forthcoming journal.

B. Journal

Nursing Diagnosis, the Official Journal of the North American Nursing Diagnosis Association, will make its debut at the Ninth Conference of the Association. During the past two years, the Committee has worked to establish the journal in the market place. The Chair wishes to acknowledge the outstanding contributions made by Committee members including the efforts of Kris Gebbie and

Mary Hurley, early promoters of a journal for the Association.

Leading nursing publishers responded to letters of inquiry concerning the possible development of a journal. The Committee met with each publisher and reviewed extensive marketing and planning material. Three publishers were forwarded to the Board. The J. B. Lippincott Company was selected as the official publisher of the NANDA *Journal.*

A call for editor in the *Newsletter* resulted in five candidates. Each applicant was reviewed by the Committee according to specific criteria and three names were sent to the Board for final selection. Rose Mary Carroll-Johnson (California) was chosen as the Editor.

Rose Mary brings a strong publishing background to this role as well as editorial experience. Her talent, nursing knowledge, and leadership have influenced the early beginning of this publication. The Committee acknowledges her patience as well as her perseverance during the journal's initial growth. We look forward to her continued presence as this publication grows.

The Publications Committee met in Boston during 1989 with representatives from Lippincott as well as Rose Mary Carroll-Johnson. At that meeting, the initial design, format, and early content decisions were made. In addition, a proposed organizational structure was drafted that created a link among the journal, editor, and NANDA. This structure was approved by the Board.

An Editorial Advisory Board was established to oversee the journal development; participate in policy formation; review manuscripts; and advise the editor on matters of content, design, and potential authors. Dorothy Jones currently serves as liaison between the NANDA Board of Directors, Publications Committee, and the Advisory Board for the *Journal.*

From the more than 50 individuals who submitted applications to the Committee, 13 names were approved by the Board. They are

Gloria Bulechek, Iowa
Joan Fitzmaurice, Massachusetts
Jean Jenny, Ontario, Canada
Dorothy Jones, Massachusetts
Margaret Lunney, New York
Brenda Lyon, Indiana
Elizabeth McFarlane, Washington, DC
Audrey McLane, North Carolina
Elizabeth Mottet, California
Joan Norris, Nebraska
Joyce Shoemaker, Ohio
Mariah Snyder, Minnesota
M. Anne Woodtli, Arizona

In addition to the Editorial Advisory Board, the Editor continues to seek reviewers for journal manuscripts. A growing list of interested participants has already begun. Persons interested in serving as a reviewer or journal author should contact Rose Mary Carroll-Johnson at P.O. Box 801360, Santa Clarita, CA 91380 for more information.

In-House Publications

In-house publications have been expanded over the past year and resulted in *Taxonomy I Revised* (1989). In addition, Proceedings from the Invitational Research Conference held in April 1989 are currently being prepared and will be available for purchase in Spring 1990. It is anticipated that NANDA will increase its publication of materials in concert with the growing activities of the Association.

Archives

The Publications Committee is attempting to create a structure for preserving the Association's history. A call for a nurse historian was placed in the *Newsletter* with limited response. The Committee is still accepting applications for this role and has contacted the National Nurse Historians Group to solicit further interest.

In addition, the Committee is attempting to generate funds for the development of a video about the Association and its leaders. The video would be both informational and income generating and could be used at all NANDA conferences and other conventions when NANDA is in attendance.

Proceedings

The *Proceedings* of the Eighth NANDA Conference were edited by Rose Mary Carroll-Johnson and published by the J. B. Lippincott Company. The Proceedings for the Ninth NANDA Conference will also be edited by Rose Mary Carroll-Johnson and published by J. B. Lippincott.

Goals for 1990–1992

During the next two years, the Committee will

1. Continue to monitor the *Journal* development and evaluate its impact on the market place
2. Foster the development of an Association video
3. Continue to pursue the organization of NANDA's history
4. Foster the production of in-house publications, and
5. Add new holdings to our listings.

The Committee has enjoyed the opportunity to serve NANDA during the past two years. We welcome continued input from the Association's members.

Public Relations/Membership Committee Report

Submitted by Joanne McCloskey, Chairperson
Joseph Burley
Elizabeth Gerety
Anne LeGresley
Susan Ruppert
Lynn Wieck

The only time the Committee has met has been at the Eighth Conference in March 1988 when it met as a committee twice and also hosted the first liaison specialty group breakfast. Due to a tight budget, work since the Conference has been mostly done by mail, with the Chair and the Executive Director of NANDA assuming most of the responsibility. One conference call was held in January 1990 to discuss nominations for awards and to select recipients.

Accomplishments

1. **Liaison Groups.** Formal liaison relationships have been established with 40 specialty groups. A purpose and responsibilities statement has been written and there are regular communications with liaison persons appointed by their organizations. There will be a panel presentation by representatives of five liaison organizations on their nursing diagnosis activities at the Ninth Conference. A second liaison group breakfast will be held at the Ninth Conference.

2. **Awards.** The criteria and process for awards were reviewed and rewritten. The changes were implemented with the October request for nominations and the new process and criteria used to select the 1990 recipients.

3. **Membership Card.** A membership card for new and renewing members was designed and purchased and is being used. In addition, the membership renewal form was updated.

4. **NANDA Pin.** A nursing diagnosis pin and NANDA guard were designed and are for sale through Balfour. Advertisements have been included in the NANDA *Newsletter* and sent to liaison and

regional groups. As of January 1990, NANDA has made $211 on royalties from the sale of pins.

5. **Bookmarks.** A bookmark with all the diagnoses was designed and a quantity purchased by NANDA for resale to members. The first ad for the bookmark was included in the Summer NANDA *Newsletter.* Letters advertising the availability of the bookmarks as inexpensive gifts for staff were sent to a national sample of nurse executives both in April for National Nurses' Day and in November for the holidays. As of January 1990, NANDA had made $5,317 from the sale of bookmarks.

6. **Promotional Letter.** An open letter entitled "Benefits of Membership" was written and is now included with all requests for organization and membership information.

7. **Nonrenewal Membership Survey.** In Fall 1988, a survey of previous members who did not renew membership was completed. This resulted in many renewals and on the basis of this survey, a second and third renewal notice (not previously done) has been implemented. There was discussion of a lesser dues category for student members and retired members but this was not approved by the Board due to questions of definition.

8. **NANDA Brochure and Membership Mailing.** A NANDA promotional brochure was developed in Fall 1989. At that time two mailings were also completed to promote membership in the organization. The first was to all NANDA members with a letter from Jane Lancour, President, asking them to assist in the recruitment of new members. Two sets of membership information, including the new brochure, were included for distribution. The second mailing was to targeted groups of nurses who might be interested in joining NANDA. For this and for the mailing of ads for the bookmarks, mailing lists had to be purchased.

9. **Booth.** Research and cost estimates for a NANDA conference booth and travel/registration were done. At the January 1990 Board meeting a booth purchase was approved. The booth will be available at the ANA convention in June 1990.

10. **Response to Members' Concerns.** The routine requests for information are handled by the Executive Director. However, on three to four occasions when a troublesome (e.g., angry or complicated) letter has arrived, it has been forwarded to the Chair of Public Relations/Membership Committee, and she has responded to it.

11. **Appointment of a Canadian Member.** In Fall 1989, a Canadian member was appointed to the Committee. This was viewed as one mechanism to help recruit new members in Canada.

Despite the implementation of several mechanisms to retain and recruit, membership in the organization has fallen considerably.

Membership in January 1990 was 1,231, compared to membership in July 1989 of 1,440 and in June 1987 of 1,900. Members come from all states in the United States and from all provinces of Canada. The following states have over 100 members in NANDA: California, Michigan, Illinois, Ohio, Wisconsin, New York, Pennsylvania, and Massachusetts.

A reason for the drop in membership is the increase in dues in January 1989 from $25 to $65 (which includes $15 for the *Journal*). Since the dues increase in January 1989, 430 people did not renew membership; as of January 1990, 198 new members have joined with 53 known to result from the Fall 1989 membership mailings, which were coded.

Diagnosis Review Committee Report

Submitted by Lynda Juall Carpenito, Chairperson
Joseph Davie
Joann Maklebust
Ann McCourt
Brooke Randell
Karen Vincent
Joyce Fitzpatrick, Ad Hoc

Activities

1. Received 45 proposed diagnoses (see Table 1). The following tabulation represents the status of the total diagnoses submitted.
   a. 10 returned for failure to include required components for submission and not resubmitted to date
   b. 35 reviewed by DRC and secondary reviewers
   c. 29 rejected for the following reasons
      1) duplicated an approved NANDA diagnosis
      2) represented a medical diagnosis
      3) represented a medical treatment
      4) did not represent a response
      5) did not defend the need for a syndrome diagnosis versus using one or more NANDA-approved diagnoses
      6) defining characteristics for a proposed actual diagnosis were not signs and symptoms
      7) research population was not representative for conclusions drawn
      8) inadequate literature support for proposed diagnosis
         a) 4 held for revision by submitter and additional reviews
         b) 2 accepted and forwarded to the Board
         c) 2 accepted by the Board to be forwarded to the membership
2. Revised guidelines for submission of a new nursing diagnosis.
3. Developed guidelines for revision or deletion of an approved NANDA nursing diagnosis.
4. Created an Expert Advisory Panel to serve as secondary reviewers.
5. Created a permanent review cycle with deadline for submission of March 1 the year prior to the NANDA National Conference.
6. *Diagnosis to be Developed (TBD)*: Submitted diagnoses that represent promising work but require substantive devel-

opment will be placed on a TBD list. These diagnoses have a rejection status with a TBD qualifier. TBDs will not be represented on NANDA's approved list. They will have to be resubmitted to the Diagnosis Review Committee. It is hoped that designating a diagnosis on the TBD list with the submitter identified will prompt nurses to collaborate on joint development.

7. Created a Translation Ad Hoc Committee to the Diagnosis Review Committee to review proposed nursing diagnoses. The Association of North American Nursing Diagnosis—Montreal section and Saguenay–Lac Saint-Jean regional group met and reported to the Diagnosis Research Committee regarding the translation of proposed diagnoses.

Committee Goals/Projected Activities

1. Collaborate with Research Committee to develop a proposal for soliciting researchers for validation of existing approved NANDA nursing diagnoses.
2. Collaborate with Taxonomy Committee regarding taxonomic issues as they relate to diagnosis development.
3. Explore the possibility of NANDA developing official translations of its work into, e.g., Spanish, French.

Table 1: DRC Review Cycle 1988–1990

Diagnosis	Returned for Resubmission	Reject	Hold for Revisions	Accept
Potential Altered Maintenance of Patent Access		X		
Altered Maintenance of Pregnancy		X		
Altered Protection (resubmission)				X
Altered Immune Response: Actual/Potential		X		
Decreased Venous Return: Central		X		
Decreased Venous Return: Peripheral		X		
Potential for Injury, Altered Response to Medications		X		
Alteration in Glucose Metabolism		X		
Parenting: Potential for Growth (proposed change in Altered Parenting)	X			
Distressful Life-Death Transition		X		
Non-Alliance (proposed change in Noncompliance)	X			
Nausea & Vomiting		X		
Altered Comfort: Nausea		X		
Alcohol Abuse		X		
Inability to Sustain Spontaneous Ventilation			X	
Interruption of Breastfeeding		X		
Effective Breastfeeding				X
Ineffective Breastfeeding		X		
Apathy		X		
Impaired Resource Management: Time		X		
Altered Nutrition (Revision)		X		
Altered Comfort: Itching		X		
Relocation Syndrome		X		

(continued)

Table 1: (*Continued*)

Diagnosis	DRC Decision			
	Returned for Resubmission	Reject	Hold for Revisions	Accept
Failure to Thrive		X		
Altered Feeding Pattern		X		
Decreased Adaptive Capacity: Intracranial		X		
Ineffective Management of Therapeutic Regimen (Individual)			X	
Ineffective Management of Therapeutic Regimen (Community)		X		
Ineffective Management of Therapeutic Regimen (Family)			X	
Effective Management of Therapeutic Regimen		X		
Loneliness		X		
Alteration in Family Caregiving		X		
Ineffective Coping (Community)		X		
Parenting: Potential for Growth Parent/Infant Attachment		X		
Dysfunctional Ventilatory Weaning Response			X	

Research Committee Report

Submitted by Elizabeth McFarlane, Chairperson
Cynthia Dougherty
Jacqueline Fortin
Connie Higgins-Vogel
Phyllis Jones
Audrey McLane, Board Liaison

Members of the Committee, 1988–1989

Betty Chang
Mi Ja Kim
Gertrude McFarland

Meetings, March 1988–March 1990

- March 17 and 18, 1990 (at the Ninth Conference)
- April 28 and 30, 1989 (at Methodologies Conference)
- April 6, 1989 (conference call)
- November 14, 1988 (conference call)
- September 30–October 2, 1988
- March 14, 1988 (at the Eighth Conference)

Committee Purpose and Goals

Purpose

The Research Committee shall promote nursing diagnosis research.

Goals

1. To stimulate collaboration among nurses interested in conducting research relevant to the development and application of nursing diagnoses by
   a. Maintaining a data bank containing such information as researchers involved in nursing diagnosis research, nature of research being conducted, methodology used, and tools utilized.
   b. Developing appropriate relationships with organizations of importance to or with interest in nursing diagnosis research.
2. To stimulate nursing diagnosis research by
   a. Consulting with other nursing professional organizations in the planning of research activities.
   b. Developing a research section in NANDA's *Newsletter* and editing or publishing research articles.
   c. Developing position papers and

meetings on critical issues relevant to nursing diagnosis research.

d. Reviewing and funding nursing diagnosis research proposals.

Committee Activities 1988–1989

1. Prepared the "Research Column" for the *Nursing Diagnosis Newsletter* (Goal 1b)
   - Spring 1988 (14:4), Joanne McCloskey
   - Summer 1988 (15:1), Phyllis Jones
   - Fall 1988 (15:2), Gertrude McFarland
   - Winter 1989 (15:3), Gertrude McFarland
   - Spring 1989 (15:4), Elizabeth McFarlane
   - Summer 1989 (16:1), Elizabeth McFarlane
2. Prepared and distributed to seven nursing journals a list of NANDA members who were interested in and qualified to review nursing diagnosis research manuscripts. The list was comprised of members who had responded to a request made through the *Nursing Diagnosis Newsletter* (Goal 1b).
3. Reviewed the second cycle of research proposals submitted for consideration of funding through NANDA. The first grant was awarded in May 1987 and the second in May 1988. The 1988 award was funded over two years due to budgetary constraints. No award was made in 1989. The Committee has recommended that the annual grant be reinstituted. The purpose of the grant is to provide seed money for research endeavors concerning nursing diagnosis (Goal 2d).
4. Planned and implemented the Invitational Conference on Research Methods for Validating Nursing Diagnoses (Goals 1a, 2b, 2c). The conference, held on April 28–30, 1989, was co-sponsored by NANDA and Case Western Reserve University, Frances Payne Bolton School of Nursing. The objectives for the conference were (a) to analyze existing research methodologies for the development and validation of nursing diagnoses and (b) to generate new research methodologies for the development and validation of nursing diagnoses. Thirty-seven researchers with expertise in qualitative, quantitative, and integrated research methodologies were invited to participate. The proceedings of the conference will be available to participants attending the Ninth Conference.
5. Participated in the review of research abstracts submitted for consideration as paper or poster presentations at the Ninth Conference. Dr. McFarlane and Dr. Fortin represented the Committee in this activity (Goal 2d).

Plans 1990–1991

1. Develop a specific program of action to support NANDA's Strategic Plan: 1990–1993. The Committee will direct its efforts to the following areas identified by the Board of Directors:
   a. Generate research questions for proposals and facilitate focused research work groups
   b. Establish a plan for the development of a research data bank
   c. Direct research activities for validation of approved diagnoses.
2. Develop and implement a plan for a second research conference to be held in 1991. This conference would be financially self-supporting. Determine feasibility of applying for a NIH Conference Grant.
3. Support the establishment of a "Foundation" that will fund research efforts designated to contribute to the identification and validation of nursing diagnoses.

Finance Committee Report

Submitted by Margaret Briody, Chairperson
Georgia Griffith Whitley
Marilyn Rantz

The Finance Committee was established as a standing committee of NANDA via Bylaws changes in March 1988 and elections in June 1989.

There is no formal Committee activity to report. Our first Committee meeting is scheduled for March 1990 at the Ninth Conference.

Taxonomy Committee Report

Submitted by Joyce J. Fitzpatrick, Chairperson
Kay Avant
Lois Hoskins
Dorothea Jakob
Mary Kerr
Margaret Lunney
Winnifred Mills
Lynda Carpenito, Ad Hoc

Members of the Committee, 1988–1989

Mary Hurley
Barbara Rottkamp
Judith Warren

Meetings

Five meetings were held.

Activities

1. Prepared summary of taxonomic issues discussed at Eighth Conference for dissemination to NANDA membership.
2. Participated in preparation of *NANDA Taxonomy I Revised* (1989) for publication by NANDA.
3. Provided leadership for ICD-10 translation of NANDA nursing diagnosis, in collaboration with ANA. As a result, a document was jointly submitted to WHO from ANA and NANDA.
4. Provided leadership for *American Journal of Nursing* publication ICD-10 translation of Taxonomy I.
5. Specified rules for taxonomic placement of diagnoses.
6. Participated in planning for Ninth Conference program.
7. Organized Taxonomy Think Tank held in January 1989 in collaboration with Board of Directors.
8. Participated in Delphi Study of Definition of Nursing Diagnosis with Board of Directors.
9. Began development of Taxonomy II:
   a. Initiated development of expanded definitions of human response patterns.
   b. Delineated issues related to taxonomy development and refinement

c. Began definitions of potential axes for nursing diagnoses.
10. Prepared program on Taxonomy II developments for Ninth Conference.

2. Present draft of Taxonomy II and related issues at Ninth Conference.
3. Publish Taxonomy II and disseminate to the membership.

Projected Goals 1989–1990

1. Continue development of Taxonomy II.

Regional Affairs Committee Report

Submitted by Mary Ann Kelly, Chairperson
Eleanor Borkowski
Marilyn Hurt
Mary Kontz
Joscelyn Matthewman
Sue Popkess-Vawter, Board Liaison

Meetings

The Committee held one meeting. This meeting was held via conference call on October 5, 1989. All members participated including Sue Popkess-Vawter, NANDA Board Liaison.

Activities

The Committee has been reconstituted following the 1989 election. Two members, Marilyn Hurt and Mary Kontz, were elected to the Committee. The Chair, May Ann Kelly, was appointed by the Association President and two additional members appointed as recommended by the new Chair, Eleanor Borkowski and Joscelyn Matthewman.

Three goals have been adopted by the Committee for the two-year term, 1989–1991. These are to

1. Effect changes in NANDA Bylaws that will organize the association membership into districts.
2. Develop policy and procedures for implementation of proposed Bylaws changes.
3. Develop mechanisms/procedures for communication between districts and between the Association and districts.

Changes in the current NANDA Bylaws have been developed to facilitate the organization of the Association membership into districts (see proposed Bylaws amendments). The proposal was approved by Committee membership and forwarded to the Board for approval and inclusion on the agenda for the next Association meeting. Rationale for changes has been developed and plans made for responding to anticipated discussion points that could be raised at the time of presentation of the proposal to the Association membership for vote.

Bylaws Committee Report

Submitted by Edward Halloran, Chairperson
J. Keith Hampton

A call for Bylaws proposals was included in the Summer 1989 *Newsletter*. The Committee met via telephone conference call to discuss the proposals submitted.

Proposed Amendments to the Bylaws

The NANDA Bylaws Committee proposes the following Bylaws revisions to reflect the refinement of certain policies and procedures as the organization has developed. The Bylaws are listed below in order of (1) the present Bylaws, (2) the proposed change/addition, and (3) the rational for the change.

Article VI Committees

Section 2. j) International Committee

Proposed Amendment
Section 2. j) International Committee. The Committee will promote networking with international nurses interested in nursing diagnosis and encourage involvement of these nurses in Association activities.

Rationale: To include a purpose for this Committee as listed in Bylaws for other Committees.

Article XII Amendments

Section 1. Amendments. Amendments to these Bylaws must be submitted to the Board prior to submission to the General Assembly.

Proposed Amendment
Section 1. Amendments. Amendments to these Bylaws must be submitted to the Board for their endorsement 120 days prior to submission to the membership.

Rationale: To facilitate efficiency in the processing of Bylaws changes.

Proposal from Regional Affairs Committee for Bylaws Changes

The Regional Affairs Committee has developed the following changes in Association Bylaws to implement affiliation of regional organizations as proposed in the Committee report at the 1988 Biennial Meeting. Purposes identified for such a district organization scheme would be to

1. Facilitate communication and activities among the regional organizations and between regional organizations and NANDA.

2. Provide a structure for representation on the Regional Affairs Committee which maximizes the autonomy and integrity of the regional organizations while providing the recognized affiliation with NANDA.
3. Serve as a liaison group for individual members and regional organizations between biennial meetings.

Functions of selected district representatives would be to

1. Communicate with regional organizations within the district.
2. Serve as liaison between individual members and regional organizations and NANDA.
3. Coordinate communications from regional organizations and official NANDA publications.
4. Communicate with representatives of other districts to promote Association goals.
5. Assist Regional Affairs Committee to facilitate the orderly and timely development of regional and local nursing diagnosis organizations within the district structure of NANDA.
6. Provide for periodic review of nursing diagnosis organizations within the district structure of NANDA.

Article II Membership

Section 3. The presentation to this Association of completed application, as required by Association policy or Bylaws, together with annual dues shall establish them as a member or associate member of this Association.

Section 4. Membership Year. The membership year shall be a period of 12 consecutive months, beginning July 1 of each calendar year.

Proposed Amendment

Section 3. (new Section 3; present Section 3 to become Section 4). The membership shall be organized into seven (7) districts. These shall consist of the following:

District #1—Northeastern

- Connecticut
- Maine
- Massachusetts
- New Brunswick
- New Hampshire
- Nova Scotia
- Newfoundland
- Prince Edward Island
- Quebec
- Rhode Island
- Vermont

District #2—Central Atlantic

- Delaware
- Maryland
- New Jersey
- New York
- Ohio
- Pennsylvania
- Washington, DC

District #3—Southeastern

- Alabama
- Florida
- Georgia
- Kentucky
- Louisiana
- Mississippi
- North Carolina
- Puerto Rico
- South Carolina
- Tennessee
- Virginia
- West Virginia

District #4—North Central

- Illinois

- Indiana
- Iowa
- Manitoba
- Michigan
- Minnesota
- Montana
- Nebraska
- North Dakota
- Ontario
- Saskatchewan
- South Dakota
- Wisconsin
- Wyoming

District #5—South Central

- Arkansas
- Colorado
- Kansas
- Missouri
- New Mexico
- Oklahoma
- Texas

District #6—North Pacific

- Alaska
- Alberta
- British Columbia
- Idaho
- Oregon
- Washington
- Yukon, North West Territory

District #7—South Pacific

- Arizona
- California
- Hawaii
- Nevada
- Utah

Section 4 (new Section 4; present Section 4 to become Section 7). Individual membership in NANDA is established through pre-sentation to the Association of the completed application, as required by Association policy or Bylaws, together with annual dues.

Section 5 (new Section). Affiliate Regional Organization Membership is granted to Regional Organizations

a) whose membership is consistent with the Association criteria
b) whose purpose is consistent with the Association purpose
c) whose organization, structure, and bylaws meet such criteria as shall be determined by the Association.

Section 6 (new Section). Affiliate Regional Organization membership with the Association may be established by application to the Regional Affairs Committee. Approval of the application by the Association Board and submission of any such membership fees as may be required by the Association, shall establish regional organizations as affiliate member organizations.

Section 7 (old Section 4). Membership Year. The membership year shall be a period of 12 consecutive months, beginning July 1 of each calendar year.

Rationale: These recommended changes will provide for district organization as proposed in the report of the Regional Affairs Committee accepted at the 1988 Biennial Meeting. The wording of the proposed changes will allow for individual membership and for affiliate regional organization membership for regional organizations that are already in existence and any new groups. It does not designate the states/provinces that make up a district. This will eliminate Bylaws change as membership changes bring about a need for shifting states/provinces from one district to another. It also avoids the potential problems of regional groups that presently may have membership from states/provinces other than those proposed in the 1988 Regional Affairs Committee Report.

It should be a goal of the Regional Affairs Committee to bring about gradual change that would align existing and new regional organizations within the identified district. Individual members will be identified by district at the time dues are paid and membership cards are issued, which would assist in communication within a district to participate in the selection of district membership on the Regional Affairs Committee.

A change in Committee membership is also being proposed. Each region would have a representative on the Committee who would then serve as a liaison to NANDA and an organizer for the district.

Policies and procedures can be developed that will identify the states/provinces belonging to a district and will set the criteria for affiliate regional organization membership. The Board can determine any membership dues for an affiliate organization and other such policy and procedures as may be needed without changes in Bylaws.

Article VI Committees

Section 1. Committee appointments. The Association may have standing committees. Each committee shall be chaired by a NANDA member, as appointed by the president. The appointed chair shall name additional members with attention to geographic and clinical practice distribution with concurrence by the president. The size of the committee shall be determined by the Board. Committees shall report to the Board and to meetings of the Association as requested or as required by these Bylaws.

Section 2. h) Regional Affairs. The committee shall promote the involvement of members in affairs of the Association through activities and communication at a local or regional level, and provide a mechanism for bringing issues of regional concerns to the attention of the Board and the Association.

Proposed Amendment

Section 1. Committee appointments. The Association may have standing committees. Each committee shall be chaired by a NANDA member, as appointed by the president. The appointed chair shall name additional members with attention to geographic and clinical practice distribution with concurrence by the president. The size of the committee shall be determined by the Board unless otherwise stated by the Bylaws. Committees shall report to the Board and to meetings of the Association as requested or as required by these Bylaws.

Section 2. h) Regional Affairs. The committee shall promote the involvement of members in affairs of the Association through activities and communication at local, regional, or district level, and provide a mechanism for bringing issues of concern to the attention of the Board and the Association. The committee shall be composed of seven members, one selected from each district.

Rationale: This change in membership composition is necessary to ensure that each district is represented on the committee, a necessary condition for a committee whose major function is to promote district development and serve as a sounding board for regional organizations. If committee members are to be appointed by chairs, this plan can be followed; if members are elected, candidates can be obtained from each district.

International Committee Report

Submitted by Ann Becker, Chairperson
Susan MacLean
Elizabeth Mottet
Ann Neufeld
Virginia Saba

Members of the Committee, 1988–1989

Beatrice Turkoski
Winnifred Mills
Gertrude McFarland
Jeannette Clough

Meetings

The Committee held one meeting at the Eighth NANDA Conference and three telephone conference calls.

Activities

1. The major activity was planning and presenting the "Nursing Diagnosis Special Session" at the Congress of the International Council of Nurses in Seoul, Korea, on June 1, 1989. Presentations were given by Dr. Joyce Fitzpatrick, Dr. Lucille Joel, Dr. Beatrice Turkoski, Dr. Virginia Saba, and Dr. Mi Ja Kim. A report of the presentations may be found in the Summer 1989 issue of the *Nursing Diagnosis Newsletter*.
2. At the presentation a form was distributed to nurses interested in developing an international nursing diagnosis network. To date, 43 nurses from Australia, Denmark, Pakistan, and the Republic of China have responded.

Goals for 1990

1. Conduct a survey to determine the state of the art of nursing diagnosis in non-North American countries.
2. Develop a directory of international groups/nurses for liaison relationships with NANDA.

Projected Activities

1. Members are developing a survey questionnaire to be sent to nursing groups

and selected nurses in non-North American countries.

2. Questionnaires will be sent in April or May 1990.

3. The Committee will explore financing (funding sources) for an international nurse leader(s) to participate in the Tenth NANDA Conference in 1992.

VII

New Nursing Diagnoses

Altered Protection

Kathleen C. Sheppard, MSN, RN

Altered protection is the state in which an individual experiences a decrease in ability to guard the self from internal or external threats such as illness or injury (Lunney, 1982). Its major defining characteristics are deficient immunity, impaired healing, altered blood clotting, maladaptive stress, and neurosensory alterations. Minor characteristics include chills, perspiration, dyspnea, cough, itching, restlessness, insomnia, fatigue, anorexia, weakness, immobility, disorientation, and pressure sores. Other factors related to *altered protection* include extremes of age, inadequate nutrition, alcohol abuse, abnormal blood profiles, drug therapies, treatments, and diseases.

Persons at risk for *altered protection* can be categorized by diseases, treatments, and conditions.

Diseases

One disease that can lead to *altered protection* is cancer. Cancer alters protection because it affects resistance and immunity; this is especially true for hematologic cancers such as leukemia, lymphoma, and multiple myeloma. Immune disorders also can alter protection. A classic example is acquired immune deficiency syndrome (AIDS). Persons with immune disorders are at risk for cancers and infection. In bone marrow transplantation (BMT), the development of graft versus host disease is an example of altered protective mechanisms rejecting the host. The rejection of transplanted organs is another example of *altered protection*. Autoimmune disorders are a third type of disease that can alter protective mechanisms. Among these diseases are rheumatoid arthritis and multiple sclerosis. Coagulation disorders (e.g., hemophilia, disseminated intravascular coagulation) alter the protective mechanisms for blood clotting. Other disorders that might alter protection are sickle cell disease, idiopathic thrombocytopenia purpura, neutropenia, neuropathy (e.g., from a brain tumor or a coma), burns, and pressure sores.

Treatments

Treatments affecting the immune, hematopoietic, integumentary, and neurosensory systems are radiation, surgery, and drugs (e.g., antineoplastics, corticosteroids, immunosuppressants, biologic response modifiers, anticoagulants, thrombolytic enzymes, antibiotics).

Conditions

Among the conditions affecting protection is stress. Chronic, maladaptive stress depresses the immune system and stress-management techniques (e.g., relaxation, exercise, music) have demonstrated an ability to increase immune function. Persons at the extremes of age—the elderly and newborns—have less effective immune function than do other people. Cancer in the elderly has been linked to the decreased immune function associated with aging. Other conditions that alter mechanisms of protection are inadequate nutrition, inadequate sleep, and alcohol abuse. Obviously, the factors involved in protection are so numerous and diverse that concern for protection spans a variety of patient populations.

Literature Review

The concept of *altered protection* was developed through literature review, clinical practice, and research. Norris (1982) described basic physiologic protection mechanisms and referred to functional behavioral responses that attempt to remove threats to bodily organs or systems. These threats are perceived as needs, drives, and discomforts; they are warnings. Attributes of the macrosystem of protection include increased drive or activity, increased vigilance, ejecting activity, withdrawing, and withholding. Attributes of the microsystem include healing, immunity, clotting, stress response, and integrative nervous- and endocrine-system responses.

Griffin (1986) used the diagnosis *alterations in protective mechanisms* throughout *Hematology and Immunology. Alterations in protective mechanisms* were related to bleeding disorders, decreased immune disorders, increased immune system functions, and disorders of leukocytes. Lunney (1982) recommended diagnostic categories of com-

fort, communication, coping, elimination, nutrition, sexuality, sleep, thought, parenting, self-concept, independence, learning, oxygenation, activity, growth and development, grieving, fear, and protection (among others). The *Standards of Oncology Nursing Practice* developed by the American Nurses' Association (1987) with the Oncology Nursing Society (ONS) relate to issues in prevention and detection, information, coping, comfort, nutrition, mobility, elimination, sexuality, ventilation, circulation, and protective mechanisms defined as the immune, hematopoietic, integumentary, and sensorimotor systems. Also, at the American Association of Critical-Care Nurses and Marquette University's National Conference on Nursing Diagnoses in Critical Care, the third most frequently identified concern needing a diagnostic category was compromised immunologic defenses (Wake, McLane, & Gotch, 1985).

In addition, medical-surgical textbooks include discussions of protection. *Pathophysiological Phenomena in Nursing: Human Responses to Illness* (Carrieri, Lindsay, & West, 1986) is developed in three sections, one of which is devoted to alterations in protection. The presentation includes information on stress response, impaired immunocompetence, impaired wound healing, altered clotting, and impaired sleep. Phipps, Long, and Woods (1987) also addressed the issue of protective mechanisms, including the skin, mucous membranes, macrophages, leukocytes, thrombocytes, interferons, antibodies, lymphocytes, the thymus, the lymph modes, and the spleen.

The identification of a need for a nursing diagnosis dealing with protection began in the clinical area, specifically in oncology nursing, where the problems associated with cancer, chemotherapy, BMT, immunotherapy, and bleeding are paramount. The diagnosis oncology nurses used in many of these instances was *potential for injury*, for which three subcomponents have been defined: poisoning, suffocation, and trauma. *Potential for trauma* is defined as the risk of accidental tissue injury (e.g., from a wound, burn, or fracture). That subcategory was devised based on reports of falls and accidents, for which it is obviously useful. However, it has been extended in practice to encompass infection, bleeding, and hypokalemia. The broader interpretation becomes misleading because everything nurses do can be interpreted as preventing injury. The clinical identification of a need for a more appropriate diagnosis prompted concern, and at the Southern Regional Nursing Diagnosis Conference in 1985, the critical care interest group recommended further research on *potential for injury* and development of *altered protection*.

Research

In 1985, an identification survey was conducted at the University of Texas M. D. Anderson Cancer Center. Participants were asked to list diagnoses/problems/needs they used most often. The most frequently listed items included various labels for infection, neutropenia, injury, and bleeding (Sheppard, 1987). Protective issues clearly were a major concern.

A second identification study was conducted using oncology nurses nationwide. Results were reported at the North American Nursing Diagnosis Association (NANDA) Seventh National Conference (Sheppard, 1987). In this study, the nurses read a brief case report of a patient who had immunosuppression and myelosuppression; they then were asked to identify the most appropriate diagnosis from four choices given. The respondents chose *alterations in protective mechanisms* as most appropriate 52% of the time.

A validation study of the diagnosis was undertaken. The results were reported at NANDA's Eighth National Conference (Sheppard,

1989). A sample of 108 registered nurses belonging to ONS rated each defining characteristic of *alterations in protective mechanisms* on a scale of 1 to 5, where 1 = not at all characteristic and 5 = very characteristic. The results showed that critical indicators of the diagnosis included leukopenia, thrombocytopenia, lymphopenia, infection, bleeding, immune deficiency, antineoplastic therapy, corticosteroid therapy, and immunosuppressant therapy. Minor characteristics were erythrocytopenia, immunoglobulinemia, abnormal coagulation profile, delayed hypersensitivity reaction, anemia, extremes of age, maladaptive stress, inadequate nutrition, presence of microorganisms, anticoagulant therapy, thrombolytic enzyme therapy, antibiotic therapy, radiation therapy, surgery, and alcohol abuse.

Reaction to these results was positive and the diagnosis was submitted for ballot at the eighth conference. Based on reviewer comments, on the literature, and on the results of the validation study, the diagnosis had been revised and broadened to protection, but because the revisions were incorporated at the conference and not before it, the diagnosis was removed from the ballot. Now, however, *altered protection* is ready for implementation and clinical application.

Clinical Application

The nurse's goals when *altered protection* exists can generally be categorized as

1. *Promotion* of the patient's protection: resistance is increased through stress management, strengths are enhanced, and the patient becomes knowledgeable about protective measures.
2. *Maintenance* of the patient's protection: protecting the patient and thus preventing threats.
3. *Restoration* of the patient's protection: the institution of therapeutic ap-

proaches to protection (e.g., sleep, nutrition) that decrease symptoms.

The nurse's interventions, categorized by Bulechek and McCloskey (1985), can include but are not limited to surveillance, education, and relaxation.

Case Study

Case examples could include any persons with the characteristics previously mentioned. The example presented here is that of a patient with *altered protection* related to immunosuppression and immunomodulation.

Mr. R. had ecchymotic areas on his inner thighs and petechiae on his face. Bone marrow analyses indicated hypocellularity (to 30% of normal), and the results of blood tests indicated anemia, leukopenia, and thrombocytopenia. Mr. R. was diagnosed with aplastic anemia. Prednisone therapy was initiated but was later discontinued because of abnormal liver function. The petechiae increased and gingival bleeding began, and Mr. R. was entered on the institution's granulocyte-macrophage colony-stimulating factor protocol. Treatment was scheduled to last 14 days, but after 10 days the patient was admitted to the hospital with shaking, chills, fever, weakness, petechiae, and fatigue. Laboratory test results again indicated anemia, leukopenia, and thrombocytopenia—the symptoms of aplastic anemia and the side effects of immunotherapy.

The plan of care included many of the elements previously described:

Diagnosis:
   Altered protection related to immunosuppression and immunomodulation
Goals:
   • Prevent complications.
   • Manage symptoms.

• Protect weaknesses.
• Enhance strengths.

Interventions:
Surveillance
• Monitor signs and symptoms of disorders.
• Monitor vital signs.
• Provide nurse presence.
• Provide a safe environment.

Education:
• Teach patient to conserve energy, rest, and eat nutritious foods.
• Teach about signs and symptoms and about management of side effects.

Relaxation:
Initiate relaxation techniques to increase internal protection.

Proposal

Altered protection is proposed as a diagnostic label in and of itself. It does not take the place of *potential for infection*, which is itself clinically useful and important. *Potential for infection* is the state in which an individual is at increased risk for being invaded by pathogenic organisms, and it will still be used when the risk of infection exists. No diagnosis addresses the presence of actual infection, nor does one label cover all the situations that *altered protection* encompasses. The diagnoses may overlap somewhat. For instance, when the discharge planning nurse orders a walker for someone going home, is the diagnosis *impaired mobility, potential for injury* (falls), or *impaired home maintenance management*? All include defining characteristics that may be applicable, and only further research into the question will resolve the issue.

Altered protection guides a different plan than does *potential for infection*. Interventions for *potential for infection* focus on the environment and organisms (e.g., hygiene, hand washing, isolation, decreasing invasive procedures). Interventions for *altered protection* focus not only on protecting and preventing but also on restoring and on the potential for growth. *Potential for infection* has a limited focus and a potential focus (at risk); *altered protection* has a broad focus (guard, prevent, and enhance) and an actual focus.

Protection was viewed in Taxonomy I as being on the same level of abstraction as nutrition and circulation. In Taxonomy II it would be considered as belonging on Level 2—as are, for example, coping and social isolation. So, both diagnoses are valuable and useful in practice, just as both levels of diagnoses are clinically useful and valuable.

Summary

The nursing literature has long used the term protection. Therefore, in theory at least, protection is in our body of knowledge. For nursing diagnoses to reflect the needs of clinical practice, I recommend that the term protection be used consistently.

Clinically, protection needs have been found to cross the strata of individual, family, and community; of age; and of wellness/illness. The diagnosis is holistic with interventions directed at the interconnectedness of the person, and it is clinically useful. Several institutions have implemented this diagnosis, and their positive feedback should be respected.

For research, a consistent database enables studies and findings to be compared and replicated. The impetus to conduct such studies is enormous because protecting patients from complications that extend the length of hospitalization is a major economic concern in today's health care environment. The use of the label *altered protection* could provide a consistent database.

Knowledge of the implications of a depressed immune system is increasing. The area of interventions in psychoneuroimmunology such as stress management, music, exercise, and relaxation techniques to increase protection is an exciting and rich field. It tells us that people in support groups live longer, and that patients allowed out on pass increase their platelet counts sooner. We do not yet have a nursing diagnosis to label this important area of nursing practice and nursing research. Perhaps the gap can be filled with *altered protection*.

I once wrote that the term protection is also applied to the protective coloring that some animals such as chameleons use to hide themselves from their enemies. The protective interventions of guarding, safekeeping, defending, and promoting work similarly, if not quite to the extent of the chameleon's abilities. Further research will give us the answers we need, and the way to study this diagnosis is to have it on our list. I recommend we adopt *altered protection* as a nursing diagnosis to be tested and evaluated.

Discussion

Margaret Kiss: I support the diagnosis *altered protection*. I am in the clinical setting at Memorial-Sloan Kettering Cancer Center. Nurses in practice at Memorial have found great utility with the use of this diagnosis. We've been working with it for over five years. I feel we need an opportunity to work with the diagnosis and perform validation studies. I see wide applicability in its use in the nursing care of groups well described by Kathy Sheppard. Because of our experience with the use of this diagnosis and its applications for individual, family, and community, I strongly support the acceptance of this diagnosis.

Liz Hiltunen: I'm speaking as a representative of the Massachusetts Conference Group for Nursing Diagnosis. At our February meeting, we broke into groups and discussed the two diagnoses, so I'm bringing some consensus types of comments. We felt that there were some problems with this diagnosis in that it needed a lot more specificity. The title seemed to be a broad category. The label *altered protection* looked like a broad category now in Taxonomy I, *altered physical regulation*. We also felt, and I think the speaker spoke to this this morning, that perhaps we already have a more specific label such as *potential for infection* or *potential for injury*. In the definition there was a phrase of internal and external threats and we felt that this needed to be more clearly defined. We didn't know what external and internal threats were. Moving down to the major characteristics, they looked like they could all be risk factors if you used the label *potential for infection* or *potential for injury*. Also, the major characteristics as they were listed at that point were not operationally defined. And we also felt that nurses could not assess these major characteristics independently. The minor characteristics looked to us maybe like a syndrome, and I'm anxious to hear Ann Court's talk to see if that's in fact what we are looking at there. Finally, we needed clarification with the information we were given about nursing treatment. I think that would have been helpful to have that when we reviewed the diagnosis to see what the treatments were. We were not able to really focus on that with the lack of specificity in the paper.

KATHY SHEPPARD: I appreciate what you're saying about the level. I would say with further research, maybe we'll find we can specify the diagnosis further. The diagnosis was broadened based on the reviewers' comments in the review cycle and based on the literature.

MARGARET LUNNEY: Needless to say I'm speaking in favor of the diagnosis. I've been using it for many years. In contrast to Kathy Sheppard and Peggy Kiss, it comes out of my community health practice. I see it as somewhat related to safety. I have identified those differences in other papers, but I don't have them with me. We use this diagnosis for many vulnerable populations and I'd like to just speak very briefly to the issue of specificity. I know there is a swell of need for specific diagnoses and I would, again, implore the members of NANDA [that] although we need those diagnoses, not to preclude the use of broad level diagnoses. Some nurses at the competent, proficient, and expert level really can see the broader picture and can integrate many clusters of diagnoses in order to make a broad level diagnosis which is much more efficient to guide their practice and their interventions of surveillance and all of those other broad level interventions than to have many different specific diagnoses. Some of the diagnoses that would be specified have not been accepted by NANDA perhaps because of some of the issues related to physiological diagnoses that have been mentioned before. Immunocompromise, for example, might be a subdiagnosis of protection; one that, combined with many other types of specific diagnoses, would lead you to *altered protection* because it's more efficient to talk about one thing that's encompassing than it is to talk about all the different specific things in detail. So I would just ask for the population to try it and see. I really resent the fact that some of us who use diagnoses cannot get them on the list because a lot of people are not using them and are not familiar with them. I would like us to be open and inclusive.

ROSEMARIE HOGAN: I have some questions about the defining characteristics and the etiologies and their relationships. The major defining characteristics seem to be pathophysiological states, and the minor defining characteristics are, for want of better things, a syndrome or signs and symptoms. And then when you look at the etiological factors, there is an overlap between the major defining characteristics and some of the etiological factors. And I guess my concern is that we need some clarity and differentiation between major defining characteristics and etiological factors.

KATHY SHEPPARD: The major defining characteristics have the validity from the study and textbooks and literature written on protection. To be consistent with that literature, that's how it was defined and [those] would be the major characteristics. On related factors, there is some overlap. But instead of calling it physiological, I guess I like to say it's holistic because there are interventions that affect the interconnectedness, the mind over the body, so physiological only tells half the story.

ROSEMARIE HOGAN: I think for the novice nurse, in terms of teaching someone the diagnosis and etiological factors, I think there'll be a problem in terms of which comes first, the chicken or the egg. In other words, altered immunity is a major defining characteristic but also, in your etiology, there are some of the same ideas. I just like to see that developed and clarified a little bit.

BETTY GERETY: I'm a clinical nurse specialist and consultation liaison—psychiatry. I'm supportive of the diagnosis, but I have reservations about the defining characteristic of disorientation. Restlessness, insomnia, and disorientation make me look for delirium confusion, and I think this could be misleading. Many times staff nurses don't recognize that this potentially life-threatening situation is existing. I don't think disorientation fits as well with the rest of the definition's major and minor characteristics.

KATHY SHEPPARD: I think it's going to be an individual assessment and the disorientation [means the patient has] protection needs and that'll be the deciding factor. We need more research for specificity.

PAT IYER: I have used this diagnosis for a number of years and have taught it to a number of nurses. I think that it's sufficiently broad that it applies to a variety of settings.

And I have found that staff nurses are easily able to use it and apply it to their work.

BARBARA TAPTICH: I strongly support this diagnosis. I supported it two years ago for one specific population. My specialty is cardiovascular nursing and we have patients who undergo invasive procedures with large doses of radiopaque dye who are at high risk for dire reactions following that. Since that time we've seen the advent of thrombolytic therapy and this diagnosis gives a wonderful opportunity to group things that we're considering under multiple diagnoses into one.

References

American Nurses' Association. (1987). *Oncology Nursing Society standards for oncology nursing practice.* Kansas City, MO: Author.

Bulechek, G. M., & McCloskey, J. C. (1985). *Nursing interventions: Treatments for nursing diagnoses.* Philadelphia: Saunders.

Carrieri, V. K., Lindsay, A. M., & West, C. M. (1986). *Pathophysiological phenomena in nursing: Human responses to illness.* Philadelphia: Saunders.

Griffin, J. (1986). *Hematology and immunology: Concepts for nursing.* Norwalk, CT: Appleton-Century-Crofts.

Lunney, M. (1982). *Nursing diagnosis: Refining the system. American Journal of Nursing, 82,* 456–459.

Norris, C. (1982). Synthesis of concepts: Evolving an umbrella concept-protection. In C. M. Norris (Ed.), *Concept clarification in nursing* (pp. 385–411). Rockville, MD: Aspen.

Phipps, W. G., Long, B. C., & Woods, N. F. (1987). *Medical-surgical nursing concepts and clinical practice* (3rd ed.). St. Louis, MO: Mosby.

Sheppard, K. C. (1987). Alterations in protective mechanisms. In A. M. McLane (Ed.), *Classification of nursing diagnoses: Proceedings of the seventh national conference* (pp. 239–246). St. Louis, MO: Mosby.

Sheppard, K. C. (1989). Validation of the diagnosis alterations in protective mechanisms. In R. M. Carroll-Johnson (Ed.), *Classification of nursing diagnoses: Proceedings of the eighth national conference* (pp. 281–283). Philadelphia: Lippincott.

Wake, M. M., McLane, A. M., & Gotch, P. M. (1985). Nursing diagnosis in critical care: Reflections and future directions. *Heart & Lung, 14,* 444–448.

Effective Breastfeeding

Mary L. Henrikson, MN, RNC, ARNP
Ginna Wall, MN, RN
Dona Lethbridge, PhD, RN
Vicki E. McClurg, MN, RN

Definition:

The state in which a mother–infant dyad/family exhibits adequate proficiency and satisfaction with breastfeeding behaviors

Defining Characteristics:

Major

- Mother able to position infant at breast to promote a successful latch-on response
- Infant appears content after feedings
- Regular and sustained suckling at the breast
- Adequate infant weight gain

Minor

- Signs and symptoms of oxytocin release (let-down milk or milk ejection reflex)
- Adequate elimination by infant
- Eagerness of infant to nurse
- Maternal verbalization of satisfaction with the breastfeeding process

Related Factors:

- Basic breastfeeding knowledge
- Normal breast structure
- Normal infant oral structure
- Infant gestational age greater than 34 weeks
- Support sources
- Maternal confidence

Substantiating/Supportive Materials

Breastfeeding is an intricate process that is both physiologic and psychologic in nature. The ultimate measure of successful breastfeeding is a well-fed infant measured by adequate weight gain and, on a daily basis, stool and urine output (DeCarvalho, Robertson, Merkatz, & Klaus, 1982; Neifert & Seacat, 1986a). In the literature, success is also measured by length of time (weeks or months) a mother breastfeeds her baby (Auerbach & Avery, 1980; Cadwell, 1981; DeChateau, Holmberg, Jakobeson, & Winberg, 1977). This time period is related to how effectively the mother and her family learn and adapt to breastfeeding behaviors that lead to a well-nourished infant.

Validation of Breastfeeding Nursing Diagnoses

The study to be reported here was aimed at the validation of the following nursing diagnoses by nurses expert in the care of breastfeeding mothers and infants:

1. *Effective breastfeeding*
2. *Ineffective breastfeeding*
3. *Interruption in breastfeeding*

Background

This study is part of a larger program of research aimed at validating nursing diagnoses that will enable the organization and documentation of nursing care for breastfeeding mothers and infants. The North American Nursing Diagnosis Association (NANDA) has compiled a list of nursing diagnoses that are essentially problem oriented. Many nurses working in parent and child nursing, however, have expressed the need for wellness- and health promotion-oriented nursing diagnoses.

During 1988, of four breastfeeding diagnoses submitted to NANDA, two (*effective breastfeeding* and *termination of breastfeeding*) were rejected, and two (*interruption in breastfeeding* and *ineffective breastfeeding*) were merged into *impaired breastfeeding*. A defense of the original wording was given at the seventh conference in March 1988, and in August 1988 NANDA accepted the diagnosis of *ineffective breastfeeding* for the approved list.

Sample

Three hundred nurses were randomly selected from the NAACOG list of certified postpartum and normal newborn nursery nursing, and 100 nurse lactation consultants were randomly selected from the membership of the International Lactation Consul-

tant Association. Participants were dispersed throughout the United States and Canada. Of the 134 (33%) who returned completed instruments, 66 were selected as having expertise in both breastfeeding nursing care and nursing diagnoses.

Methods

Defining characteristics were formulated by the authors using the nursing research and clinical literature and clinical experience. These defining characteristics were submitted to five nursing experts for a general evaluation of their suitability and for judgment as to clarity. Additionally, several incorrect items were added to each instrument to verify that participants were not just responding randomly.

The Delphi technique was used to obtain consensus from nurse experts on the validity of the three nursing diagnoses. Initially, instruments were compiled consisting of the nursing diagnosis definition, related factors, and defining characteristics. Respondents were asked to indicate agreement or disagreement with the definition and related factors, and to comment. The defining characteristics were rated on a five-point Likert scale from 1 to 5, where 1 = not at all representative and 5 = very representative. After analysis of data, results were returned to the 66 nurse experts for their agreement or disagreement.

Data Analysis

Ratios were calculated for each defining characteristic. Responses were weighted so that the total score could reach only 1.0; no value was given to a defining characteristic that the experts judged to be not at all indicative. Then the characteristics with mean weighted ratios of less than 0.05 were discarded.

Written comments were subjected to content analysis. Suggested definitions, related factors, and defining characteristics were added to instruments for the second round of the Delphi technique.

Findings

When defining characteristic scores were weighted, all incorrect items were weighted less than 0.5. For *effective breastfeeding*, all defining characteristics were weighted as "retain." Added comments supported a change in the diagnosis definition.

After the second round of Delphi analysis, there was further refinement of related factors and definitions. Participants in the Delphi analysis agreed with all decisions resulting from the weights assigned to defining characteristics.

Clinical Implications

Before use of this diagnosis is warranted, it must be tested with another group of experts—breastfeeding women. Formulation of nursing diagnosis instruments using lay language is now in progress. In addition, testing with nurse experts is planned for the diagnoses *effective termination of breastfeeding* and *difficulty with termination of breastfeeding*. Finally, suggested modifications in the use of the Delphi technique with nursing diagnosis validity studies will be discussed.

Discussion

ANGELA NICOLETTI: My comments reflect some of the deliberations at the last meeting of the Massachusetts Conference Group. I am also a maternal-child health nurse and though I have some comments which I think reflect changes that I think should be made, I do want to see a diagnosis that reflects the normal process of breastfeeding accepted. I want it to be a good one, and that's where the comments come from. I have a problem with the name effective and I think you, also, will

see that in that your comments on changes in the characteristics and relating it to the axes indicated that this is a process and "effective" kind of connotes a goal, an end point. And my suggestion would be something like, *breastfeeding—initiated; breastfeeding—sustained*, or perhaps something like *breastfeeding, stage one, stage two* because your diagnosis really reflects initiation of breastfeeding in the hospital, in the very early postpartum period, and we want something useful beyond that. I don't see any need for putting family in the definition, although family support certainly belongs in the related factors. The eagerness to nurse could be measurable, e.g., something exhibits rooting behavior. I want to see [this diagnosis] modified, [but] I do want to see something like this accepted.

KATHLEEN POWERS: I have some concerns in that I understand that everybody wants the wellness diagnoses, and I see this as an attempt to do that, but I have a problem differentiating this from an outcome. You have *ineffective breastfeeding* and you want to have *effective breastfeeding*. It's hard for me to realize what the difference in my interventions are going to be for this diagnosis as opposed to a problem. And I have a real hard time with it. I understand the concept but I'm not sure that this is the mechanism in which to do it.

VICKI MCCLURG: If you think back to the history of the program: I needed to document why I was in [a room] for 45 minutes with a mother that was effectively breastfeeding. I wasn't just teaching; I was positioning, I was monitoring her skill, and I was evaluating the baby's whole picture.

KATHLEEN POWERS: But if you were repositioning, you were doing things; there was a problem that you were dealing with.

VICKI MCCLURG: I understand how you're grappling because we've grappled, too. And I think that in many ways, this is a mirror image or the flip side of *ineffective breastfeeding*. But we need a label for it.

KATHLEEN MCMILLAN: I'm bringing reviews

from the clinical nurse specialist who's the lactation expert at Mt. Sinai Hospital in Toronto, Annemarie de Jardin, and Barb Sangieri, who is the nursing unit administrator in the nursery. First, they'd like to compliment the submitters on the wellness-oriented focus because they do feel that this diagnosis has utility. The concerns that they expressed were that the definition of regular and sustained suckling may not be the equivalent of regular and sustained feeding, i.e., suckling may not necessarily mean milking the breast. It was interesting to hear Judith Warren's presentation on axis because it became very clear as they were reading this, there was a definite need to separate out the initiation phase of the newborn and the established phase of the infant. So I would strongly recommend that we look at a developmental axis definition for this diagnosis. The only other issue that they had, which will probably be covered again by looking at a developmental axis, was whether meconium would be considered a stool. And also the comment that breastfed infant stools are primarily liquid rather than soft, and there was a concern about whether perhaps it should be identified under frequency of stooling rather than consistency.

LINDA MIERS: I would have to speak against this particular diagnosis. I think we have to once again put in a plea for what is a definition of a response. In the materials that we received in the mail, you say that breastfeeding is a process. And according to our definition that was accepted two days ago, we're looking for responses to processes. The next thing you say is that the ultimate parameter of successful breastfeeding is a well-fed infant measured by adequate weight gain on a daily basis, stool and urine output. So, consequently, to me, the well-fed baby is the response. You know whether they're well-fed by the defining characteristics of urine, stool, and a satisfied infant. The process is feeding. I would have to think that you could have a similar diagnosis for *effective bottlefeeding.*

And you could look at the position of the mother and the infant with the bottle. But the process is feeding, not the *effective* or *ineffective breastfeeding* as the response that you're dealing with. I think it's also important that we define the client that we're assessing, because your defining characteristics include characteristics for both the parent and for the infant. The soft stools and the wet diapers would apply to the infant whose response [is] nutrition. The positioning and particularly the oxytocin release would be looking at lactation as a response in the mother. So I think you have to again analyze these concepts more clearly and I once again put in my plea for clearer definitions of what it is that we're classifying and accepting concepts into a list for.

VICKI MCCLURG: We believe that lactation is the process. *Effective breastfeeding* is the interaction between the mother and the infant, and requires a great deal of support both by family members, as well as the nursing and medical profession. We believe that an outcome is a well-fed baby.

CONNIE PINCKLEY: I would like to speak in support of the diagnosis. I bring comments from our specialists at University Hospitals of Cleveland. The comments that I would make relate to particularly the wording. Number one, breastfeeding was looked at as a much broader issue than just feeding, and it was looked at as a process. Because of that, we felt that it was important to use the word process and not behaviors in the definition. The second thing that we felt was very important as the diagnosis was reviewed was to look at not using words like adequate proficiency. In the old definition, it said exhibits adequate proficiency, and much of the work of the nurse is very early in the process. We came up with a diagnosis [of] *establishing breastfeeding process.* In further review, we did come up with *effective breastfeeding* as being the state in which a mother and her infant learn the process of breastfeeding and develop proficiency and satisfaction with breastfeeding. The point being that it is very difficult to establish between effective and ineffective very early in the breastfeeding process and that by broadening out the definition, it was much easier for our clinicians to distinguish at what point breastfeeding became ineffective. The one other comment is to look in defining characteristics. If you don't look at it simply as feeding, there probably need to be characteristics that deal with that interaction, such as productive mother-infant communication patterns, that are currently not there. The only thing that we have for satisfaction is the infant being content; there's nothing about the mother-infant relationship.

ANGELA NICOLETTI: I think now that we've included life processes in the definition [of nursing diagnosis], we're not going to be able to so clearly conceive of it as a response to a life process as much as an experience of a life process. I think the comments reflect that what the diagnosis label needs is to be staged so that people can see that in stage one you do this, and then you plan for achieving what you want in stage two, and so on, and I think that will make it much more acceptable.

GINNA WALL: And that would fit very nicely into axis number two as I understand it.

DOROTHEA JAKOB: As a long-term proponent for conceptual room for wellness diagnoses, I'd like to just raise a small point of information that's useful for me. I see and hear many people when they think about wellness diagnoses stumble on the terminology "related to." I would like to share with you a mechanism that is really useful for me and I might add it was coined by Mi Ja Kim in a taxi cab going to two conferences ago when we were talking about this. As we now know, potential nursing diagnoses have listed risk factors. Well, it makes an amazing amount of sense for wellness diagnoses to have listed enhancing factors so that something is "enhanced by." In my experience with breastfeeding women, I noticed that many of the breastfeeding women offer an openness to identify-ing their gaps in breastfeeding knowledge. I don't perceive that as a problem, I perceive that as an enhancing factor.

GINNA WALL: And they're really glad to have somebody there that can help them.

JEAN JENNY: For the majority of nurses who are not yet comfortable with the health-oriented diagnoses in the label, may I suggest—to indicate, to clarify—that a nursing diagnosis represents a state of patient needing nursing intervention; would you consider inserting "potential for effective breastfeeding"? For the majority of us who are not there yet, that, I think, would indicate the direction, the movement, the interventions globally for the nurse. "Breastfeeding" per se says nothing to me. But if we use potential for, I think the nurse knows what her goal is.

References

Auerbach, K., & Avery, J. L. (1980). Relactation: A study of 366 cases. *Pediatrics, 65*, 236–242.

Boggs, K. R., & Raw, P. K. (1983). Breastfeeding the premature infant. *American Journal of Nursing, 83*, 1437–1439.

Bose, C. L., D'Ercole, A. J., Lester, A. G., Hunter, R. S., & Barrett, J. R. (1981). Relactation by mothers of sick and premature infants. *Pediatrics, 67*, 565–569.

Cadwell, J, (1981). Improving nipple graspability of success at breastfeeding. *Journal of Obstetric, Gynecologic & Neonatal Nursing, 10*, 277–279.

Choi, M. W. (1978). Breast milk for infants who can't breastfeed. *American Journal of Nursing, 78*, 852–855.

DeCarvalho, M., Robertson, S., Merkatz, R., & Klaus, M. (1982). Milk intake and frequency of feeding in breast-fed infants. *Early Human Development, 7*, 155–163.

DeChateau, P., Holmberg, H., Jakobeson, K., & Winberg, J. (1977). A study of factors promoting and inhibiting lactation. *Developmental Medicine and Child Neurology, 19*, 525–534.

Feher, S., Berger, L., Johnson, J., & Wilde, J. (1989). Increasing milk production for premature infants with a relaxation/imagery audiotape. *Pediatrics, 83*, 57–60.

Grassley, J., & Davis, K. (1978). Common concerns of mothers who breastfeed. *MCN: The American Journal of Maternal Child Nursing, 7* 370–375.

Gulick, E. (1982). Informational correlates of successful breast feeding. *MCN: The American Journal of Maternal Child Nursing, 7*, 347–351.

Hall, J. M. (1978). Influencing breastfeeding success. *Journal of Obstetric, Gynecologic & Neonatal Nursing, 7, 28–32.

Henderson, K., & Newton, L. (1978). Helping nursing mothers maintain lactation while separated from their infants. MCN: The American Journal of Maternal Child Nursing, 3, 352–356.

Herrera, A. (1984). Supplemented versus unsupplemented breastfeeding. Perinatology-Neonatology, 8, 70–71.

Hopkinson, J., Schanler, R., & Garza, C. (1988). Milk production by mothers of premature infants. Pediatrics, 81, 815–820.

Howard, M. M. (1986). Factors associated with the success of breastfeeding the premature infant. Unpublished master's thesis, University of Washington School of Nursing, Seattle.

McNeilly, A., Robinson, I., Houston, M., & Howie, P. (1983, January 22). Release of oxytocin and prolactin response to suckling. British Medical Journal, 286, 257–259.

Morgan, J. (1986). A study of mother's breastfeeding concerns. Birth, 13, 104–108.

Morse, J., & Harrison, M. (1987). Social coercion for weaning. Journal of Nurse Midwifery, 32, 204–210.

Neifert, M., & Seacat, J. (1986a, July). A guide to successful breastfeeding. Contemporary Pediatrics, 26–45.

Neifert, M., & Seacat, J. (1986b). Practical aspects of breastfeeding the premature infant. Pediatric Clinics of North America, 33, 743–762.

Neifert, M, & Seacat, J. (1988). Practical aspects of breastfeeding the premature infant. Perinatology-Neonatology, 12, 24–31.

Newton, M., & Newton, M. (1948). The letdown reflex in human lactation. Journal of Pediatrics, 33, 1179–1188.

Pereira, G. R., Schwartz, D., Gould, P., & Grim, N. (1984). Breastfeeding in neonatal intensive care—beneficial effects of counseling. Perinatology-Neonatology, 8, 24–31.

Riordan, J., & Countryman, B. (1980). Basics of breastfeeding, Part V: Self-care for continued breastfeeding problems and solutions. Journal of Obstetric, Gynecologic & Neonatal Nursing, 9, 357–366.

Rumsey, S., Tully, M., & Overfield, M. (1983). Breastfeeding low birth weight babies—how to help. NAACOG update series (Lesson 11, Vol. 1). Princeton, NJ: NAACOG.

Salaryia, F., Easton, P., & Carter, J. (1980). Breastfeeding and milk supply failure. Maternal Child Health, 5, 38–42.

Starling, J., Fergusson, D., Horwood, L., & Taylor, B. (1979). Breastfeeding success and failure. Australian Paediatric Journal, 15, 271–274.

Stewart, D., & Gaiser, G. (1978). Supporting lactation when mothers and infants are separated. Nursing Clinics of North America, 132, 47–61.

Stone, C. S. (1988). Breastfeeding the premature infant. Pediatric Nursing Forum, 3, Ross Labs.

Tully, J., & Dewey, K. (1985). Private fears, global loss: A cross-cultural study of the insufficient milk syndrome. Medical Anthropology, 9, 225–243.

Verronen, P. (1982). Breastfeeding: Reasons for giving up and transient lactational crisis. Acta Paediatric Scandia, 71, 447–450.

Verronen, P., Voscospi, J. K., Lammi, A., et al. (1980). Promotion of breastfeeding: Effect on neonates change of feeding routines at a maternity unit. Acta Paediatric Scandia, 69, 279–282.

Winikoff, B., & Baer, E. (1980). The obstetricians opportunity: Translating "breast is best" from theory to practice. American Journal of Obstetrics and Gynecology, 138, 105–117.

Winikoff, B., Laukaran, V., Meyers, D., & Stone, R. (1986). Dynamics of infant feeding: Mothers, professionals and the institutional context in a large urban hospital. Pediatrics, 77, 357–365.

Wolfe, S. (1986). Breastfeeding success and support systems. ICEA News, 25, 10.

VIII

Group Meetings

Eight Special Interest Groups met during the Ninth Conference. Minutes of each meeting have been included here for your interest. Primarily NANDA members interested in a particular focus or subject area met to exchange information, network, and discuss current concerns in the area of nursing diagnosis.

Two Regional Groups met to discuss their mutual concerns. On the agenda of both meetings were the proposed Bylaws changes dealing with Regional Group establishment.

Special Interest Groups

Community Health

Leader Dorothea Jakob
Recorder Patricia Kucharski
Number of participants 11
Discussion The following topics were addressed:

1. Criteria for acceptance of diagnoses identifying community as client

The group expressed concern that the current criteria used by the Diagnostic Review Committee (DRC) do not accommodate concepts that are in the initial stages of development. Margaret Lunney shared her work on community diagnoses and the difficulty encountered in the review process. The group decided to introduce either a resolution or motion at the business meeting that would charge the Board to critically examine the diagnostic review process. Specific suggestions include a call for conceptual papers to stimulate a critical mass in the literature, a plan to review existing diagnoses for utility to the community as a unit of analysis, a call for case studies that include community diagnostic formulations, and a clarification by the DRC of the criteria and guidelines for submission of community diagnoses.

2. Proposed definition of community

The group expressed pleasure with the inclusion of community in the proposed working definition of nursing diagnosis and suggested that although the definition of community could be broadened to include the concept of aggregate, it was a positive beginning. The possible inclusion of a community axis in the Taxonomy should encourage development of current diagnoses for the community as client. It was suggested that a study group be formed to begin the process of examining the current diagnoses.

3. Integration of other diagnostic classification systems into the NANDA system

There was discussion about the Omaha classification system as an example of other work that was not being integrated into the NANDA system and how the group might stimulate the integration process.

Computerization

Leader Peg Mehmert
Recorder Laura Strange
Number of participants 27
Discussion The following topics were addressed:

1. A communication problem exists between clinical nursing and hospital information system (HIS) vendors. Is it

possible to develop a system based on nursing diagnosis that is not "canned"?

Requirements from nursing departments are so varied, there is difficulty developing a system to fulfill everyone's needs.

Gerber Alley, IBM, SMS, and 3M are just a few of the systems that currently support nursing diagnosis. Vendors want to hear from the profession what the clinical needs are.

There is a need for greater standardization of clinical nursing data. Research is being conducted at the University of Iowa to develop a taxonomy of interventions. Werley's work on the minimum data set may be a start toward satisfying this need. The proposed inclusion of the NANDA Taxonomy in ICD-10 may be another forward step.

2. Are there any databases for the collection of data for quality-assurance analysis?

Some systems enable one to examine which nursing diagnoses are being used and how frequently. Other systems are looking at keywords or phrases.

JCAHO requirements continue to focus on target dates for outcomes, measurables, specific interventions, and compliance with the hospital's own policy/procedure requirements for care plans.

3. What is/are the purpose(s) of care plans?

Care plans can reflect the patient's total care requirements or may identify specific patient problems. There are data that need to be documented but do not necessarily belong in the care plan. Some care plans outline the tasks of a specific standard of care and only contain a nursing diagnosis when a patient problem develops outside that standard of care. There is a need for thorough documentation with this use.

4. Are there any studies that examine how much time a computerized system saves?

At the University of Iowa, a study has shown that it takes 50 minutes to manually plan a patient's care versus 15 minutes using the computer.

5. Are bedside terminals being used successfully?

The 3M system's bedside terminals are installed at the Hospital of Latter Day Saints in Salt Lake City on a 65-bed ICU and on two 48-bed nursing units. The following experiences have been observed there and at other locations:

- Nurses like the bedside terminals, but have difficulty breaking the habit of "sitting down to chart."
- Physicians do not want to use the bedside terminals.
- Sometimes it is difficult for the nurse to input data while the patient is talking to him/her, asking questions, etc.
- Patients do not appear threatened by having their data entered in the system.

6. Are there links between assessment and care planning? Are there systems whose assessment module supports the functional health patterns model?

There are systems that support the functional health patterns model, as well as systems that "recommend" certain diagnoses based on the assessment. Some participants feel that the nurse should make an independent decision regarding the nursing diagnoses made for his/her patient. Could a legal issue arise if the suggested diagnosis(es) was/were not chosen?

Critical Care

Leader Cindy Dougherty
Recorder Beth Anderson
Number of participants 10
Discussion The following topics were addressed:

1. Beth Anderson shared work on the ongoing project of identifying a nursing diagnosis for patients having difficulty weaning from the ventilator. She has been working with a NANDA-formed group on this concern and has developed a tool to identify defining characteristics/risk factors. Concern was expressed about problems with the physiologic diagnosis and difficulty with acceptance by NANDA. Cindy Dougherty noted that with the proposed definition of nursing diagnosis this may become more of a concern.
2. Molly Tyler informed the group about completion of AACN's *Outcome Standards for Critical Care*. The publication will be ready for release in May and will be available at the NTI in San Francisco. This document includes the outcome standards for the 30 nursing diagnoses/problems that were rated of highest value by survey. Molly also reminded the group that a presentation by Rebecca Kuhn during the conference will share more information on the specific diagnoses reviewed.
3. Colleen O'Brian informed the group of work she has been doing in her hospital on revision of critical orientation according to the functional health patterns. This work is to be published in *Focus on Critical Care*.
4. Diane Roberts shared work being done on her unit with clinical documentation and changing nursing care plans by use of the Marker system. She also dis-

cussed the development of a home ventilator program.
5. Juracy Farias from Brazil stated that nursing diagnosis was in early development in her country and she needed help getting started. The group offered suggestions about whom to contact and what books to review.
6. Additional topics discussed were:
   a. The validation study that Marjorie Gordon is conducting nationwide with critical care nurses who are NANDA members.
   b. The use of symptoms as diagnostic labels (e.g., *nausea*).
   c. Concerns about where the diagnoses were placed within the Taxonomy and how the bedside nurse will use the Taxonomy. Mary Hurley, a member of the Taxonomy Committee, responded to these questions and reminded the group that the Taxonomy would be discussed at length on Sunday.
   d. Is this the positive or negative connotation of the modifier Alteration?
   e. NANDA's three-year development plan.
   f. The need for more qualitative research for nursing diagnosis in critical care.

The group was encouraged to share feelings during the conference and to consider submission of a paper at the next conference outlining issues related to use of nursing diagnosis in critical care. NANDA is still a very young organization and members must "hang in there" and offer input while NANDA is developing. A suggestion was made that NANDA develop a timetable.

Curriculum/Education

Leader Georgia Whitley
Recorder Chris Layhon

Number of participants 19
Discussion The following topics were addressed:

1. Need for a definition of nursing diagnosis.
2. Need for a data-collection tool that steers students toward appropriate nursing diagnoses; many recommended Guzetta's *Clinical Assessment Tools for Use with Nursing Diagnoses.*
3. Use of etiologies: treated by nursing or medicine?
4. Teaching using a medical model or a nursing model, especially in the areas of assessment (body systems versus functional health patterns).
5. Function health patterns versus nine human response patterns identified in the Taxonomy. All agreed that pluralism is acceptable but may be confusing to students.
6. Faculty consensus is important, especially as students go from one faculty member to another while progressing through a program and need consistent information. Varied instructor backgrounds make this a difficult goal to achieve.
7. Some facilities are using interactive videos to teach staff nurses nursing diagnosis.
8. Janet Weber, Southeast Missouri State University, summarized her experience with a nursing diagnosis-based curriculum (Frisch, Ellis, & Weber. [1988]. Nursing diagnosis: A curricular model based on the NANDA list. *Nurse Educator, 13*[5].)
   a. Advantages:
      • Students are sold on nursing diagnosis.
      • Faculty collaborates with practice agencies.
      • Agencies use faculty as consultants.
   b. Disadvantages:
      • Students inadequately prepared to deal with collaborative problems
      • Increasing numbers of nursing diagnosis-crowded curricula.
   c. Preparation for curriculum integration:
      • Faculty were willing and committed.
      • A Care Plan Committee was formed.
      • Inservices about nursing diagnosis were held for faculty.
      • The curriculum module was written by Weber.
      • Guest speakers included Carpenito and Guzetta.
   d. Nursing diagnosis and collaborative problems are used by area hospitals so content is reinforced.
   e. Course content arranged by nursing diagnosis according to areas discussed (e.g., adult health, OB, psych). Nursing diagnoses are presented by definition, defining characteristics, etiologies, interventions with rationale and evaluation, followed by case studies related to course population.
   f. Future directions:
      • Incorporating more collaborative problems.
      • Looking at other frameworks (e.g., Functional Health Patterns) rather than NANDA's Taxonomy.
9. Discussed etiology portion of diagnostic statements. Agreed the "related to" is more accurately something that influences diagnosis rather than causes it. Can "related to" be another diagnosis (e.g., *pain*)? What does *pain* interfere with (e.g., *activity intolerance* related to pain)?
10. Is the taxonomy a structure for education and practice? The abstract taxonomy needs to be made more specific to apply to clinical practice.

11. Studies have shown up to 97% of nurses surveyed said they use nursing diagnosis. The question remains: How are they using nursing diagnosis? Are nursing diagnoses being used correctly?
12. The process of identifying and integrating nursing diagnosis is ongoing and always evolving.

Nurse Practitioner

Leader   Nancy Ridenour
Recorder   Arlene Brennon
Number of participants   2
Discussion   The following topics were addressed:

1. Discussion of why so few nurse practitioners attend the meeting.
2. Need nursing diagnoses that pertain to
   a. Wellness
   b. Health promotion
   c. Health maintenance
   d. Disease prevention
   e. Health restoration
   f. Chronic problem maintenance.
3. Need positively stated nursing diagnoses.
4. How to involve nurse practitioners.
   a. Survey nurse practitioners on use of nursing diagnosis.
   b. Encourage nurse practitioners to propose nursing diagnoses.
   c. Discuss issue with ANA's Councils of Clinical Specialists and Primary Health Care Nurse Practitioners.
5. Need to work out collaborative diagnoses. Nurse practitioners are accountable for many interventions and diagnoses thought to be needed by some nurses.

Psychiatric/Mental Health

Leader   Margaret D. McComb
Recorder   Marga S. Coler

Number of participants   14
Discussion   The following topics were addressed:

1. ANA phenomena of concern

The group will prepare and submit a position statement to the NANDA Board of Directors. The concern is that psychiatric nurses should work under the NANDA system and that the ANA system should be incorporated into NANDA. A task force will work on this. We will ask the Board to address this with appropriate ANA person(s).

2. Psychiatric/mental health special interest group-sponsored workshop on off year of NANDA scheduled meetings

A national workshop will be planned by members of this group focusing on intervention via Standards of Care as impacted by nursing diagnoses in psychiatric/mental health nursing. We will request help from NANDA to sponsor this invitational conference.

3. Roles in psychiatric/mental health nursing

Roles were outlined in the following areas: education, consulting, clinical, administration, private practice, writing, research, forensics, neuropsychology.

4. Other issues

- Prescription writing
- Admitting privileges
- Role blurring with other psychiatric/mental health professionals
- Third-party payments
- Differences/similarities between psychiatry and mental health
- Networking for research

Quality Assurance

Leader Deanna Stover
Recorder Carol Vestal Allen
Number of participants 19
Discussion The following topics were addressed:

The participants discussed the problems and outcomes of implementing quality-assurance (QA) programs.

Changing from centralized to decentralized QA monitors through the implementation of unit-based QA programs increased the effectiveness and efficiency of monitoring quality care. Individual nursing units wrote standards of care for the nursing process applicable to the unit's population. The nursing staff on a unit agreed to outcomes and interventions related to a nursing diagnosis and incorporated these into the unit-based QA monitor. Nursing diagnosis was the basis for the QA monitors.

Clearly defined standards of care ensured consistency of performance among nurses as each nurse approached a client differently. A review of the literature assisted nurses in validating the unit's nursing care plans. Nursing diagnoses related to the standard were listed on the back of each written standard of care. Reviewing and adapting standards of care developed by professional organizations facilitated the generation of standards for a nursing unit.

Increasing the respect for each other's input into the nursing care plan and the care of the client strengthens nursing care. Participants recommended that nurses on a unit function as if in private practice together. At one hospital, each nurse assumed the role of the manager for a three-month period. Each nurse audited three charts and three nursing care plans per month. All the nurses worked toward measuring the client's achievement of outcomes.

A monthly compliance rate of 85%, as demonstrated on the QA monitor, was deemed acceptable. Units failing to comply with the 85% were advised to use a generic QA tool. A participant stated that one person spent 28 hours per week auditing records for QA. A 94-bed hospital used 60 different monitors that resulted in an overabundance of data. Collecting data from other QA monitors (e.g., infectious disease) consolidated the data-collection tools and led to effective auditing and use of the nurse's time.

At one participant's hospital, each unit conducted monthly conferences to evaluate the quality of care. One nurse presented a nursing care plan for a client. After the conference, another nurse on the unit audited the chart for evidence of the nurse's actions. One chart per month was reviewed. This approach led to increased growth by the nurses in achieving QA.

At another hospital, one nurse was appointed the QA nurse for the unit and designated a member of the QA committee for the division (e.g., surgery, medicine). Each educator assisted with the QA monitor for assigned units. Sharing information among the units, divisions, and the entire hospital resulted in a collaborative effort that increased control of quality care throughout the hospital.

One participant testified as an expert nursing witness in medical malpractice suits. The participant recommended the elimination of standardized nursing care plans, because it was considered a legal standard and obligated the nurse to complete all nursing interventions listed. The participant recommended (1) use of the word guideline, and the development of guidelines for nursing care to replace the standardized nursing care plans; and (2) identify minimum standards of nursing care and list on the guidelines for nursing care.

If a procedure manual indicates specific actions by the nurse, the nurse's notes should reflect implementation of these actions.

Focus charting is not tied to a nursing diagnosis and participants were advised not to use this format for documentation.

Computerization of nursing care plans and documentation expedited the monitoring of QA. The Eleven Points of Care system was launched on the market. The Shared Medical Systems (SMS) is currently used by numerous hospitals. Orem's Model was developed into a software package. Symposium Computer Applications in Medical Care (SCAMC) was published by the IEE Society. SCAMC office is located at George Washington University. The Unitary Pattern Assessment tool has been published.

Changing the delivery of nursing practice will facilitate the use of bedside computers. The bedside computer reflects the actual time the nurse spends in delivering client care.

The majority of the participants advised their nursing staff to limit the nursing diagnoses to NANDA's approved list. If nurses encountered difficulty arriving at a nursing diagnosis, they conducted a review of the literature for current research on nursing diagnosis. The participants encountered difficulties in auditing charts when nurses created their own nursing diagnoses. The use of NANDA-approved nursing diagnoses leads to consistency in monitoring QA.

The effect of the number of registered nurses to the client census on the unit impacted QA. One participant stated her hospital maintained a 100% registered nurse staff. The majority of participants stated their hospitals upheld 1:4 or 1:5 ratios of registered nurses to clients.

Of the participants present, no hospital charged separately for nursing care. The participants agreed that increased worth would be placed on nursing care if nurses were paid separately.

The majority of hospitals conducted quarterly QA monitoring. Several hospitals conducted a centralized review on a quarterly basis. The majority of participants stated their hospitals conducted unit-based monitors. Weekly monitoring was considered an inefficient and ineffective method. The information gathered from the audit was shared with the unit. All nurses were aware of their compliance rates and areas requiring improvement. Several participants noted that as the acuity level of the clients decreased, the number of errors increased.

One participant introduced the QA monitor during orientation and sent the orientees to the units. The orientees audited charts for one morning. This experience markedly increased their awareness of QA and the ramifications of monitoring.

In summary, unit-based QA tools proved effective in measuring the impact of nursing care. Each nursing unit developed minimum standards of care agreed upon by the staff. The nursing diagnoses provided the basis for the QA tool. Quarterly QA monitors proved effective in evaluating the status of care. Sharing the unit and individual compliance rates with the nurses aided in the identification of unit problems and the nurse's strengths and weaknesses. Computerization of nursing care plans and documentation expedited the monitoring of nursing care. Collaboration with other disciplines resulted in increased quality of care.

Wellness

Leader Sue Popkess-Vawter
Recorder Ginna Wall
Number of participants 3
Discussion The following topics were addressed:

1. Introductions

Participants introduced themselves and described how they were using nursing diagnoses in their settings. Jan Ander, who works with a county health department outside Chicago, stated that they have developed a "health concerns" list based on the NANDA Taxonomy; Sue Popkess-Vawter is working on developing a handbook that describes wellness diagnoses as mirror images of the problem diagnoses.

2. Wellness

Concern was expressed about the proposal from the 1988 Wellness Interest Group. Sue Popkess-Vawter explained that a national survey was done (using Delphi technique) to refine/expand the definition of nursing diagnoses. The group was referred to the Taxonomy Committee materials for discussion at this convention. Wellness is listed as an axis, allowing for the concept of health in nursing practice.

3. Nursing diagnosis definition

Sue Huether felt that the current new definition is still inadequate; Sue Popkess-Vawter suggested that she write up a revision. The group discussed various changes. It was agreed that certain words have medical implications (e.g., diagnosis, therapy, prescriptions). Using a thesaurus and a dictionary, the group developed the following revisions:

A nursing diagnosis is a clinical judgment about an individual, family, or community response to life processes and potential or actual health problems, which provides the basis for definitive actions toward achievement of outcomes for which the nurse is accountable.

Changes made and rationale:

   a. Life processes comes first on the list because of the order of nursing priorities: i.e., to prevent health problems whenever possible and secondly to restore.

   b. The word actions is used instead of therapy because of the illness-orientation of that word ("the treatment of a disease or disorder as by some remedial or curative process"). The word actions does not discriminate between wellness or illness, and implies a proactive, action-oriented approach.

Victoria Cole Schonlau agreed to bring these suggested changes to the General Assembly at L. Carpenito's session "Development of the NANDA Definition of Nursing Diagnosis" and to the business meeting.

4. The need for a two-step process in proposing new nursing diagnoses

It was suggested that ideas for diagnoses could be presented, voted upon, and then researched. Findings would then be brought back to the next conference. Requiring research first might intimidate some submitters and thereby diminish interest/work on developing nursing diagnoses.

Regional Groups

Mid-Atlantic Nursing Diagnosis Association (MANDA)

Call to Order Joan Crosley, President
Minutes Barbara Vassallo, Secretary
Number of Members Attending 14

Report of the Districts

1. Upper New York State (Margaret Briody, Representative). The informal group is keeping in touch by networking through correspondence and informal meetings.
2. New York Long Island Nursing Diagnosis Association (NYLINDA) (Barbara Rottkamp, Representative)
   a. NYLINDA and MANDA cosponsored a successful 5th Regional Conference, "Nursing Diagnosis: Nurses Claiming Nursing," in November 1989 at Rockville Centre, NY. There were 105 participants and the program included paper and poster presentations as well as invited papers and guest speakers. Profits from the conference were equally divided between the two sponsoring associations.
   b. Two of the posters at the regional conference are part of the poster presentations at this NANDA conference.
   c. The group is preparing a NYLINDA banner.
   d. The next meeting will be in June 1990.
3. Staten Island Nursing Diagnosis Association (SINDA) (Margaret Lunney, Representative)
   a. This group began by finding nurses interested in nursing diagnosis by writing to directors in health care agencies, hospitals, and long-term care agencies in the Staten Island area. In October 1988, the interested people met and in nine months had developed a set of bylaws and were an established group. At present they have 25 paid members. Dues are $10/year. The group met 6 times during 1989 and plans to meet six times in 1990. During each meeting an accepted nursing diagnosis is discussed in depth, using a 10-step guideline that includes title, meaning of definition, interventions, defining characteristics, history of the development of the diagnosis, bibliography.
   b. A June 1990 program is planned.
4. Eastern Pennsylvania Nursing Diagnosis Association (EPANDA) (Paula Rich, Representative)
   a. The group is beginning its sixth year. Current membership numbers 46 members. This is a decline from pre-

369

vious years, which is a concern to the district group.

b. There are three special interest groups within this district: a psychiatric/mental health group, which is presently conducting a nurse validation study on *potential for violence toward self and others*; an education group; and an implementation and quality-assurance group.

c. A program is planned for April 26 1990, focusing on patient education and nursing diagnosis, and a tentative fall program using an interactive video package is in preparation.

d. EPANDA publishes a quarterly newsletter.

5. Southern New Jersey Nursing Diagnosis Association (Barbara Vassallo, Representative). An informal group structure is in place. They are looking to establish a traveling inservice/continuing education program that a survey of the health care institutions in the Southern New Jersey area indicated was a priority need.

6. Washington Area Nursing Diagnosis Association (WANDA) (Sheila Sparks, Representative)

a. Presently there is a stable group membership of 28 to 30.

b. A February program had to be canceled because of lack of interest. The group plans to reevaluate the goals of the Association and how best to meet the needs of nurses in the area after this NANDA conference.

c. The annual dinner meeting is scheduled for June 1990.

d. The published newsletter continues to be well received.

7. Delaware Nursing Diagnosis Association (DENDA) (Ellen McFadden, Representative, unable to attend but sent this report). Due to the change in work places of major officers of the Association, there has been a lack of sustaining

interest. The group plans to regroup and reorganize shortly.

Discussion regarding the trends of decreased interest and participation in the nursing diagnosis movement followed. Some points that were raised were:

1. Many institutions are under financial constraints that did not exist a few years ago. Time and economic pressures on the nurses are very real factors.

2. The newness of the idea of nursing diagnosis may have worn off and people may have gone on to other activities.

3. Some of the original members have gone beyond the basic implementation phase, and may not feel the need for group support. Nurses have progressed from the introductory level and now are at, perhaps, an advanced level. Therefore, there may be a need to redefine the purpose of the organization.

4. Would the creation of specialty interest groups at the district level, e.g., research, attract more members?

Discussion of Regional Group linkage with NANDA

Concerns and questions raised by the participants included:

1. Would changes in terminology be needed if the new Bylaws are accepted? Would MANDA become a district and would present districts become chapters?

2. Would there be a fee to establish an affiliation with NANDA? How would the cost be calculated?

3. What would be the benefits of belonging to NANDA?

4. Would membership in the Regional Group be more of a benefit to the group rather than for the individual?

5. What can be the advantage of belonging

to MANDA and NANDA on the local level of nursing practice? How can districts/regions and NANDA bring an impact to nursing function at the grassroots level?

a. Recent automation has led hospitals to count tasks to determine what nurses do and to use this method for calculating the financial cost of patient care.

b. The use of a nursing diagnostic framework makes more sense as the basis of estimating how much it costs to prepare a patient for discharge.

c. Nursing diagnosis is a way of looking at the economics and politics of health care.

6. Would a three-level membership structure be a feasible method of leading from the local into the regional and then to the national organization? A selling point for local membership is the viewpoint that the local group is a subgroup of NANDA and MANDA.

7. How would MANDA pay for its membership in NANDA?

8. J. Crosley summarized the points to be considered as follows:

a. Costs would be reasonable for affiliation with NANDA.

b. Three-level membership should be considered.

c. Clarity in describing the relationship with NANDA is needed.

d. Need to know more about the ramifications of the implications of the Regional Affairs Committee.

e. Regional Affairs Committee is in a transition phase.

Bylaws proposal

Sue Popkess-Vawter, NANDA Regional Affairs Committee Board liaison, clarified the Bylaws proposal and discussed various aspects of the function of NANDA and Regional Groups:

1. The states that comprise District #2 are Delaware, Maryland, New Jersey, New York, Ohio, Pennsylvania, and Washington, DC. The proposed grouping of states was done taking time zones into consideration.

2. The new regional representative on the Regional Affairs Committee would address fee structure.

3. The Regional Group would pay a fee, probably on a sliding scale, to be formally recognized by NANDA.

4. Present and future benefits for groups who are affiliated with NANDA are:

a. Executive Director can assist Regional Groups.

b. NANDA can provide mailing labels for a nominal fee.

c. Placement of notices such as programs, meetings, etc., in *Nursing Diagnosis* free of charge.

d. Space for the regional meetings at the NANDA conference.

e. A table for display of regional materials free of charge at NANDA conference.

f. Access to major speakers through a speakers bureau.

g. Discount on NANDA conference registration for regional officers.

h. Discount to Regional Groups for NANDA publications

i. Discounts to Regional Groups to advertise in *Nursing Diagnosis.*

j. Co-sponsorship of programs between the Regional Groups and NANDA.

k. Vehicle to increase correspondence between Regional Groups via newsletters.

l. Assistance producing newsletters.

Northeast Nursing Diagnosis Association (NENDA)

Call to Order Beverly Bartlett, Vice-Chair
Minutes Suzanne MacAvoy, Secretary

Number of Members Attending 10

Beverly Bartlett called the meeting to order and announced that Carol Soares-O'Hearn (Chair) was unable to attend.

1. Mary Ann Kelly, Chair of the Regional Affairs Committee, addressed the proposed Bylaws changes regarding membership and representation on the Regional Affairs Committee. She requested our reaction to the list of states and provinces in the proposed districts and our ideas regarding what we would expect from NANDA if we were an affiliate member. We agreed with the district designations and would expect NANDA to
   a. Communicate via newsletter.
   b. Run the election of the district representative.
   c. Provide district mailing list.
   d. Co-sponsor district conferences.
      The group thanked Mary Ann for her input and supports the idea of the districts. Beverly agreed to communicate the above to Mary Ann.
2. Beverly gave an update of the NENDA meeting held last fall.
3. We discussed having a conference in 1990. A sign-up sheet was circulated for those who would be able to help plan the conference.
4. Old Business: Nominating Committee Report
   Need candidates for vice-chair and secretary (1 each) and nominating committee (2). Beverly is going to run for Chair.

A

Nursing Diagnosis Submission Guidelines and Diagnostic Review Cycle

I. Newly Proposed Diagnosis

The North American Nursing Diagnosis Association (NANDA) solicits newly proposed nursing diagnoses for review by the Association. Such proposed diagnoses undergo a systematic review process for inclusion in NANDA's approved list of diagnoses. Approval indicates that NANDA endorses the diagnoses for clinical testing and continuing development by the discipline.

To assist with submission of proposed diagnoses, the NANDA Diagnosis Review Committee has prepared a set of guidelines. These guidelines are designed to promote the consistency, clarity, and quality of submissions. Diagnoses that are submitted but do not meet the guidelines will be returned to the submitter for appropriate revision. Questions regarding the submission process may be forwarded to the NANDA office.

Nursing Diagnosis Defined (Approved at the Ninth Conference)

A nursing diagnosis is a clinical judgment about individual, family, or community responses to actual or potential health problems/life processes. Nursing diagnoses pro-

vide the basis for selection of nursing interventions to achieve outcomes for which the nurse is accountable.

Actual Nursing Diagnosis

1. Label

The label provides a name for the diagnosis, a concise phrase or term which represents a pattern of related cues. Diagnostic labels may include but *are not limited* to the following qualifiers:

Altered—A change from baseline

Impaired—Made worse, weakened; damaged, reduced, deteriorated

Depleted—Emptied wholly or partially; exhausted of

Deficient—Inadequate in amount, quality, or degree; defective; not sufficient; incomplete

Excessive—Characterized by an amount or quantity that is greater than is necessary, desirable, or useful

Dysfunctional—Abnormal; incomplete functioning

Disturbed—Agitated; interrupted, interfered with

Ineffective—Not producing the desired effect

Decreased—Lessened, lesser in size, amount, or degree

Increased—Greater in size, amount, or degree

Acute—Severe but of short duration

Chronic—Lasting a long time; recurring; habitual; constant

Intermittent—Stopping and starting again at intervals; periodic; cyclic

2. Definition

The definition of the diagnosis provides a clear, precise description. The definition delineates its meaning and helps differentiate this diagnosis from similar diagnoses.

3. Defining Characteristics

Defining characteristics are clinical cues that cluster as manifestations of a nursing diagnosis. Diagnostic cues are clinical evidence that describe a cluster of behaviors or signs and symptoms that represent a diagnostic label. Diagnostic cues are concrete and measurable through observation or client/group reports. Diagnostic cues are separated into major and minor.

Major diagnostic cues are critical indicators of the diagnosis. Minor diagnostic cues are supporting indicators that are not always present but they complete the clinical picture and increase the diagnostician's confidence in making the diagnosis (Gordon, 1982). Differentiation of major from minor characteristics should be logically defended. If appropriate, the submitter may designate major as occurring 80% to 100% of the time and minor as occurring 50% to 79% of the time.

4. Related Factors

Related factors are conditions or circumstances that can cause or contribute to the development of a diagnosis. Related factors that are associated with the proposed diagnosis must be listed and supported by an accompanying literature review.

5. Literature/Clinical Validation

A narrative review of the relevant literature is required to support the rationale for the diagnosis, the defining characteristics, and the related factors. If the diagnosis is similar to an approved NANDA diagnosis, the reason for its usefulness must be addressed. Literature citations for defining characteristics are required and should be cited for each cue. If defining characteristics are not supported by the literature, an explanation for their inclusion is required. In addition, the designation of major versus minor defining characteristics must be supported by clinical data. These data can be derived from case studies, nurse consensus, retrospective chart reviews, or other appropriate validation methods. A sample three-part (label, related factors, and signs and symptoms) nursing diagnostic statement with the associated outcome criteria and nurse-prescribed interventions must accompany the submission.

Sample

Activity intolerance related to deconditioned status as evidenced by inability to wash body or body parts without tachycardia, dyspnea, and fatigue.

Outcome Criteria

Bathes independently without tachycardia or dyspnea

Interventions

Position to minimize energy requirements; assist to recondition; teach energy-conservation/pacing techniques; provide assistance as indicated.

II. High-Risk Nursing Diagnosis (NANDA-approved diagnoses currently designated as "Potential" will be labeled "High Risk for" in 1992)

A high-risk nursing diagnosis is a clinical judgment that an individual, family, or community is more vulnerable to develop the problem than others in the same or similar situation. High-risk nursing diagnoses are supported by risk factors that guide nursing interventions to reduce or prevent the occurrence of the problem.

1. Label

The label provides a name for the diagnosis, a concise phrase or term which represents a pattern of related cues. Diagnostic labels may include but are not limited to the following qualifiers:

Altered—A change from baseline

Impaired—Made worse, weakened; damaged, reduced, deteriorated

Depleted—Emptied wholly or partially; exhausted of

Deficient—Inadequate in amount, quality, or degree; defective; not sufficient; incomplete

Excessive—Characterized by an amount or quantity that is greater than is necessary, desirable, or useful

Dysfunctional—Abnormal; incomplete functioning

Disturbed—Agitated; interrupted, interfered with

Ineffective—Not producing the desired effect

Decreased—Lessened, lesser in size, amount, or degree

Increased—Greater in size, amount, or degree

Acute—Severe but of short duration

Chronic—Lasting a long time; recurring; habitual; constant

Intermittent—Stopping and starting again at intervals; periodic; cyclic

2. Definition

The definition of the label provides a clear, precise description. The definition delineates its meaning and helps differentiate this diagnosis from all others.

3. Risk Factors

Risk factors identify behaviors, conditions, or circumstances that render an individual,

family, or community more vulnerable to a particular problem than others in the same or similar situation. There are no signs and symptoms for high-risk diagnoses.

4. Literature/Clinical Validation

A narrative review of literature is required to support the rationale for the diagnosis and the risk factors. Literature citations for each risk factor are required. If the diagnosis is similar to an approved NANDA diagnosis, the reason for its usefulness must be addressed. The submission must include a sample two-part (including label and risk factors) high-risk nursing diagnostic statement with related outcome criteria and nursing-prescribed interventions.

Sample
   High risk for injury: fall related to fatigue and altered gait
Outcome Criteria
   Describes or demonstrates necessary safety measures
Interventions
   Teach measures to prevent falls; instruct to request assistance when needed.

III. Wellness Nursing Diagnosis

A wellness nursing diagnosis is a clinical judgment about an individual, family, or community in transition from a specific level of wellness to a higher level of wellness.

1. Label

The term "Potential for Enhanced" will be the designated qualifier. Enhanced is defined as made greater, to increase in quality, or more desired. Wellness diagnoses will be one-part statements.

2. Definition

The definition of the label provides a clear, precise description. The definition delineates its meaning and helps differentiate this diagnosis from all others.

3. Literature/Clinical Validation

A narrative review of literature is required to support the rationale for the diagnosis. A sample one-part wellness nursing diagnostic statement with related outcome criteria and nursing-prescribed interventions must accompany the submission.

Sample
Potential for enhanced parenting
Outcome Criteria
Will practice listening without advice-giving with children.
Interventions
Describe active listening; differentiate between listening and advice giving.

IV. Revision of NANDA-Approved Nursing Diagnoses

Changes can be proposed for the label, the definition, and/or the defining characteristics. In order for any NANDA-approved nursing diagnosis to be refined or revised, the proposal must contain

1. A narrative describing the rationale for the proposed changed.
2. Research findings to support the proposed changes. These findings can be the results of research by the submitter or from research reported in the literature.

V. Deletion of NANDA-Approved Nursing Diagnoses

Proposals can be submitted to delete a NANDA-approved nursing diagnosis. The proposal must contain a narrative describing the rationale for the proposed deletion. The rationale must be supported by

1. Logical justification, and
2. Research findings or relevant literature review.

VI. Diagnosis Review Committee Review Cycle

1. Submission Deadline: March 1 of year prior to conference (e.g., 1991, 1993, 1995).
2. Initial review by DRC Chairperson for inclusion of required components.
3. Incomplete submissions returned with a resubmission deadline date of July 1.
4. Submissions with all the required components will be reviewed by the Diagnosis Review Committee. One of the following decisions will be made for each submission:
   a. *Not Accepted:* The proposed diagnosis has not been accepted for review by the Expert Advisory Panel. Reasons for "not accepted" are
      • represents a medical diagnosis.
      • represents a treatment or procedure.
      • did not represent a human response.
      • defining characteristics for actual nursing diagnosis are not cues or signs/symptoms.
      • defining characteristics for high-risk nursing diagnosis are not risk factors.
   b. *Hold for Revisions:* The proposed diagnosis will be returned to the submitter for revisions. Examples of needed revisions are
      • research population was not representative for conclusions drawn.
      • inadequate literature support for proposed diagnosis.
   c. *Accepted for Expert Advisory Panel Review*
5. After the Expert Advisory Panel and the DRC review, each proposed diagnosis or

proposal (revisions or deletions) will receive one of the following designations:

a. *Returned To Be Developed (TBD):* This decision delineates submitted work as promising but requiring substantive development. This work will require resubmission in its entirety to the DRC. This category acknowledges promising work in need of substantive revisions.

b. *Conditional Accept:* This category indicates a provisional acceptance of the submitted work pending receipt of revisions agreed on by the Committee and the submitter.

c. *Accepted:* This category indicates the submitted work is accepted.

6. Accepted diagnoses or proposals for revisions/deletions will be forwarded to the Board of Directors for approval.

7. Board-approved proposed diagnoses or proposals for revisions/deletions will be represented at the NANDA Conference and will be subject to membership mail vote.

Reference

Gordon, M. (1982). *Nursing diagnosis: Process and application.* New York: McGraw-Hill.

B

Taxonomy I Revised (1990)

Introduction

Taxonomy I Revised (1990) includes the nursing diagnoses accepted for clinical testing and use at the ninth conference. The bracketed items and blank spaces found within the Taxonomy represent areas that are yet to be named, described, or voted on.

Approved nursing diagnoses are placed by the Taxonomy Committee based on the following considerations:

1. Level of abstraction
2. Consistency with current theoretic views in nursing
3. Consistency with basic definitions within each pattern area

The order of numbers within a level is determined by the order in which the diagnoses were received, not by priority or importance.

I. EXCHANGING

1.1. Altered nutrition
  1.1.1.
  1.1.2. [Systemic]
    1.1.2.1. More than body requirements
    1.1.2.2. Less than body requirements
    1.1.2.3. Potential for more than body requirements
  1.2. [Altered physical regulation]
    1.2.1. [Immunologic]
      1.2.1.1. Potential for infection
    1.2.2. [Temperature]
      1.2.2.1. Potential for altered body temperature
      1.2.2.2. Hypothermia
      1.2.2.3. Hyperthermia
      1.2.2.4. Ineffective thermoregulation
    1.2.3. [Neurologic]
  1.3. Altered elimination
    1.3.1. Bowel
      1.3.1.1. Constipation
        1.3.1.1.1. Perceived
        1.3.1.1.2. Colonic
      1.3.1.2. Diarrhea
      1.3.1.3. Bowel incontinence
    1.3.2. Urinary
      1.3.2.1. Incontinence
        1.3.2.1.1. Stress
        1.3.2.1.2. Reflex
        1.3.2.1.3. Urge
        1.3.2.1.4. Functional
        1.3.2.1.5. Total
      1.3.2.2. Retention
  1.4. [Altered circulation]
    1.4.1. [Vascular]
      1.4.1.1. Tissue perfusion
        1.4.1.1.1. Renal

1.4.1.1.2. Cerebral
1.4.1.1.3. Cardiopulmonary
1.4.1.1.4. Gastrointestinal
1.4.1.1.5. Peripheral
1.4.1.2. Fluid volume
1.4.1.2.1. Excess
1.4.1.2.2. Deficit
1.4.1.2.2.1. Actual (1) Actual (2)
1.4.1.2.2.2. Potential
1.4.2. [Cardiac]
1.4.2.1. Decreased cardiac output
1.5. [Altered oxygenation]
1.5.1. [Respiration]
1.5.1.1. Impaired gas exchange
1.5.1.2. Ineffective airway clearance
1.5.1.3. Ineffective breathing pattern
1.6. [Altered physical integrity]
1.6.1. Potential for injury
1.6.1.1. Potential for suffocation
1.6.1.2. Potential for poisoning
1.6.1.3. Potential for trauma
1.6.1.4. Potential for aspiration
1.6.1.5. Potential for disuse syndrome
1.6.2. Altered protection
1.6.2.1. Impaired tissue integrity
1.6.2.1.1. Oral mucous membranes
1.6.2.1.2. Skin integrity
1.6.2.1.2.1. Actual
1.6.2.1.2.2. Potential

2. COMMUNICATION

2.1. Altered communication
2.1.1. Verbal
2.1.1.1. Impaired

3. RELATING

3.1. [Altered socialization]
3.1.1. Impaired social interaction
3.1.2. Social isolation
3.2. [Altered role]
3.2.1. Altered role performance
3.2.1.1. Parenting
3.2.1.1.1. Actual
3.2.1.1.2. Potential
3.2.1.2. Sexual
3.2.1.2.1. Dysfunction
3.2.2. Altered family processes
3.2.3. [Altered role conflict]
3.2.3.1. Parental role conflict
3.3. Altered sexuality patterns

4. VALUING

4.1. [Altered spiritual state]
4.1.1. Spiritual distress

5. CHOOSING

5.1. Altered coping
5.1.1. Individual coping
5.1.1.1. Ineffective
5.1.1.1.1. Impaired adjustment
5.1.1.1.2. Defensive coping
5.1.1.1.3. Ineffective denial
5.1.2. Family coping
5.1.2.1. Ineffective
5.1.2.1.1. Disabled
5.1.2.1.2. Compromised
5.1.2.2. Potential for growth
5.2. [Altered participation]
5.2.1. [Individual]
5.2.1.1. Noncompliance
5.3. [Altered judgment]
5.3.1. [Individual]
5.3.1.1. Decisional conflict
5.4. Health seeking behaviors (specify)

6. MOVING

6.1. [Altered activity]
6.1.1. Physical mobility
6.1.1.1. Impaired
6.1.1.2. Activity intolerance
6.1.1.2.1. Fatigue
6.1.1.3. Potential activity intolerance
6.2. [Altered rest]
6.2.1. Sleep pattern disturbance
6.3. [Altered recreation]
6.3.1. Diversional activity
6.3.1.1. Deficit
6.4. [Altered ADL]
6.4.1. Home maintenance management
6.4.1.1. Impaired
6.4.2. Health maintenance
6.5. Self care deficit
6.5.1. Feeding
6.5.1.1. Impaired swallowing
6.5.1.2. Impaired breastfeeding
6.5.1.3. Effective breastfeeding
6.5.2. Bathing/hygiene
6.5.3. Dressing/grooming
6.5.4. Toileting
6.6. Altered growth and development

7. PERCEIVING

7.1. Altered self-concept
  7.1.1. Body image disturbance
  7.1.2. Self-esteem disturbance
    7.1.2.1. Chronic low self-esteem
    7.1.2.2. Situational low self-esteem
  7.1.3. Personal identity disturbance
7.2. Altered sensory/perception
  7.2.1. Visual
    7.2.1.1. Unilateral neglect
  7.2.2. Auditory
  7.2.3. Kinesthetic
  7.2.4. Gustatory
  7.2.5. Tactile
  7.2.6. Olfactory
7.3. [Altered meaningfulness]
  7.3.1. Hopelessness
  7.3.2. Powerlessness

8. KNOWING

8.1. [Altered knowing]
  8.1.1. Knowledge deficit (specify)
8.2. [xxxxxxxxx]
8.3. Altered thought processes

9. FEELING

9.1. Altered comfort
  9.1.1. Pain
    9.1.1.1. Chronic
9.2. [Altered emotional integrity]
  9.2.1. Grieving
    9.2.1.1. Dysfunctional
    9.2.1.2. Anticipatory
  9.2.2. Potential for violence
  9.2.3. Post-trauma response
    9.2.3.1. Rape-trauma syndrome
      9.2.3.1.1. Compound reaction
      9.2.3.1.2. Silent reaction
9.3. [Altered emotional state]
  9.3.1. Anxiety
  9.3.2. Fear

DIAGNOSIS QUALIFIERS

CATEGORY 1

Actual: Existing at the present moment; existing in reality.
Potential: Can, but has not as yet, come into being; possible.

CATEGORY 2

Ineffective: Not producing the desired effect; not capable of performing satisfactorily.
Decreased: Smaller; lessened; diminished; lesser in size, amount, or degree.
Increased: Greater in size, amount, or degree; larger, enlarged.
Impaired: Made worse, weakened; damaged, reduced; deteriorated.
Depleted: Emptied wholly or partially; exhausted of.
Deficient: Inadequate in amount, quality, or degree; defective; not sufficient; incomplete.
Excessive: Characterized by an amount or quantity that is greater than is necessary, desirable, or usable.
Dysfunctional: Abnormal; impaired or incompletely functioning.
Disturbed: Agitated; interrupted; interfered with.
Acute: Severe but of short duration.
Chronic: Lasting a long time; recurring; habitual; constant.
Intermittent: Stopping and starting again at intervals; periodic; cyclic.

C

Proposed ICD-10 Version of NANDA Taxonomy I Revised: Conditions That Necessitate Nursing Care

Prepared by NANDA Board of Directors, Taxonomy Committee, and ANA Liaison, January 28, 1989

Human Response Pattern: Choosing

*Y00 Family Coping, Impaired
   Y00.0 Compromised
   Y00.1 Disabled
 Y01 [Health Seeking Behavior]
   Y01.0–9 Health Seeking Behaviors (Specify)
 Y02 Individual Coping, Impaired
   Y02.0 Adjustment, Impaired
   Y02.1 Conflict: Decisional
   Y02.2 Coping: Defensive
  *Y02.3 Denial, Impaired
   Y02.4 Noncompliance

Human Response Pattern: Communicating

Y10 [Communication, Impaired]
   Y10.0 Verbal

Human Response Pattern: Exchanging

Y20 [Bowel Elimination]
   Y20.0 Bowel Incontinence

   Y20.1 Constipation: Colonic
   Y20.2 Constipation: Perceived
   Y20.3 Diarrhea
*Y21 Cardiac Output, Altered
 Y22 [Fluid Volume, Altered]
   Y22.0 Deficit
   Y22.1 Deficit: Risk
   Y22.2 Excess
*Y23 Injury: Risk
  *Y23.0 Aspiration
  *Y23.1 Disuse Syndrome
  *Y23.2 Poisoning
  *Y23.3 Suffocation
  *Y23.4 Trauma
 Y24 [Nutrition, Altered]
   Y24.0 Less than Body Requirement
   Y24.1 More than Body Requirement
  *Y24.2 More than Body Requirement: Risk
 Y25 [Physical Regulation, Altered]
   Y25.0 Dysreflexia
   Y25.1 Hyperthermia
   Y25.2 Hypothermia
  *Y25.3 Infection: Risk
  *Y25.4 Thermoregulation, Impaired
 Y26 [Respiration, Altered]

*Y26.0 Airway Clearance, Impaired
*Y26.1 Breathing Pattern, Impaired
Y26.2 Gas Exchange, Impaired
Y27 Tissue Integrity, Altered
 *Y27.0 Oral Mucous Membrane, Impaired
 Y27.1 Skin Integrity, Impaired
 Y27.2 Skin Integrity, Impaired: Risk
Y28 [Tissue Perfusion, Altered]
 Y28.0 Cardiopulmonary
 Y28.1 Cerebral
 Y28.2 Gastrointestinal
 Y28.3 Peripheral
 Y28.4 Renal
Y29 Urinary Elimination, Altered
 Y29.0 Incontinence: Functional
 Y29.1 Incontinence: Reflex
 Y29.2 Incontinence: Stress
 Y29.3 Incontinence: Urge
 Y29.4 Incontinence: Total
 *Y29.5 Retention

Human Response Pattern: Feeling

Y30 Anxiety
Y31 [Comfort, Altered]
 Y31.0 Pain, [Acute]
 Y31.1 Pain, Chronic
Y32 Fear
Y33 [Grieving]
 Y33.0 Anticipatory
 Y33.1 Dysfunctional
Y34 Post-Trauma Response
 Y34.0 Rape Trauma Syndrome
 Y34.1 Rape Trauma Syndrome: Compound Reaction
 Y34.2 Rape Trauma Syndrome: Silent Reaction
*Y35 Violence; Risk

Human Response Pattern: Knowing

Y40 [Knowledge Deficit]
 Y40.0–9 Knowledge Deficit (Specify)
Y41 Thought Processes, Altered

Human Response Pattern: Moving

Y50 [Activity, Altered]
 Y50.0 Activity Intolerance
 Y50.1 Activity Intolerance: Risk
 Y50.2 Diversional Activity Deficit
 Y50.3 Fatigue
 Y50.4 Physical Mobility, Impaired
 Y50.5 Sleep Pattern Disturbance
*Y51 Bathing/Hygiene Deficit
*Y52 Dressing/Grooming Deficit
*Y53 Feeding Deficit
 *Y53.0 Breastfeeding, Impaired
 Y53.1 Swallowing, Impaired
Y54 Growth and Development, Altered
Y55 Health Maintenance, Altered
Y56 Home Maintenance Management, Impaired
*Y57 Toileting Deficit

Human Response Pattern: Perceiving

Y60 [Meaningfulness, Altered]
 Y60.0 Hopelessness
 Y60.1 Powerlessness
Y61 [Self Concept, Altered]
 Y61.0 Body Image Disturbance
 Y61.1 Personal Identity Disturbance
 Y61.2 Self-Esteem Disturbance: Chronic Low
 Y61.3 Self-Esteem Disturbance: Situational
*Y62 [Sensory Perception, Altered]
 Y62.0 Auditory
 Y62.1 Gustatory
 Y62.2 Kinesthetic
 Y62.3 Olfactory
 Y62.4 Tactile
 Y62.5 Visual
 Y62.6 Unilateral Neglect

Human Response Pattern: Relating

Y70 Family Processes, Altered
Y71 Role Performance, Altered
 Y71.0 Parental Role Conflict
 Y71.1 Parenting, Altered
 Y71.2 Parenting, Altered: Risk

Y71.3 Sexual Dysfunction
Y72 Sexuality Patterns, Altered
Y73 [Socialization, Altered]
Y73.0 Social Interaction, Impaired
Y73.1 Social Isolation

Human Response Pattern: Valuing

Y80 [Spiritual State, Altered]
Y80.0 Spiritual Distress

Notes

- Items in brackets are not NANDA-accepted diagnoses.
- Items with an asterisk (*) are changes in terminology from NANDA diagnostic labels.
- NANDA diagnoses not specifically identified are embedded in the coding system.

D

Awards for Unique Contributions to the Advancement of Nursing Diagnosis

NANDA's Award for Unique Contribution to the Advancement of Nursing Diagnosis was initiated in 1984. Previous award winners were: in 1984—Marjory Gordon, Christine Gebbie, Sister Theresa Noth, Sister Callista Roy, Mary Ann Lavin; in 1986—Ellen Barkowski, Lucy Field, Audrey McLane; and in 1988—Lynda Carpenito, Phyllis Kritek, and Paula Rich.

Each awardee was presented with a plaque to take home, and each had her name added to the large award plaque that is kept in the NANDA office.

Gail Marculescu

Current Position: Enterstomal Clinical Nurse Specialist
Education and Training Department
El Camino Hospital
Mountain View, California

Gail has uniquely contributed to the advancement of nursing diagnosis by her leadership in the dissemination and use of nursing diagnosis in clinical practice. Gail is dedicated in her efforts to expand others' knowledge of nursing diagnosis through workshops, continuing education presentations, and in-service presentations. She founded and is a board member of BANDA, the Bay Area Nursing Diagnosis Association. As president of the group she helped expand initial membership from 12 to 150 in a short period of time.

Gail's efforts to promote nursing diagnosis are also reflected in her publications. She is co-author of a very successful nursing diagnosis book, *Care Planning Pocket Guide: A Nursing Diagnosis Approach*, now in its 3rd edition.

Gail was nominated for this award by the Bay Area Nursing Diagnosis Association, whose members note her enthusiasm that always motivates others to greater achievement.

Peg Mehmert

Current Position: Assistant Director of Nursing
Mercy Hospital
Davenport, Iowa

Mention the words "computerized nursing diagnoses" in the Midwest and you mention Peg Mehmert. She led her hospital and the country in the development of one of the first, and still one of the few, computerized care planning pathways based on NANDA-defined nursing diagnoses. The system today, which integrates staffing, acuity, and documentation features, is at the heart of the hospital's patient care system. Visitors, who often drive hours to see the model system, are never disappointed.

Peg's expertise in nursing diagnosis, however, extends beyond her own institution. She is a leader of the Midwest Nursing Diagnosis Task Force, serving as Secretary of this group since 1985. Her more than 25 presentations on nursing diagnosis and nine publications have encouraged many others to begin what she has accomplished.

More recently, Peg and colleagues have begun to use the nursing diagnosis clinical data set that her system generates to validate select nursing diagnoses and to research costs of nursing care. As a dedicated user and promoter of NANDA's work, Peg represents the best of NANDA members.

Mi Ja Kim

Current Position: Professor and Dean
College of Nursing
The University of Illinois
Chicago, Illinois

Mi Ja is well known for her many contributions to nursing diagnosis and to NANDA. Since 1976, she has been providing leadership to NANDA and the nursing diagnosis movement. From 1985 to 1989 she was a member of the Board of Directors of NANDA and she has chaired NANDA's Program Committee, which planned an outstanding conference in 1988.

Mi Ja was the lead editor in 1982, and again in 1984, of NANDA's conference proceedings. She is also the editor, with McFarland and McLane, of the well-used *Pocket Guide to Nursing Diagnosis*, which in 1984 was awarded an AJN Book-of-the-Year Award and which is now in its 3rd edition. Included in her more than 30 publications related to nursing diagnosis are a symposium issue of *Nursing Clinics of North America* in 1987 on Ineffective Breathing Patterns and Airway Clearance, and a 1989 *Annual Review of Nursing Research* chapter on research on nursing diagnosis.

Through her own research and that of her students, Mi Ja has been influential in helping the rest of us understand the role of physiologic nursing diagnoses. She has presented more than 60 talks and workshops on nursing diagnosis in such faraway places as Beijing, China, and Seoul, Korea. It's hard to imagine the nursing diagnosis movement without Mi Ja. For all your efforts, Mi Ja, we salute you.

Doris Carnevali

Last Position: Associate Professor, Emeritus Community Health Care Systems Department
School of Nursing, University of Washington
Seattle, Washington

Doris Carnevali is recognized by NANDA for her pioneering work in concept development and the diagnostic process, which has provided a foundation for the nursing diagnosis movement.

Doris Carnevali is a scholar with more than 45 publications, several of which have also been published in other languages. She has conducted numerous research projects and made over 300 presentations and approximately 60 consultations in the United States, Sweden, and Australia.

Many of us figuratively cut our teeth on Little and Carnevali's *Nursing Care Planning*, first published in 1969. The 3rd edition, published in 1983, was authored solely by Carnevali and entitled *Nursing Care Planning: Diagnosis and Management.* The six-step diagnostic framework described in the third edition formed the basis of another book, *Diagnostic Reasoning in Nursing*, co-authored and published in 1984. Her newest book, *The Cancer Experience: Nursing Diagnosis and Management*, is to be published this year.

In the last 15 years, Doris Carnevali's consultations and presentations have been largely focused on helping others to understand and apply the diagnostic process within a nursing model for practice. The model that she developed, the Daily Living-Functional Health Status Model, provides a framework for the diagnostic process within the nursing domain. One of the outcomes of her work in Sweden is a magnet nursing home of 210 beds that offers planned learning experiences for nurses who wish to work for a short time in a setting where nursing diagnosis and treatment plans are the norm.

A tribute to Doris Carnevali's influence in nursing practice is that she has been invited to share her work with nurses in all types of settings in approximately 20 states of the United States. Selected examples of scholarly presentations on nursing diagnosis include her keynote addresses for the Geriatric Conference for Nursing Faculty, the University of Maryland, 1980; for the Second Northwest Conference on Nursing Diagnosis in Portland, Oregon, in 1982; and for the Second Annual Gerontologic Nursing Research and Clinical Conference in South Carolina in 1987.

Doris L. Carnevali has provided an example of scholarly work for the advancement of nursing diagnosis that inspires many. NANDA is pleased to recognize one who has dedicated her career to the advancement of nursing knowledge.

E

Bylaws of the North American Nursing Diagnosis Association

Article I   Title, Purpose and Function

Section 1. Title. The name of this Association shall be the North American Nursing Diagnosis Association, Inc.

Section 2. Purpose. This Association is organized to develop, refine and promote a taxonomy of nursing diagnostic terminology of general use to professional nurses.

Section 3. Restrictions. The Association qualifies as a tax exempt organization within the meaning of section 501(c)(6) of the U.S. Internal Revenue Code. The affairs of the Association shall be conducted in such a manner as to qualify for tax exemption under that provision.

Section 4. Equal Rights. The purposes of this Association shall be unrestricted by consideration of nationality, race, creed, life style, color, sex, or age.

Section 5. Functions. The function of the Association shall be to develop and promote a taxonomy of nursing diagnoses, including but not limited to:

a) conducting conferences
b) publishing documents
c) facilitating research
d) serving as an information resource

Article II   Membership

Section 1. Member. A member is one:

a) who has been granted a license to practice as a registered nurse and who does not have a license under suspension or revocation, or
b) whose dues are not delinquent.

Section 2. Associate Member. An associate member is one who does not qualify as a member, who shares an interest in the purposes of the Association and whose dues are not delinquent. Associate members do not have a vote, but may actively participate in all other affairs of the Association.

Section 3. The membership shall be organized into seven (7) districts. These shall consist of the following:

District #1—Northeastern
District #2—Central Atlantic
District #3—Southeastern

District #4—North Central
District #5—South Central
District #6—North Pacific
District #7—South Pacific

Section 4. Individual membership in NANDA is established through presentation to the Association of the completed application, as required by Association policy or Bylaws, together with annual dues.

Section 5. Affiliate Members. Affiliate membership is granted to a regional organization:

a) whose membership is consistent with the Association criteria
b) whose purpose is consistent with the Association purpose
c) whose organization, structure and bylaws meet such criteria as shall be determined by the Association.

Section 6. Affiliate membership with the Association may be established by application to the District Affairs Committee. Approval of the application is made by the Association Board. Benefits for affiliate membership and membership fees required will be established by the District Affairs Committee and approved by the Association Board.

Section 7. Membership Year. The membership year shall be a period of 12 consecutive months, beginning July 1 of each calendar year.

Article III   Financial Administration

Section 1. Fiscal Year. The fiscal year of this Association shall commence on the first day of July of each year.

Section 2. Dues. The dues of this Association shall be set by the Board of Directors with the approval of two-thirds of the General Assembly. Any member who fails to pay the dues within four (4) months after they become payable shall be dropped from the membership rolls.

Section 3. Change of Dues. No monies shall be refunded nor additional monies collected when a change of dues category is made within a membership year.

Section 4. Budget. A biennial budget with an annual review/revision shall be adopted by the Board of Directors prior to the beginning of the fiscal year.

Section 5. Executive Director's Duties. The Executive Director shall have the authority to direct and maintain the headquarters of the Association; insure that all funds, physical assets and other property of the organization are safeguarded and administered, as directed by the Board of Directors.

Article IV   Officers and Duties of Officers

Section 1. The officers of this Association shall be a president, a vice-president, a secretary, and a treasurer who shall be elected as hereinafter provided.

Section 2. Duties. The officers of the Association shall constitute an Executive Committee, and are authorized to transact the business of the Association between meetings of the Board, and assist the president as needed. They shall also perform the duties usually performed by such officers as specified in these Bylaws or as designated by the Board.

Section 3. Term of Office. The term of office for all officers shall commence at the beginning of the Association's fiscal year and shall continue until the expiration of their respective terms of office or until their successors are elected. No officer shall be eligible to serve more than two consecutive terms in the same office. A member who has served more than half a term shall be deemed to have served a term. The term of office shall be four years.

Section 4. President. The president shall be chairman of the Board of Directors; shall be an ex officio member of all committees and task forces except the Nominating Committee; shall preside at all meetings of the Association; appoint special committees or task forces as outlined by these Bylaws or the Board; serve as the Association's representative; and perform all other duties of the office.

Section 5. Vice-President. The vice-president shall assume the duties of the president in case of that officer's absence or inability to serve.

Section 6. Secretary. The secretary shall keep minutes of all proceedings of this Association and the Board; shall report at meetings of this Association or Board; shall be familiar with procedures of the headquarters of this Association relating to notification of elections or appointments, notices of time and place of meetings, records of members, and policies of the Board and the Association. The secretary shall perform such other duties as may be assigned by the Board.

Section 7. Treasurer. The treasurer shall have custody of the funds and securities of this Association; shall see that full and accurate financial reports are made to the Board and at Association meetings. The treasurer shall perform such other duties as may be assigned by the Board.

Section 8. Compensation. Elected officers shall not receive any compensation for their services as such but may be reimbursed for their expenses.

Article V Board of Directors

Section 1. Composition. The Board of Directors of the Association shall be the officers plus seven directors, who shall be elected as hereinafter provided.

Section 2. Terms of Office. The term of office for all directors shall commence at the beginning of the Association's fiscal year, and shall continue until the expiration of their respective terms of office or until their successors are elected. No Board member shall be eligible to serve more than two consecutive terms. A member who has served more than half a term shall be deemed to have served a term. The term of office shall be four years.

Section 3. The Board of Directors shall meet at least annually during the fiscal year of the Association.

Section 4. Special Meetings. Special meetings of the Board may be called by the president on 10 days' notice to each member and shall be called by the president on like notice upon the written request of four or more members of the Board.

Section 5. Automatic Vacancy of Office. If any member of the Board is absent from two regular meetings in succession, unless excused by the Board for valid reasons, the office shall automatically become vacant and the vacancy shall be filled as provided in these Bylaws.

Section 6. Powers of the Board. The Board of Directors shall have power and authority over the affairs and business of this Association between regular Association meetings, except that of modifying any action taken by the members. It shall perform the duties prescribed in these Bylaws and such others as may be delegated to it by the Association. The Board in addition shall:

a) appoint an executive director and fix compensation for the position.
b) establish administrative policies governing the affairs of the Association.
c) develop a master plan allowing the accomplishment of the Association's purposes and for the growth and prosperity of the Association.
d) transact the general business of the Association.
e) report business transacted at regular meetings of the Association and give an annual report to the membership at regular meetings of the Association.
f) act as custodian of the property, securities and records of the Association; select a place for deposit of funds of the

Association; provide for the audit of the books of the Association; provide for bonding of Association officials as it may deem necessary and provide for payment of authorized expenses.

g) establish and dissolve committees, task forces and appointments for such to accomplish the purposes of this Association.

h) have the power to fill vacancies except the offices of president and vice-president.

i) decide on the date and place of Association meetings.

j) perform such other duties as may be assigned elsewhere in these Bylaws or by the Association.

Section 6. Retiring Members. All retiring members of the Board shall deliver to the Association within one month all Association properties in their possession.

Article VI   Committees

Section 1. Committee Selection. The Association may have standing committees. Each committee shall be chaired by a NANDA member, as appointed by the president. Committee members shall be elected or appointed by the committee chairperson with attention to geographic and clinical practice distribution. The size of the committee shall be determined by the Board unless otherwise stated by the Bylaws. Committees shall report to the Board and to meetings of the Association as requested or as required by these Bylaws.

Section 2. Committees. The Association may have, but shall not be limited to, the following committees:

a) Program Committee. The Program Committee shall plan the General Assembly meetings of the Association and provide consultation to regional groups and special interest groups desiring to conduct programs of interest to members of the Association.

b) Publications Committee. The Publications Committee shall oversee the publications of the Association including but not limited to a regular newsletter, official proceedings of the General Assembly, and nursing diagnoses. Recommendations for the editors of these documents shall be submitted to the Board.

c) Public Relations/Membership Committee. The Public Relations/Membership Committee shall disseminate information about NANDA to the nursing community, promote relationships between NANDA and other nursing and health-related organizations, establish annual objectives for the recruitment of new members, recommend and implement strategies for the recruitment of new members, recommend strategies for the retention of members, and make awards at the meetings of the General Assembly for outstanding contribution to the advancement of nursing diagnosis.

d) Diagnosis Review Committee. The Diagnosis Review Committee shall review proposed diagnoses and recommend acceptance/modification/rejection to the Board. The Committee shall appoint specialized clinical/technical review task forces in specific clinical areas to review diagnoses prior to Committee action; shall designate the format for submission of proposed diagnoses or changes to existing diagnoses; and following meetings of the General Assembly shall prepare proposed diagnoses in final form as recommended for membership voting.

e) Research Committee. The Research Committee shall promote conducting research studies and review research papers for the publications of the Association.

f) Finance Committee. The Finance Committee will develop and monitor the annual budget, monitor salaries for the Executive Director and staff, and recommend policies and procedures of the fiscal management of the organization.

g) Taxonomy Committee. The Taxonomy Committee shall develop and regularly review a taxonomic system for the diagnoses, and submit to the Board for review and action; promote its (taxonomy) use, and promote collaboration with groups supporting other established health-related taxonomies.

h) Districts Affairs Committee. The Committee shall promote the involvement of members in affairs of the Association through activities and communication at a local, regional or district level, and provide a mechanism for bringing issues of concern to the attention of the Board and the Association. The Committee shall be composed of seven members, one elected from each district.

i) Bylaws Committee. The Bylaws Committee will review the Bylaws every two years and recommend changes to be presented for approval of the General Assembly.

j) International Committee. The Committee will promote networking with international nurses interested in nursing diagnosis and encourage involvement of these nurses in Association activities.

Section 3. Term of Office. The term of office shall be four (4) years. One-half of the membership shall be selected every two years. A member may be elected or reappointed one time with no more than eight successive years of service on a Committee.

Section 4. Automatic vacancy of office. If any member of a Committee is absent from two regular meetings in succession, unless excused by the Board for valid reasons, the office shall automatically become vacant and the vacancy shall be filled as provided in these Bylaws.

Section 5. Retiring Members. All retiring members of the Committees shall deliver to the Association within one month all Association properties in their possession.

Article VII Elections

Section 1. Nominating Committee. The president shall appoint a chair and one (1) member to a Nomination Committee. No member of the Committee may be a member of the Board of Directors. In addition, three (3) members shall be elected by the membership during the regular elections. All terms shall be four (4) years.

Section 2. Ballot and Election. All elections shall be in accordance with written Board policy and these Bylaws. An election is constituted by a plurality of voting members and in case of a tie, the choice shall be by lot.

Section 3. Tellers. The president shall appoint tellers one month in advance of elections, who shall serve as inspectors of the election.

Article VIII General Assembly

Section 1. Composition. The composition of the General Assembly shall be the voting members and associate members who are in attendance at the meetings of the Association.

Section 2. Authority. The General Assembly shall approve policies and Bylaws to govern the Association; shall review and comment on proposed diagnoses for the Diagnosis Review Committee's actions prior to the submission to the membership for acceptance.

Article IX   Meetings

Section 1. Regular Meetings. Regular meetings of the General Assembly shall be at least once every thirty (30) months.

a) With regard to regular meetings, receipt of a copy-written notice setting the time and place of each regular meeting shall be deemed sufficient notice of the meeting. With regard to any special meeting, each member shall be sent written notice at least ten (10) days prior to the date of the meeting. Said notice shall set forth the time and place of the meeting. It shall not be required that any such notice set forth the purpose for which the meeting is being called.
b) Waiver of Notice. Whenever any notice is required to be given under the provision of these Bylaws or under the provisions of the Articles of Incorporation or under the provisions of the laws of the State of Missouri, a waiver in writing signed by the person or persons entitled to such notice, whether before or after the time stated therein, shall be deemed equivalent to the giving of such notice. Further, the notice may be published in the Association's newsletter, which is mailed to all members, and the notice therein shall be deemed to meet any notice requirements.

Section 2. Special Meetings. Special meetings of the General Assembly may be called by the president upon majority vote of the Board or upon the written request of five (5) members each from twenty states.

Article X   Quorum

Section 1. General Assembly. Two hundred of the voting membership of the Association shall constitute a quorum at any regular or special meeting of the General Assembly.

Section 2. Board of Directors. A majority of the members of the Board shall constitute a quorum at any meeting of the Board.

Article XI   Parliamentary Authority

The rules contained in "Robert's Rules of Order, Newly Revised" shall govern meetings of this Association in all cases to which they are applicable and in which they are not inconsistent with these Bylaws.

Article XII   Amendments

Section 1. Amendments. Amendments to these Bylaws must be submitted to the Board 120 days prior to submission to the membership.

Section 2. Previous Notice. These Bylaws may be amended at any regular or special meeting of the General Assembly by a two-thirds vote of the members present and voting, provided the proposed amendments have been sent to all members at least two months prior to the meeting.

Section 3. No Notice. These Bylaws may be amended without previous notice at any regular or special meeting of the General Assembly by a ninety-nine percent vote of those members present and voting.

Article XIII   Dissolution

The Association may be dissolved by a two-thirds vote of the members upon recommendation of the General Assembly. Upon dissolution after payment of all liabilities, the remaining assets shall be distributed to any nursing organization provided that no distribution shall be made to any organization not then covered by Section 501(c)(3) of the

Internal Revenue Service Code of 1954 or the corresponding provisions of any future federal or applicable tax law.

THE NORTH AMERICAN NURSING DIAGNOSIS ASSOCIATION ADOPTED ITS BYLAWS IN APRIL, 1982. THE ORGANIZATION REPLACED THE NATIONAL GROUP FOR THE CLASSIFICATION OF NURSING DIAGNOSIS WHICH WAS ESTABLISHED IN 1973. THE ORGANIZATION INCORPORATED IN FEBRUARY, 1985 AND THE BYLAWS WERE AMENDED IN MARCH 1986, MARCH 1988, AND MARCH 1990.

APPENDIX

F

Participants in the Ninth Conference

Marilyn E. Abraham, Alcester, SD
Marsha H. Adams, Tuscaloosa, AL
Cathy Aden, Omaha, NE
Dianna Aideuis, Chapel Hill, NC
Shirley Aizenstein, Skokie, IL
Rosalinda Alfaro-Lefevre, Malvern, PA
Nagia S. Ali, Muncie, IN
Dorothy Allison, Charlotte, NC
Janice Ander, Hanover Park, IL
Donna Anderson, Danvers, IL
Beth Anderson, Bellbrook, OR
Sally K. Arner, Tampa, FL
Ann Ashbaugh, APO, NY
Samar Assousa, West Roxbury, MA
Virginia Aukamp, Columbia, MO
Kay Avant, Waco, TX
Mary Nealon Aymar, Wanamassa, NJ
Carol Ann Baer, Medfield, MA
Erma M. Bahrenburg, Largo, FL
Laurie Baker, New York, NY
Kathleen Miller Baldwin, Lewisville, TX
Elaine Mary Barrett, Cleveland, OH
Vivian J. Barry, Chicago, IL
Beverly J. Bartlett, Kingston, RI
Valerie J. Bayliss, Dover, OH
Martha A. Beaudry, Ann Arbor, MI
Ann Becker, St. Louis, MO
Deborah A. Berkshire, Navarre, OH
Donna Bernocch, Redwood, CA

Jackie Berry, Jacksonville, FL
Suzanne Beyea, Gilford, NH
Anne Bishop, Lynchburg, VA
Virginia Blackmer, Franklin, NH
Kathy Bloom, Jacksonville, FL
Lenore Boles, Norwalk, CT
Eleanor Borkowski, Redlands, CA
Barbara Branson, Tulsa, OK
Lawrence Brennan, Syracuse, NY
Arlene Brennan, Traverse City, MI
Ruthann Brinthall, Grand Rapids, MI
Margaret Briody, Webster, NY
Barbara Briscoe, Yorba Linda, CA
Mary H. Brown, New York, NY
Barbara A. Brown, Wexford, PA
Genee Brukwitzki, Glendale, WI
Patricia McKay Bufalino, Riverside, CA
Gloria Bulechek, Solon, IA
Catherine Burns, Sherwood, OR
Shannon Burton, Farmington, UT
Joan M. Caley, Vancouver, WA
Mary Judy Campbell, Murfreesboro, TN
Suzanne Canale, Eugene, OR
Doris Carnevali, Seattle, WA
Lynda Carpenito, Mickleton, NJ
Rose Mary Carroll-Johnson, Valencia, CA
Patricia Casey, White Plains, NY
Carol Casto, Jacksonville, FL
Nan K. Chandler, Bozeman, MT

Betty L. Chang, Los Angeles, CA
Melodie Chenevert, Washington, DC
Ken Cianfrani, Waukegan, IL
Pat Cipriani, Cleveland, OH
Carla Clark, Phoenix, AZ
Claudia Cline, Akron, OH
Jeanette Clough, Wakefield, MA
Ellan Cole, Pelham, MA
Marga Coler, Storrs, CT
Janet Colville, Pittsburgh, PA
Mary Kay Conway, Charlotte, NC
Valerie Cook, Omaha, NE
Margaret Copley, Tahlequioh, OK
Marie E. Cox, Uniondale, NY
Helen Cox, Lubbock, TX
Carol A. Craft, St. Louis, MO
Nancy Creason, Urbana, IL
Patricia Cremins, Milton, MA
Betty Croonquist, Kandiyohi, MN
Joan Marie Crosley, Babylon, NY
Janet Cuddigan, Omaha, NE
Lynne Ann Dapice, South Burlington, VT
Donna David, Omaha, NE
Joseph Kevin Davie, San Diego, CA
Carolyn B. Deer, Raleigh, NC
Carol Delage, Eagan, MN
Carol A. Dickel, Davenport, IA
Shirley Dickinson, Jacksonville, FL
Jacqueline Dietz, Chicago, IL
Pauline Dion, Williamstown, MA
Janet Dobrzyn, Van Nuys, CA
Marilynn E. Doenges, Colorado Springs, CO
Suzanne Donaldson, Longwood, FL
Nancy Donaldson, Newport Beach, CA
Cindy Dougherty, Seattle, WA
Joyce M. Dungan, Honolulu, HI
Karen Faircloth, Leeds, AL
Ruth Ann Farley, Philadelphia, PA
Arlene Farren, Staten Island, NY
Richard J. Fehring, Wauwatosa, WI
Lucy Feild, Brighton, MA
LuAnne F. Fenderich, Peoria, IL
Nancy B. Fisk, Amherst, MA
Joan Fitzmaurice, Newtonville, MA
Joyce J. Fitzpatrick, Cleveland, OH
Nancy M. Flynn, Hacerton, PA
Patricia W. Foley, Kansas City, MO

Jane Freeman, Marion, OH
Sandra Frick, Columbia, SC
Candice Friestad, Sioux Falls, SD
Noreen Frisch, Arcata, CA
Ellen F. Garneau, Meredith, NH
Kathrine Garthe, Northport, MI
Karen Gattie, Fresno, CA
Kristine Gebbie, Olympia, WA
Elizabeth Gerety, Boring, OR
Roxanne C. Gillis, Kalamazoo, MI
Nancy Glenn, Charlotte, NC
Susan M. Glover, Baltimore, MD
Elaine Goehner, Los Angeles, CA
Karla Good, Richland, MI
Marjory Gordon, Brighton, MA
Patricia Gossett, Shrewsbury, NJ
Cheryl Graham-Eason, Sewickley, PA
Jesse E. Greene, Columbia, SC
Libby Greene, Columbia, SC
Bill Greenfield, North Bay Village, FL
Catherine Greenlee, Racine, WI
Barbara Haas, Yarmouth, ME
Edward J. Halloran, Chapel Hill, NC
J. Keith Hampton, Ann Arbor, MI
Doris Hancock, Louisville, KY
Mary V. Hanley, West Roxbury, MA
Marika Wowk Hartman, Philadelphia, PA
Rose Mary Harvey, Lexington, MA
Gwendolyn M. Harvey, Rochester, MN
Haneh Hattar, Toluca Lake, CA
Barbara Haight, Charleston, SC
Marilyn Hennings, Elm Grove, WI
Mary L. Henrikson, Bellingham, WA
Linda Hensley, El Cajon, CA
Linda M. Herrick, Rochester, MN
Marge Herzog, Bremerton, WA
Doris A. Hill, Chicago, IL
Sharon Hilton, Walnut, CA
Elizabeth Hiltunen, Ipswich, MA
Deborah Hinson, Salt Lake City, UT
Kim S. Hitchings, Allentown, PA
Tracy J. Hoeft, Omaha, NE
Doris Hoerdeman, Peoria, IL
Rosemarie Hogan, Cleveland, OH
Norma S. Holbrook, Topeka, KS
Lois Hoskins, Ashton, MD
James E. Hovey, Oxford, ME

Donna Hovey, Oxford, ME
Verna Hubbard, Westerville, OH
Sue E. Huether, Salt Lake City, UT
Lou Ella Humphrey, Texarkana, AR
Anne L. Hunt, Scituate, MA
Mary Hurley, Basking Ridge, NJ
Marilyn Hurt, Houston, TX
Bev Iceman, Polk, OH
Suzanne C. Irvin, Marietta, GA
Patricia W. Iyer, Stockton, NJ
Janice K. Janken, Charlotte, NC
Jean Jarosz, Arcadia, CA
Barbara Jarrow, Glenco, IL
Joanne M. Johnson, Cincinnati, OH
Sharon E. Johnson, Wayne, PA
Dickey Johnson, Murray, UT
Dorothy Jones, Braintree, MA
Arlene Kahn, Oakland, CA
Jane Kelley, Cape Girardeau, MO
Mary Ann Kelly, Seneca, SC
David J. Kelly, Tucson, AZ
Mitzi Kerr, Polk, OH
Mary E. Kerr, Evans City, PA
Sharon Dill Kerr, Winston-Salem, NC
Mi Ja Kim, Chicago, IL
Marguerite R. Kinney, Birmingham, AL
Mary Kontz, Miami, FL
Phyllis Kritek, Whitefish Bay, WI
Patricia Kucharski, Gales Ferry, CT
Rebecca Kuhn, Newport Beach, CA
Susan Labarthe, Montpelier, VT
Susan Lampe, Minneapolis, MN
Jane Lancour, Irvine, CA
Judy Lapora, Oxnard, CA
June Larson, Vermillion, SD
Christine M. Layhon, Federal Way, WA
Patricia Leigh, Jonesboro, IL
Leva J. Lessure, Rockville, MD
Rona Levin, Westbury, NY
Christina M. Lewis, Los Angeles, CA
Margaret Lindsay, Hesperia, CA
Karen J. Lourence, Waban, MA
Margaret Lunney, Staten Island, NY
Louette Lutjens, Plainwell, MI
Brenda L. Lyon, Nineveh, IN
Suzanne MacAvoy, Ridgefield, CT
Morris A. Magnan, Ferndale, MI

Margaret Magnussen, Albuquerque, NM
Margaret Kiss Magyar, Bayside, NY
Debra Sue Mahoney, Rusk, TX
Regina M. Maibusch, Milwaukee, WI
Jo Ann Maklebust, Livonia, MI
Deborah B. Mangan, Rochester, MN
Anne Manton, Westwood, MA
Gail Marculescu, Sunnyvale, CA
Carol Matz, Boyertown, PA
Geraldine McCarthy, Cleveland Heights, OH
Kay McCash, Tijeras, NM
Joanne McCloskey, Iowa City, IA
Vicki E. McClurg, Edmonds, WA
Margaret D. McComb, Portland, OR
Ann McCourt, Ormond Beach, FL
Gertrude K. McFarland, Clifton, VA
Elizabeth A. McFarlane, Fairfax Station, VA
Frances A. McHolm, Kent, OH
Audrey M. McLane, Hendersonville, NC
Susan McLoughlin, Prairie Village, KS
Susan L. Mease, Springhouse, PA
Peg A. Mehmert, Davenport, IA
Victoria L.C. Meissner, Rancho Palos Verdes, CA
Maria A. Mendoza, Baldwin, NY
Sharon Merritt, Hinsdale, IL
Norma Metheny, St. Louis, MO
Risa Mettberg, West New York, NY
Linda J. Miers, Birmingham, AL
Barbara K. Miller, Garden City, NY
Emmy Miller, Richmond, VA
Mary Mirch, Tujunga, CA
Julie L. Mirkin, Cedarhurst, NY
Carol Ann Mitchell, Garden City, NY
Mary K. Moberg, St. Paul, MN
Karen L. Mokros, Duluth, MN
Joseph Molinatti, E. Patchogue, NY
Linda Mondoux, Farmington, MI
Martha Montgomery, Farmington Hills, MI
Mary Frances Moorhouse, Colorado Springs, CO
Derry Ann Moritz, New Haven, CT
Elizabeth A. Mottet, San Diego, CA
Terese Mullen, Palmer, MA
Karen Mulvey, Oceanport, NJ
Mary Beth Myers, Urbana, IL

Marie Neaton, Ann Arbor, MI
Brenda Nichols, Henderson, KY
Angela Nicoletti, Newton, MA
Lucyanne E. Nolan, Martinez, GA
Ruena Norman Williams, Tallahassee, FL
Joan Norris, Omaha, NE
Barbara Norwitz, Albany, NY
Julie Mirkin, Babylon, NY
Margaret O'Brien, Huntington Beach, CA
Colleen M. O'Brien, Denmark, WI
Jean A. O'Neil, Watertown, MA
Rita Olivieri, Winchester, MA
Anna Omery, Los Angeles, CA
Elinor Parsons, West Chicago, IL
Peggy L. Pelish, Omaha, NE
Cynthia Peltier-Coviak, Ada, MI
Judith Perron, Fiskdale, MA
Debra Pettit, North Liberty, IA
Connie Pinkley, University Heights, OH
Sue Popkess-Vawter, Overland Park, KS
Kathleen L. Powers, Upland, CA
Marilyn S. Price, Seattle, WA
Nancy Pullen, San Rafael, CA
Patricia K. Rackstein, Belleair Bluffs, FL
Jan M. Radoslovich, Seattle, WA
Brooke P. Randell, Pacific Palisades, CA
Michael Reedy, Orlando, FL
Toni Tripp Reimer, Iowa City, IA
Tamara Rice, Irvine, CA
Paula L. Rich, Philadelphia, PA
Stephanie Richardson, Salt Lake City, UT
Nancy Ridenour, Lubbock, TX
Diane J. Roberts, Columbus, OH
Anita L. Robertson, Martinsville, IN
Susan Robertson, New Hyde Park, NY
Marie Rohan, Springfield, MA
Beverly Ross, Indianapolis, IN
Paula Ross, Colonia, NJ
Laura Rossi, Walpole, MA
Barbara C. Rottkamp, Ridge, NY
Frances Rowley, Greenfield, WI
Terry Ruane, West New York, NY
Louise Rupp, Glendale, CA
Susan Ruppert, Sugar Land, TX
Virginia Saba, Arlington, VA
Carol Sarokas, Clarks Summit, PA
Nancy Schappler, Brighton, MA
Connie Schmidt, Sioux Falls, SD

Joanne Schneider, Derby, KS
Mary Ann Schroeder, Columbia, SC
Susan Schwegler, Delano, MN
Leann Scroggins, Rochester, MN
Elizabeth Sergent, East Williston, NY
Kim Shaffer, Bremerton, WA
Doreen Shephard, Nacogdoches, TX
Kathy Sheppard, Katy, TX
Joyce K. Shoemaker, Toledo, OH
Janice Shoultz, Kaneohe, HI
Mary Sieggreen, Northville, MI
Lina Sims, Shorewood, IL
Lo Rae Skalski, Devore, CA
Jane E. Smith, Philadelphia, PA
Anna Marie Smith, Schenectady, NY
Deborah Soholt, Aberdeen, SD
Susan Sorenson, Green Bay, WI
Sheila Sparks, Sterling, VA
Barbara Spillers, Torrance, CA
Barbara Stachowiak, Leverett, MA
Paulette Stirewalt, Clinton, MA
Dorothy Stitzlein, Ashland, OH
Sandra L. Stockton, Upper Marlboro, MD
Kathleen M. Stolzenberger, Mahwah, NJ
Deanna Stover, Riverside, CA
Laura B. Strange, Norcross, GA
Catherine Strauss, Holbrook, NY
Susanne Nancy Suchy, Southgate, MI
Sharon Summers, Overland Park, KS
Chris Szabo, Powhatan, VA
Barbara Taptich, Mercerville, NJ
Anne Taylor-Loughran, Laguna Hills, CA
Nancy Thompson, Chesterfield, VA
Marita Titler, Alburnett, IA
Mary C. Townsend, Derby, KS
Catherine A. Tracey, Nashua, NH
Sally Tripp, Amherst, MA
Doris Tucker, Cabot, AR
Martha Tyler, Seattle, WA
Susan Ulrich, Eugene, OR
Barbara M. Vassallo, Willingboro, NJ
Donna F. Ver Steeg, Pacific Palisades, CA
Carol Vestal-Allen, Birmingham, AL
Karen Vincent, Randolph, MA
Bonnie Wakefield, Iowa City, IA
Merri D. Walkenstein, Blue Bell, PA
Elaine Walker, Amelia, VA
Virginia R. Wall, Seattle, WA

Rosemary Wang, Barrington, NH
Judy J. Warren, Bellevue, NE
Jacquelyn Warren-Smith, Gaylord, MI
Evelyn Wasli, Laurel, MD
Janet Weber, Jackson, MO
Sylvia Weber, Cranston, RI
Barbara Weber, Jacksonville, FL
Harriet H. Werley, Milwaukee, WI
Bonnie Wesorick, Grand Rapids, MI
Peggy A. Wetsch, Orange, CA
Roger Whiting, Chippewa Falls, WI
Georgia Whitley, Plainfield, IL
Lynn Wieck, Katy, TX
Geraldine Williamson, Atlanta, GA
Nina Wilson, Nahant, MA
Sharon Wing, Oregon, OH
M. Anne Woodtli, Tucson, AZ
Judy Wooldridge, Columbia, SC
Jacqueline Wylie, Kalamazoo, MI
Mararet Wyman, Coralville, IA
Kathy Wyngarden, Grand Rapids, MI
Maria T. Zickuhr, Cleveland, OH
Shirley Melat Ziegler, Dallas, TX

CANADIAN ATTENDEES

Janet Anderson, Willowdale, Ontario
Baerbel Anderson, Unionville, Ontario
Dawne L. Barbieri, Maple, Ontario
Claire Beaudin, Laval, Quebec
Marie Bell, New West Minster, British Columbia
Gisele Besner, Dorion, Quebec
Nancy Bol, London, Ontario
Anne Brackstone, Nepean, Ontario
Ann Brokenshire, Scarborough, Ontario
Beverley A. Bryan, London, Ontario
Louise Chartier, Sherbrooke, Quebec
Hazel Chuck, Unionville, Ontario
Enid Collins, North York, Ontario
Linda D. Cooper, Toronto, Ontario
Betsy Dalton, Scarborough, Ontario
Lenore Duquette, Mississauga, Ontario
Brenda Dutil, Jonquiere, Quebec
Marj Gammel, Saskatoon, Saskatchewan
Dorothea Jakob, Toronto, Ontario
Jean Jenny, Nepean, Ontario
Phyllis E. Jones, Toronto, Ontario

Gratienne G. Lamarche, Ville St. Laurent, Quebec
Cecile Lambert, Outremont, Quebec
W. Lee, Saskatoon, Saskatchewan
Anne LeGresley, Etobicoke, Ontario
Jo Logan, Ottawa, Ontario
Kathleen MacMillan, Scarborough, Ontario
Joscelyn Matthewman, Toronto, Ontario
Kathy McGilton, Scarborough, Ontario
Carmen Millar, Pierre Fonds, Quebec
Winnifred Mills, Edmonton, Alberta
Mary Moulds, Scarborough, Ontario
Margaret Patricia Netzer, Edmonton, Alberta
Linda O'Brien-Pallas, Toronto, Ontario
Karen Perkin, London, Ontario
Monica J. Poole, London, Ontario
Lina Rahal, Blainville, Quebec
Dorothy Reynolds, Edmonton, Alberta
Denyse Rousselet, Dollard-des-Oreaux, Quebec
Vivianne Saba, Montreal, Quebec
Danielle Schmouth, Bellefeville, Quebec
H. Luella Sinha, Winnipeg, Manitoba
Micheline Ulrich, Longueil, Quebec
Janice Wiberg, Lacombe, Alberta
Susanne Williams, Toronto, Ontario
Bonnie Zwack, Calgary, Alberta

INTERNATIONAL ATTENDEES

Cecile Boisvert, St. Aubin, France
Claude Drouard, St. Maximin, France
Juracy Farias, Joao Pessoa, Brazil
Jean Griffiths, Ballina, NSW, Australia
Maria Gudmundsdottir, Reykjavik, Iceland
Sigridur Johannesdottir, Reykjavik, Iceland
Teresa Miralles, Madrid, Spain
Randi Annikki Mortensen, Copenhagen, Denmark
Gunnar Haase Nielsen, Copenhagen, Denmark
Piera Poletti, Padua, Italy
Luis F. Ramos, Arecibo, PR
Birgit Holritz Rasmussen, Copenhagen, Denmark
Renzo Zanotti, Padua, Italy

Author Index

Subject Index

Wellness nursing diagnosis, NANDA Guidelines
 for Submission, 375–376
Woodtli Nursing Diagnosis Model Within the
 Nursing Process, 149
World Health Organization (WHO). *See also* In-
 ternational Classification of Diseases
 (ICD)
 American Association of Critical-Care Nurses
 (AACN), 213
 cultural factors, diversional activity defi-

cit/altered health maintenance, Brazilian
 study, 255–256
diagnostic axes, discussion of, 60
International Classification of Diseases,
 Tenth Revision (ICD–10), 45–46
International Classification of Diseases (ICD)
 and, 14, 15, 16, 19, 22, 23
Society for Education and Research in Psychi-
 atric Nursing/Mental Health Nursing
 (SERPN), 218

DATE DUE

6/2/93 ILL			
OC 2 1 '93			
AP 6 '94			
OC 3 1 '94			
30 Dec 94			
APR 2 9 1997			
APR 2 9 1997			
NOV 0 3 2003			

DEMCO 38-297